Study Guide to Accompany

Roach's Introductory Clinical Pharmacology

NINTH EDITION

P9-AZX-986

SUSAN M. FORD, MN, RN, CNE
Nursing Tenured Faculty
Tacoma Community College
Tacoma, Washington

SALLY S. ROACH, MSN, RN, AHN-BC
Associate Professor
University of Texas at Brownsville and Texas Southmost College
Brownsville, Texas

Wolters Kluwer | Lippincott Williams & Wilkins
Health

Philadelphia · Baltimore · New York · London
Buenos Aires · Hong Kong · Sydney · Tokyo

Acquisitions Editor: Elizabeth Nieginski
Project Manager: Michelle L. Clarke
Director of Nursing Production: Helen Ewan
Art Director: Brett MacNaughton
Senior Designer: Joan Wendt
Manufacturing Coordinator: Karin Duffield
Senior Manufacturing Manager: William Alberti
Production Service: Spearhead Global

9th Edition

9 8 7 6 5

ISBN-13: 978-1-60547-634-6
ISBN-10: 1-60547-634-X

RRS1204

Preface

This study guide has been designed to help you get the most benefit from the ninth edition of *Introductory Clinical Pharmacology*. Completely updated, this study guide provides current and comprehensive coverage of the newest pharmacological aspects as well as basic nursing skills needed in administering medications and caring for patients.

Additionally, as you read your textbook, this guide will be an important tool in helping you discover whether your reading and study habits are allowing you to identify the most important ideas in each chapter. To help you accomplish this goal, the following types of exercises are provided in this study guide:

ASSESSING YOUR UNDERSTANDING

This section includes fill-in-the-blank questions as well as matching exercises. The types of questions included will follow the same format in each study guide chapter.

- Fill-in-the-Blanks
  These questions correlate very closely with the textbook and focus on important information in each chapter.

- Matching Exercises
  Matching exercises help you to distinguish among several key terms, drugs, or adverse reactions.

- Dosage Calculations
  These problems give you practice in solving common medication dosage problems related to the specific medications in each chapter. Doing these calculations reinforces your ability to solve dosage problems and allows you to gain practice as well as confidence in preparation for the clinical setting.

- Short Answer Questions
  Requiring more critical thinking than the exercises in the Assessing Your Understanding section, these short answer questions offer an exciting and practical means to challenge you and "stretch" your application of the concepts.

APPLYING YOUR KNOWLEDGE

These case studies challenge you to reflect on the critical thinking and blended skills developed in the classroom and apply them to your own practice.

PRACTICING FOR NCLEX

Each chapter contains a section of multiple choice questions presented in NCLEX exam format.

Enjoy your studies, and know that this study guide is a tool that will help you better understand the sometimes complicated world of pharmacology.

Contents

CHAPTER 1

General Principles of Pharmacology

Learning Objectives

- Define pharmacology
- Identify the different names assigned to drugs
- Distinguish between prescription drugs, non-prescription drugs, and controlled substances
- Discuss drug development in the United States
- Discuss the various types of drug activity and reactions produced in the body
- Identify factors that influence drug action
- Define drug tolerance, cumulative drug effect, and drug idiosyncrasy
- Discuss the types of drug interactions that may be seen with drug administration
- Discuss the nursing implications associated with drug actions, interactions, and effects
- Discuss the use of herbal medicines

SECTION I: ASSESSING YOUR UNDERSTANDING

Activity A MATCHING

1. *Match the drug reactions given in Column A with their actions in Column B.*

Column A	Column B
B 1. Additive drug reaction	A One drug interferes with the action of another, causing neutralization or a decrease in the effect of one drug
C 2. Synergistic drug reaction	B Combined effect of two drugs is equal to the sum of each drug given alone
A 3. Antagonistic drug reaction	C Drugs interact with each other and produce an effect that is greater than the sum of their separate actions

2. *Match the terms given in Column A with their process in Column B.*

Column A	Column B
C 1. Absorption	a. Changes a drug to a more or less active form
d 2. Distribution	b. Eliminates drugs from the body
a 3. Metabolism	c. Moves drug particles within the gastrointestinal tract
b 4. Excretion	d. Dispenses drugs to various body tissues or target sites

Activity B FILL IN THE BLANKS

1. When a drug is given orally, food may impair or enhance its _absorption._

2. _Intravenous_ administration of a drug produces the most rapid drug action.

3. A/An _antagonist_ drug reaction occurs when one drug interferes with the action of another.

4. Drug _synergism_ occurs when drugs interact with each other and produce an effect that is greater than the sum of their separate actions.

5. A/An _pharmacogenetic_ disorder is a genetically determined abnormal response to normal doses of a drug.

Activity C SHORT ANSWERS

The role of a nurse is to educate patients about a prescribed drug, its adverse reactions, signs and symptoms of those adverse reactions, and any implications thereof. Briefly answer the following questions that involve the nurse's role in managing such situations.

1. A nurse is educating a patient about how drugs act on the body by altering the cellular environment. What are the changes that occur due to alteration of cellular environment?

   Some drugs act on the body by changing the cellular environment physically and chemically. Physical changes include changes in osmotic pressure, lubrication, absorption or the conditions on the surface of the cell membrane. Chemical changes include inactivation of cellular functions or alterations of the chemical components of bodily fluid.

2. Which organization is responsible for approving new drugs? How long does the process of drug development take?

   Drug development is a long and arduous process that can take from 7-12 yrs and sometimes longer. The FDA has the responsibility of approving new drugs and monitoring drugs currently in use for adverse or toxic reactions.

Activity D

1. List the processes that take place during the pre-FDA phase of drug development.

   Vitro testing on an artificial environment such as a test using animal and human cells. This testing is done by studies in live animals. The manufacture then makes application to the FDA for investigation of drug states.

2. A teaching plan for a pregnant patient includes information about the harmful effects of smoking and alcohol consumption on the fetus. What should the nurse tell the patient?

   No women should drink or smoke while pregnant. There are risks involved such as low birth weight, premature birth, fetal alcohol syndrome. Pregnant women should not take herbal supplements be these products can act like drugs.

SECTION II: APPLYING YOUR KNOWLEDGE

Activity E CASE STUDY

A patient with digestion problems visits the health care center to obtain information about certain herbs and dietary supplements. The patient is already taking prescription drugs for indigestion.

What are some of the adverse reactions of consuming botanicals that the nurse will have to update the patient about?

Botanicals may produce toxic substances in the body and many botanicals have strong pharmacological activity that interact with prescription drugs that the patient takes.

How can a nurse ensure that the patient does not misuse herbs and natural supplements?

Nurse should explain that "natural" does not mean the supplement is safe or without harmful effects. Herbal supplements can act the same way as drugs and can cause medical problems if not used correctly or if taken in large amounts.

SECTION III: PRACTICING FOR NCLEX

Activity F NCLEX-STYLE

Answer the following questions.

1. At times it is very confusing for the nurse to recognize a drug by its name because there are different categories of drug names. To which of the following categories of drug names should the nurse refer to avoid confusion?
   a. Official name
   b. Scientific name
   c. Trade name
   d. Generic name

2. What is the purpose of the Controlled Substances Act of 1970? Select all that apply.
   a. Report adverse effects of drugs
   b. Regulate manufacture of drugs
   c. Organize distribution of drugs
   d. Control dispensing of drugs
   e. Encourage drug development

3. A patient wants to know what happens to the liquid medication that he has been taking for an illness. How should the nurse explain the process to the patient?
   a. Disintegrates in the gastrointestinal tract
   b. Is quickly absorbed by the body system
   c. Disintegrates in the small intestine
   d. Disintegrates into small pieces

4. A patient is admitted to a local health care center with severe dehydration. Which route of drug administration would the nurse apply to counter the dehydration quickly?
   a. Oral route
   b. Subcutaneous route
   c. Intravenous route
   d. Intramuscular route

5. A nurse explains to a patient who is not allergic to drugs that drugs alter the functions of the body's cells. Which of the following symptoms will the nurse monitor for altered cellular function in the patient? Select all that apply.
   a. Blood pressure
   b. Impaired vision
   c. Urine output
   d. Slurred speech
   e. Heart rate

6. A cancer patient requests information from the nurse on the activity of drugs that have been prescribed. Which of the following should the nurse reply as the method of action of cancer drugs? Select all that apply.
   a. Acts on the cell membrane
   b. Causes change in the pH
   c. Acts on cellular processes
   d. Causes chemical change in bodily fluids
   e. Causes cell starvation and death

7. A primary health care provider prescribes reduced doses of a drug to be administered at lengthened durations between doses to a patient with kidney disease. Which of the following are reasons for such a prescription? Select all that apply.
   a. Patient could exhibit drug toxicity
   b. Drug action is of longer duration
   c. Patient could exhibit drug tolerance
   d. Prescription prevents accumulation of the drug
   e. Patient could become drug dependent

8. When assessing a patient for an illness, the nurse takes note of certain factors that influence drug response. Which of the following factors should the nurse note? Select all that apply.
   a. Patient's age
   b. Existing disease
   c. Patient's weight
   d. Patient's appetite
   e. Patient's height

9. A patient is to undergo frequent diagnostic tests during the course of treatment at the health care facility. In which of the following conditions should the nurse perform frequent diagnostic tests?
   a. Impaired vision
   b. Impaired speech
   c. Impaired liver function
   d. Impaired hearing

10. Administration of a drug is primarily the responsibility of which health care provider?
    a. Nurse
    b. Physician
    c. Pharmacist
    d. Physician's assistant

11. The study of drugs and their action on living organisms is known as which of the following?
    a. Microbiology
    b. Pharmacology
    c. Biology
    d. Immunology

12. Which of the following agencies is responsible for the approval of new drugs in the United States?
    a. Food and Drug Administration
    b. *National Formulary*
    c. *U.S. Pharmacopeia*
    d. American Medical Association

13. Legend drugs refer to which of the following?
    a. Non-prescription drugs
    b. Nutraceuticals
    c. Prescription drugs
    d. Vitamin supplements

14. If a nurse was to look up a drug in the *U.S. Pharmacopeia* the nurse would need to know which type of drug name?
    a. Generic name
    b. Trade name
    c. Chemical name
    d. Brand name

15. Which type of dependence is the habitual use of a drug, where negative physical withdrawal symptoms result from abrupt discontinuation?
    a. Physical dependence
    b. Psychological dependence
    c. Pleasurable dependence
    d. Abuse dependence.

CHAPTER 2

Administration of Drugs

- Discuss the 5 + 1 rights of drug administration
- Discuss general principles of drug administration
- Identify the different types of medication orders
- Describe general guidelines the nurse should follow when preparing a drug for administration
- Discuss how the Joint Commission's National Patient Safety Goals and Institute for Safe
- Medication Practices website helps nurses reduce medication-related errors
- Describe the various types of medication-dispensing systems
- Discuss the administration of oral and parenteral drugs
- Discuss the administration of drugs through the skin and mucous membranes
- Discuss nursing responsibilities before, during, and after a drug is administered

SECTION I: ASSESSING YOUR UNDERSTANDING

Activity A MATCHING

1. *Match the administration routes in Column A with commonly used sites for administering them in Column B.*

Column A	Column B
1. Transdermal	**a.** Upper arm, hip, and thigh
2. Intradermal	**b.** Upper arms, upper abdomen, and upper back
3. Intramuscular	
4. Subcutaneous	**c.** Chest, flank, and upper arm
	d. Inner part of forearm and upper back

2. *Match the drugs in Column A with their common administration routes in Column B.*

Column A	Column B
1. Lozenges	**a.** Inhalation
2. Heparin	**b.** Transdermal
3. Scopolamine	**c.** Buccal
4. Mucolytics	**d.** Subcutaneous

Activity B   FILL IN THE BLANKS

1. Electronic infusion devices are classified as either infusion _____ or infusion pumps.

2. The Z-track method of intramuscular injection is used when a drug is highly irritating to _____ tissues.

3. In the _____ dose system of dispensing medications, the pharmacist dispenses each dose in a package that is labeled with the drug name and dosage.

4. Nitroglycerin is commonly given by the _____ route.

5. The nurse should instruct the patient to place the _____ drugs against mucous membranes of the cheek.

6. Escape of fluid from a blood vessel into surrounding tissues while the needle or catheter is in the vein is known as _____.

Activity C   SHORT ANSWERS

The administration of a drug is a fundamental responsibility of the nurse. An understanding of the basic concepts of administering drugs is critical if the nurse is to perform this task safely and accurately. Briefly answer the following questions, which involve the nurse's role in the administration of drugs.

1. The physician has asked a nurse to administer a drug to a patient. How can the nurse identify the patient prior to administering the medication?

   _____

   _____

2. After administering a drug to the patient, the nurse realizes that an incorrect dosage has been administered. Why should the nurse report drug errors?

   _____

   _____

Activity D

1. A nurse is required to administer a drug through the transdermal route to a patient. What are the nurse's responsibilities with regard to the administration of a drug using this route?

   _____

   _____

SECTION II: APPLYING YOUR KNOWLEDGE

Activity E   CASE STUDY

1. A nurse is caring for a group of patients. The physician has asked the nurse to administer different drugs to each. The nurse is confused in finding some drug names that sound similar, and a few spelled almost similarly. How can the nurse ensure that the right drug is administered to the right patient?

   _____

   _____

   _____

2. After administering a drug to a patient, the nurse has been asked to record the process immediately. Why is it important to document the administration of drugs?

   _____

   _____

   _____

SECTION III: PRACTICING FOR NCLEX

Activity F NCLEX-STYLE

Answer the following questions.

1. A nurse administers a drug on an as-needed (PRN) basis. Which of the following interventions should the nurse perform immediately after administering the drug to the patient? Select all that apply.

   a. Record administration of the drug

   b. Evaluate patient's response to the drug

   c. Record the site used for parenteral administration

   d. Inform physician about the drugs administered

2. What nursing intervention should be performed to minimize risk of skin irritation when administering drugs by the transdermal route?

   a. Shave the area before applying the patch

   b. Always apply patches on the same site

   c. Moisten skin before applying patches

   d. Remove the old patch for next dose

3. A nurse is caring for a patient with a superficial skin infection. What information should the nurse obtain from the primary health care provider before administering the prescribed topical drug to the patient?

   a. Cause of the skin infection

   b. Instructions for drug application

   c. Reasons for selecting the drug

   d. Composition of the drug

4. While assessing a patient, a nurse is required to perform the tuberculin test. The drug is to be administered by an intradermal injection. Which of the following sites is ideal for administering the intradermal injection to the patient?

   a. Thigh

   b. Hairy areas

   c. Inner forearm

   d. Upper arm

5. A nurse has been assigned to perform venipuncture for a patient. Three attempts to perform venipuncture have been unsuccessful. Which of the following steps should the nurse perform in this situation?

   a. Keep trying until venipuncture is successful

   b. Ask for assistance from a skilled nurse

   c. Inject the drug intramuscularly

   d. Shift the patient into a more conducive position

6. A nurse is required to administer 5 mL of a drug intramuscularly to an adult patient. Which of the following interventions should the nurse perform while administering the drug?

   a. Divide the drug and give it as two separate injections

   b. Use a half-inch long needle for the injection

   c. Administer the drug at the upper back

   d. Insert the needle at a 45-degree angle

7. The physician has asked a nurse to administer a subcutaneous injection to a patient. The nurse observes that the patient is very thin. Which of the following sites should the nurse select to administer the injection to this patient?

   a. Upper arm

   b. Lower back

   c. Upper abdomen

   d. Thigh muscle

8. A nurse is caring for a patient with a nasogastric feeding tube. The nurse is required to administer drug tablets to the patient. Which of the following interventions should the nurse perform during the administration of the drug? Select all that apply.

   a. Ensure that the tablet is completely dissolved

   b. Put the tablets in water without crushing them

   c. Flush the tube with water to clear the tubing

   d. Mix the drug after the tube is fixed

   e. Check the tube for placement

9. A nurse should use how many methods to identify the client before administering the medication?
   a. 2
   b. 1
   c. 3
   d. 4

10. A physician writes an order for a client to receive a Proventil HFA inhaler with the directions to inhale 2 puffs every 4 to 6 hours as need for wheezing. What type of order does this represent?
   a. STAT order
   b. Standing order
   c. PRN order
   d. Single order

11. Which of the following drugs are often associated with errors? Select all that apply.
   a. Humalog
   b. Heparin
   c. Potassium chloride
   d. Furosemide
   e. Promethazine

12. Nurses need to keep up with changes made by the Joint Commission to the National Patient Safety Goals (NPSG). How frequently does the Joint Commission update NPSG?
   a. Semiannually
   b. Annually
   c. Quarterly
   d. Monthly

13. Which of the following organizations is responsible for the Medication Errors Reporting Program?
   a. The Institute for Safe Medication Practices
   b. The Joint Commission
   c. The National Patient Safety Institute
   d. The Food and Drug Administration

14. Nurses are responsible for which part of the drug distribution process?
   a. Dispensing
   b. Ordering
   c. Dosing
   d. Administering

15. A Pyxis machine is an example of which type of drug distribution system?
   a. Automated medication management system
   b. Bar-coded point-of-care medication systems
   c. Unit dose system
   d. Multidose system

Calculation of Drug Dosages and Mathematical Review

Learning Objectives

- Describe how safety is provided by the multiple-check system in drug administration
- Identify information on a drug label used for calculating drug dosages
- Describe the importance of zero (0) placement in writing drug doses
- Accurately perform mathematical calculations when they are necessary to compute drug dosages

SECTION I: ASSESSING YOUR UNDERSTANDING

Activity A MATCHING

1. *Match the terms in Column A with the descriptions given in Column B.*

Column A

1. Proper fraction
2. Improper fraction
3. Mixed number
4. Lowest common denominator

Column B

a. A whole number and a proper fraction

b. Part of a whole or any number less than a whole number

c. The lowest number divisible by all the denominators

d. Fraction having a numerator the same as or larger than the denominator

2. *Match the computations in Column A with the procedures given in Column B.*

Column A

1. To change a mixed number to an improper fraction

2. To add fractions with like denominators

3. To add mixed numbers or fractions with mixed numbers

4. To divide a whole number by a fraction

Column B

a. Add the numerators and place the sum of the numerators over the denominator

b. First change the mixed number to an improper fraction

c. Change the whole number to an improper fraction by placing the whole number over 1

d. Multiply the denominator of the fraction by the whole number, add the numerator, and place the sum over the denominator

Activity B FILL IN THE BLANKS

1. When fractions with like _____ are compared, the fraction with the largest numerator is the largest fraction.

2. To compare fractions with unlike denominators, the _____ common denominator must first be determined.

3. When _____ are multiplied, the numerators are multiplied, and the denominators are multiplied.

4. When whole numbers are multiplied with fractions, the _____ is multiplied by the whole number, and the product is placed over the denominator.

5. A fraction having a numerator the same as or _____ than the denominator is an improper fraction.

6. The _____ numbers are changed to improper fractions and then multiplied.

7. To multiply a whole number and a mixed number, both numbers must be changed to _____ fractions.

8. Part of a whole or any number less than a whole number is a _____ fraction.

9. A/An _____ is a way of expressing a part of a whole or the relation of one number to another.

10. A proportion is a method of expressing _____ between two ratios.

Activity C SHORT ANSWERS

One of the nurses on your unit states the following: "Because we use the new computer system, we don't need to do the 5 rights and 3 checks anymore." Describe how you would respond to this nurse.

_____

_____

Activity D DOSAGE CALCULATION

The dosage strength of Augmentin is 125 mg/ 5 mL solution. The primary health care provider orders Augmentin 125 mg 4 times daily. How many mL will the nurse administer in each dose?

_____

_____

SECTION II: APPLYING YOUR KNOWLEDGE

Activity E CASE STUDY

Max Jones is a Caucasian male, 24 years of age, who is admitted to the hospital for surgery to repair a torn ACL. He is in good health and does not take any medications. He weighs 215 lb and his temperature prior to surgery was 37°C.

1. Most medications are given on a mg/kg basis. How many kilograms does Mr. Jones weigh?

_____

_____

2. Convert the patient's temperature to degrees Fahrenheit.

_____

_____

SECTION III: PRACTICING FOR NCLEX

Activity F NCLEX-STYLE

1. Which of the following is the best method of error detection?
   a. Manual redundancy system
   b. Bar coding system
   c. Computerized order entry system
   d. Manual order entry system

2. Patients may refuse a medication if they do not recognize which of the following?
   a. Brand name
   b. Non-proprietary name
   c. Generic name
   d. Chemical name

3. Which of the following are systems of measurement associated with drug dosing? Select all that apply.
   a. Metric system
   b. Apothecary system
   c. Hospital measurements
   d. Nursing system
   e. Household measurements

4. Which of the following represents correct placement of a zero in a decimal?
   a. 0.75
   b. 750.0
   c. .750
   d. .075

5. How many pounds are in 1 kilogram?
   a. 5.5 lb
   b. 1.2 lb
   c. 2.2 lb
   d. 3.4 lb

6. Which of the following correctly expresses the ratio 3:100 in a fraction?
   a. 100/3
   b. 3/100
   c. 1/33.3
   d. 33.3/1

7. Which of the following correctly expresses 75% in a fraction? Select all that apply.
   a. 75/100
   b. 3/4
   c. 100/75
   d. 4/3
   e. 1 1/3

8. In the household measurement system how many teaspoons are in 1 tablespoon?
   a. 2
   b. 1
   c. 0.5
   d. 3

9. Which of the following correctly represents 3/8 in a percentage?
   a. 37.5%
   b. 3.75%
   c. 266.7%
   d. 26.7%

10. How many milligrams are in 1 gram?
    a. 100
    b. 10
    c. 1000
    d. 0.1

11. Which of the following are the steps associated with using dimensional analysis to calculate dosage problems?
    a. Express the dosage strength as a fraction with the numerator having the same unit
    b. Write the next fraction with the numerator having the same unit of measure as the denominator
    c. Write dosage strength with the numerator always expressed in the same unit that was identified before
    d. Expand the equation by filling in the missing numbers using the appropriate equivalent

12. Which of the following are the characteristics of parenteral drugs available in disposable syringes?

    a. Specific dosage strength may not be available

    b. Available as a crystal or a powder

    c. Available as ampoules or vials in dry form

    d. Must be made a liquid before administration

13. Which of the following are the units of the apothecary system?

    a. Grams

    b. Ounces

    c. Meters

    d. Liters

14. Which of the following are the characteristics of a generic name of the drug as mentioned in the label?

    a. Appears in capitalized style

    b. Written first on the label

    c. Identified by the registration symbol

    d. Written in smaller print

15. Which of the following represents a unit of weight?

    a. Liter

    b. Meter

    c. Gram

    d. Deciliter

CHAPTER 4

The Nursing Process

Learning objectives

- List the five phases of the nursing process
- Discuss assessment, analysis, nursing diagnosis, planning, implementation, and evaluation as they apply to the administration of drugs
- Differentiate between objective and subjective data
- Discuss how the nursing process may be used in daily life, as well as when administering drugs
- Identify common nursing diagnoses used in the administration of drugs and nursing interventions related to each diagnosis

SECTION I: ASSESSING YOUR UNDERSTANDING

Activity A MATCHING

1. **Match the phases of the nursing process in Column A with their functions in Column B.**

Column A	Column B
1. Assessment	a. Describing steps for carrying out nursing activities or interventions that are specific and will meet the expected outcomes
2. Nursing diagnosis (analysis)	b. Carrying out a plan of action
3. Planning	c. Collecting objective and subjective data
4. Implementation	d. Determining the effectiveness of the nursing interventions in meeting the expected outcomes
5. Evaluation	e. Identifying problems that can be solved or prevented by independent nursing actions

2. *Match the nursing diagnoses related to the administration of drugs in Column A with their meanings in Column B.*

Column A

Column B

1. Effective therapeutic regimen management   *e*

2. Ineffective therapeutic regimen management   *a*   *c*

3. Deficient knowledge

4. Noncompliance *b*

5. Anxiety *d*

a. Patient may not take the medication correctly or follow the medication regimen prescribed by the health care provider

b. Patient's behavior fails to coincide with the therapeutic plan agreed on by the patient and the health care provider

c. Patient lacks sufficient knowledge to administer the drug regimen correctly, lacks interest in learning, has cognitive limitations, or exhibits inability to remember

d. Patient experiences reduced ability to focus on details

e. Patient is willing to regulate and integrate the treatment regimen into daily living

Activity B FILL IN THE BLANKS

1. _objective_ data are facts obtained by means of a physical assessment or physical examination.

2. An _ongoing_ assessment is one that is made at the time of each patient contact and may include the collection of objective data, subjective data, or both.

3. A nursing _diagnosis_ is a description of the patient's problems and their probable or actual related causes based on the subjective and objective data in the database.

4. Planning anticipates the _implementation_ phase or the carrying out of nursing actions that are specific for the drug being administered.

5. The nursing care must be planned on a _individual_ basis after a careful collection and analysis of the subjective and objective data.

Activity C SHORT ANSWERS

A nurse's role in performing various nursing processes involves assisting patients in their treatment therapy. The nurse also helps patients to understand and effectively manage the therapeutic regime. Using the nursing process requires practice, experience, and a constant updating of knowledge. Answer the following questions related to the nursing process.

1. a. What is a nursing process?

A framework for nursing actions consisting of problem-solving steps that help members of the health care team provide effective patient care.

b. What are the 5 phases of the nursing process?

1. assessment 2. Nursing diagnosis 3. plan 4. Implementation 5. Evaluation

2. What are the initial and ongoing assessments in the nursing process?

Initial assessment is subjective or objective data collected before to obtain a thorough baseline. Ongoing assessment is one in the time of each patients contact and may include subjective objective data.

Activity D

A patient is receiving three drugs for the treatment of difficulty breathing and swelling of her legs. You are giving these drugs for the first time. Discuss what questions you would ask to obtain subjective data.

You would ask the patient if they are having cognitive deficits, mobility problems, lack of fluids, visual or hearing deficits and troublesome adverse reactions.

SECTION II: APPLYING YOUR KNOWLEDGE

Activity E CASE STUDY

Mary Black is an African American female, 32 years of age, para 2 gravida 1. She has pregnancy-induced hypertension and gestational diabetes. She presents to the physician today for follow-up.

1. What information should the nurse elicit from Mrs. Black during the initial assessment?

The nurse should obtain vitals, prescriptions taking or taken, lab results, daily weights and BGs. The nurse should also check for edema due to her diabetes.

2. Mrs. Black's physician has ordered her to do finger sticks QID. What can the nurse do to ensure that the client follows the therapeutic regimen?

The nurse can educate and teach the patient how to properly complete a fingerstick, how to use the equipment, what the pt needs to know and how to clean the equipment. Make sure pt knows why they're collecting a fingerstick and testing blood sugar.

SECTION III: PRACTICING FOR NCLEX

Activity F NCLEX-STYLE

Answer the following questions.

1. A nurse is assigned to care for a patient with a respiratory problem. During assessment, what intervention should the nurse perform to obtain subjective data from the patient?

   a. Inquire about the number of cigarettes smoked per day

   b. Monitor the patient's pulse rate and rhythm

   c. Monitor the patient's blood pressure

   d. Assess the patient's body temperature

2. A nurse is caring for a patient who is of childbearing age. Which of the following is the most relevant assessment that the nurse should perform before administering a drug to this patient?

   a. Family history

   b. Relationship with spouse

   c. Pregnancy status

   d. Menstruation history

3. What should a nurse focus on when developing expected outcomes for a patient?

   a. The type of drug administered

   b. The patient's condition or illness

   c. Dosage pattern administered to the patient

   d. The patient's ability to recuperate

4. A nurse is assigned to care for a patient in a health care facility. Which of the following should the nurse include in her nursing diagnosis?

   a. Problems that can be solved by independent nursing actions

   b. Problems that have a treatment marking a definite cure

   c. Identification of the patient's condition and criticality

   d. Problems that cannot be prevented by nursing actions

5. A nurse is assigned to care for a patient who has just been admitted to a health care facility. What is the significance of planning for nursing actions specific to the drug to be administered? Select all that apply.

   a. It allows greater accuracy in drug administration

   b. It allows absolute prevention of relapse

   c. It allows patient understanding of the drug regimen

   d. It promotes an optimal response to therapy in minimum time

   e. It promotes patient compliance with prescribed drug therapy

6. A nurse is caring for a patient who has to continue with the drug regimen on an outpatient basis. Routine assessments of the patient reveal that the patient is not complying with the medication regimen. What intervention should the nurse perform to combat the patient's non-compliant attitude?

   a. Prepare a fixed schedule for the patient to take the drug

   b. Find out the reason for non-compliance if possible

   c. Teach the patient the importance of following a drug regimen

   d. Frequently monitor the patient's condition to identify a relapse

7. The following interventions of the nursing process are given in random order. Prioritize them.

2 (a.) Analyze the data collected during assessment

4 b. Formulate one or more nursing diagnoses

1 (c.) Collect the objective and subjective data

3 (d.) Identify the patient's needs or problems

5 (e.) Develop expected outcomes for the patient

8. Facts obtained by means of a physical assessment or physical examination are considered which of the following? (Choose one)

a. Objective data

b. Subjective data

c. Initial assessment

d. Ongoing assessment

9. Facts supplied by the client or the client's family are considered which of the following?

a. Objective data

b. Initial assessment

c. Subjective data

d. Ongoing assessment

10. Which of the following is the first of the 5 steps in the nursing process?

a. Assessment

b. Documentation

c. Analysis

d. Planning

e. Evaluation

11. The collection of subjective and objective data is completed during which step of the nursing process?

a. Analysis

b. Implementation

c. Assessment

d. Planning

12. Identification of problems that can be solved or prevented by the nurse without involvement of the physician is known as which of the following?

a. Nursing diagnosis

b. Nursing assessment

c. Nursing documentation

d. Nursing evaluation

13. Which of the following organizations is responsible for the continuation of defining, explaining, classifying, and researching summary statements about health problems related to nursing?

a. The Joint Commission

b. The National Council of State Boards of Nursing

c. The individual states' nursing boards

d. The North American Nursing Diagnosis Association (NANDA)

14. After the formulation of nursing diagnoses what is the next step in the nursing process?

a. Planning

b. Implementation

c. Evaluation

d. Assessment

15. Which of the following nursing steps refers to the preparation and administration of one or more drugs to a specific patient?

a. Assessment

b. Implementation

c. Evaluation

d. Analysis

CHAPTER 5

Patient and Family Teaching

Learning Objectives

- Identify important aspects of the teaching/learning process
- Discuss the three domains of learning
- Discuss important aspects of adult learning
- Explain how the nursing process can be used to develop a teaching plan
- Identify basic information to consider when developing a teaching plan
- Discuss suggestions the nurse can make to the patient to adapt drug administration in the home

SECTION I: ASSESSING YOUR UNDERSTANDING

Activity A MATCHING

1. *Match the learning domains in Column A with the corresponding patient activities in Column B.*

Column A	Column B
B 1. Psychomotor domain	a. Decision making and drawing conclusions
C 2. Affective domain	b. Learning physical skills
A 3. Cognitive domain	c. Attitudes, feelings, and beliefs

2. *Match the nursing diagnoses in Column A with their corresponding characteristics in Column B.*

Column A

C **1.** Effective individual therapeutic regimen management

A **2.** Deficient knowledge

B **3.** Ineffective therapeutic regimen management

Column B

a. Taught to patients with deficient cognitive knowledge and psychomotor skills

b. Discharge teaching

c. Teaches adverse drug reactions and effects as well as their management

Activity B FILL IN THE BLANKS

1. The psychomotor domain involves learning physical skills or tasks.

2. The affective domain includes the patient's and the caregiver's attitudes, feelings, beliefs, and opinions.

3. It is important not to _Chew_ capsules before swallowing.

4. Exposing a drug to excessive sunlight heat, cold, or moisture may cause the drug to deteriorate.

5. A daily calendar is an inexpensive yet effective means for Scheduling drug administration.

Activity C SHORT ANSWERS

A nurse's role in determining the effectiveness of patient teaching involves evaluating the patients' knowledge of materials presented. The nurse also helps the patients answer their queries and difficulties by interacting with them. Answer the following questions, which involve the nurse's role in evaluating the effectiveness of patient teaching.

1. A patient has been taught exercises for strengthening eye muscles. How should the nurse ensure that the patient perfectly remembers all the exercises that were taught?

For the patient to show the nurse she understands the exercises, performed The nurse should have the patient demonstrate a teach back having the patient practice and teach the nurse how to efficiently complete the exercises.

It's always good to have a ptor family do a teach back to show the understanding of the procedure or exercise.

2. A patient's relative has been instructed on how to measure the patient's temperature using an electronic thermometer. How does the nurse ensure that the patient's relative has understood the procedure?

The nurse could have the relative perform a teach back and demonstra the procedure.

Activity D

In the utilization of nursing processes as a framework for patient teaching, the nursing diagnosis stage comes immediately after the assessment stage. The systematic method of nursing processes differs from the teaching plan. The systematic method encompasses all the patient health care needs, whereas the teaching plan focuses on the patient's learning needs and the learning domains. Answer the following questions, which involve the nurse's role in the preparation of a framework for patient teaching.

1. A patient admitted to a health care facility for malaria is to be trained in the administration of antimalarial drugs. The patient is deficient in cognitive knowledge and psychomotor skills.

What nursing diagnosis should the nurse use for this patient?

Nursing diagnosis would be "Deficient knowledge" because the pt is deficient to antimalarial drugs and needs to know what and why the drugs are used.

2. An asthma patient in a local health care facility is due to be discharged. The patient is to be taught how to perform breathing exercises at home.

a. What patient skills are involved in this case?

Patient skills involved are psychomotor domain because the pt needs to be able to teach back and demonstrate the breathing exercises to her nurse.

b. Which nursing diagnosis should be used to teach breathing exercises to the patient?

Since the pt is lacking information about the breathing exercises, the right nursing diagnosis would be Ineffective therapeutic regimen management.

3. An obese patient visits a local health care center for a weight loss program. The weight loss program recommends strict dietary control and regular physical exercise. However, the patient claims to be a dietician herself and expects her opinions to be respected as well.

   What learning domain comes into the picture when the patient implements the weight loss program?

   When the pt implements the weight loss program she's learning using the affective domain related to patient teaching.

SECTION II: APPLYING YOUR KNOWLEDGE

Activity E CASE STUDY

Maria Sanchez is an Hispanic female, 75 years of age, who speaks very little English. She lives with her daughter and her family. Her past medical history includes hypertension, hyperlipidemia, and s/p CVA with right-sided hemiparesis. Mrs. Sanchez has just been diagnosed with diabetes. She has been referred to you, the nurse, as the clinic-certified diabetes educator, with instruction to include proper use of the glucometer.

1. Which learning domains should the nurse pay particular attention to when developing a teaching plan for Mrs. Sanchez?

   When developing a teaching plan Mrs. Sanchez should pay particular attention to the learning domains.

2. What barriers or obstacles does the nurse face in educating Mrs. Sanchez about her glucometer and her disease state?

   Barriers or Obstacles affecting Mrs. Sanchez is her culture, language barrier and knowledge about her disease. Being uneducated about the disease and disagreements of proper foods, culture and language can be challenging.

SECTION III: PRACTICING FOR NCLEX

Activity F NCLEX-STYLE

Answer the following questions.

1. A patient admitted to a health care facility for diabetes is administered insulin injections. The patient is improving and is expected to be discharged in a couple of days. The nurse assigned to the patient needs to teach him how to administer the post-discharge doses of insulin. The patient feels that administering insulin at home could be a bit too complicated for him. For which of the following reasons should the nurse adopt the Ineffective Therapeutic Regimen Management nursing diagnosis for this patient? Select all that apply.

   a. Useful in discharge teaching
   b. Manages complicated medication regimen
   c. Helps patients in achieving positive results
   d. Informs the patient about drug reactions
   e. Teaches management of adverse effects of the drug

2. A patient is admitted to a local health care center for jaundice and is prescribed a number of drugs. The nurse in charge of the patient wants to teach him how to administer the prescribed drugs and has formulated a teaching plan. When and how should the teaching plan be implemented? Select all that apply.

   a. A day or two before the patient's discharge
   b. When the patient is alone, alert, and not sedated
   c. As soon as the patient is admitted
   d. Material should be divided/taught in sessions
   e. Material should be taught at a single stretch

3. A nurse caring for a patient with typhoid needs to formulate a teaching plan to instruct the patient on drug administration. Which of the following reasons are most important for a nurse to perform a patient assessment before formulating a teaching plan? Select all that apply.

  a. To determine barriers in the learning process

  b. To improve patient motivation

  c. To improve patient participation

  d. To choose the best teaching methods

  e. To develop an effective teaching plan

4. A nurse is assigned to care for a patient with gangrene on his toes. The nurse needs to teach the patient how to bandage the wound at home. What learning domain should the nurse employ to teach the patient?

  a. Cognitive domain

  b. Psychomotor domain

  c. Affective domain

  d. Intellectual domain

5. A patient admitted to a local health care facility for chronic acidity and heartburn is administered certain drugs. The assigned nurse formulates a teaching plan listing all the interventions to be conducted for the patient. What should the nurse do during the implementation of the teaching plan?

  a. Perform the interventions identified in the teaching plan

  b. Determine the effectiveness of patient teaching

  c. Begin with expected outcomes

  d. Use the patient's past experiences

6. A nurse preparing a teaching plan for a patient needs to identify the suitable learning domain. Which of the following learning domains are domains that patients, at any given time, might be using? Select all that apply.

  a. Intellectual domain

  b. Intuitive domain

  c. Psychomotor domain

  d. Cognitive domain

  e. Affective domain

7. A patient admitted to a health care facility for bronchial asthma is prescribed drugs in the form of spray inhalers. The patient needs to be taught how to administer the drugs. Which of the following would be the main obstacle in the learning process?

  a. Patient has low grasping power

  b. Patient is nervous about using inhalers

  c. Patient and nurse exhibit different literacy levels

  d. Patient is not aware of the drug's action

8. A gastroenteritis patient is admitted to a health care facility. The nurse in charge prepares a teaching plan to help the patient follow a restricted diet at home. The patient is moody and irritable at times and wants his opinions to be respected. What learning domain should the nurse involve when teaching the patient?

  a. Affective domain

  b. Cognitive domain

  c. Intellectual domain

  d. Psychomotor domain

9. Which of the following is true of patient teaching?

  a. Patient teaching is an ongoing process

  b. Patient teaching is a tedious process

  c. Patient teaching is an unnecessary process

  d. Patient teaching is only a discharge process

10. A patient must have which of the following to learn?

  a. Ability to read

  b. Ability to write

  c. Motivation

  d. Ability to hear

11. Which of the following can change when a patient learns? Select all that apply.

  a. Behavior

  b. Thinking

  c. Beliefs

  d. Values

12. The nurse should assure that the patient is not having which of the following because it is vital to the teaching/learning process?
    a. Pain
    b. Tachycardia
    c. Hyperglycemia
    d. Hypotension

13. Which domain may be overlooked when educating a Hispanic patient?
    a. Affective domain
    b. Cognitive domain
    c. Physical domain
    d. Psychomotor domain

14. Preprinted material such as checklists are useful for helping a nurse remember important teaching points but do not take into account which of the following domains?
    a. Cognitive domain
    b. Affective domain
    c. Psychological domain
    d. Psychomotor domain

15. Which of the following is the most important prerequisite to learning about a patient's affective behavior?
    a. Development of a therapeutic relationship
    b. Treatment of a patient's pain
    c. Development of a therapeutic plan
    d. Assessment of the patient's cognitive ability

CHAPTER 6

Sulfonamides

Learning Objectives

- Discuss the uses, general drug actions, and general adverse reactions, contraindications, precautions, and interactions of the sulfonamides
- Discuss important preadministration and ongoing assessment activities the nurse should perform on the patient taking sulfonamides
- List nursing diagnoses particular to a patient taking sulfonamides
- Discuss ways to promote an optimal response to therapy, how to manage adverse reactions, and important points to keep in mind when educating patients about the use of sulfonamides
- Identify the rationale for increasing fluid intake when taking sulfonamides. Describe the objective signs indicating that a severe skin reaction, such as Stevens-Johnson syndrome, is present

SECTION I: ASSESSING YOUR UNDERSTANDING

Activity A MATCHING

1. *Match the conditions caused by sulfonamides in Column A with their symptoms in Column B.*

Column A	Column B
1. Stomatitis	a. Crystals in the urine
2. Sulfasalazine	b. Itching
3. Crystalluria	c. Inflammation of the mouth
4. Pruritus	d. Urine and skin turn orange-yellow

2. *Match the conditions in Column A with their symptoms in Column B.*

Column A	Column B
1. Thrombocytopenia	a. Decrease in red blood cell in the bone marrow
2. Aplastic anemia	b. Decrease in number of white blood cells
3. Leukopenia	c. Formation of stone in genitourinary tract
4. Calculi	d. Decrease in platelet count

Activity B   FILL IN THE BLANKS

1. The sulfonamides are contraindicated in patients with hypersensitivity to the sulfonamides, during lactation, and in children less than _____ years old.

2. The sulfonamides are primarily _____ due to their ability to inhibit the activity of folic acid in bacterial cell metabolism.

3. To avoid the adverse effects of _____ during sulfonamide therapy, patients should be cautioned to wear protective clothing or sunscreen when outside.

4. _____ juice is a commonly used remedy for preventing and relieving symptoms of urinary tract infections (UTIs).

5. _____ is manifested by easy bruising and unusual bleeding after moderate to slight trauma to the skin or mucous membranes

Activity C   SHORT ANSWERS

A nurse's role in managing patients involves assisting the patients in answering any queries regarding the treatment that is being provided. The nurse also helps the patients by educating them about the precautions to be taken. Answer the following questions, which involve the nurse's role in management of such situations.

1. A patient has been admitted to a health care facility and the primary health care provider has prescribed sulfonamide therapy. What are the activities that the nurse is required to perform as part of the preadministration assessment?

   _____

   _____

   _____

2. A patient has been admitted to a health care facility and is on sulfonamide therapy. What should the nurse include in the teaching plan for the patient and his family?

   _____

   _____

   _____

Activity D   DOSAGE CALCULATION

1. The primary health care provider has prescribed oral sulfadiazine, 3 g per day as maintenance dose to be given in equal doses. The drug is available in the form of a 500-mg tablet. How many tablets will the nurse administer to the patient for each day?

   _____

   _____

2. A patient has been prescribed 2 g of azulfidine per day, in four equal doses. The drug is available in a 500-mg tablet. How many tablets will the nurse administer to the patient for each dosage?

   _____

   _____

3. The primary health care provider has prescribed 4 g of erythromycin-sulfisoxazole per day, to be given orally 4 times a day in equal doses. After reconstitution, the concentration of the drug in the solution is 250 mg per 5 mL. How many mL of the solution should the nurse administer to the patient for each dosage?

   _____

   _____

4. The primary health care provider has prescribed 1500 mg sulfasalazine per day. The drug is available in the form of 500-mg tablets. How many tablets should be administered to the patient in a day?

   _____

   _____

5. The primary health care provider has prescribed sulfamethoxazole-trimethoprim tablets, 2 g initially for a day. The drug is available in the form of 400-mg tablets. How many tablets should the nurse administer to the patient in a day?

   _____

   _____

SECTION II: APPLYING YOUR KNOWLEDGE

Activity E CASE STUDY

Jason Williams is an African American male, 75 years of age. He is diagnosed with an acute exacerbation of chronic bronchitis. The physician would like to give Mr. Williams a sulfonamide to treat his exacerbation.

1. What information should the nurse obtain from Mr. Williams before the physician sees him?

_____

_____

_____

After the diagnosis of acute exacerbation of chronic bronchitis, the physician prescribes Bactrim DS, one tablet every 12 hours for 14 days. What should the nurse tell Mr. Williams about the prescription before letting him leave the physician's office?

_____

_____

_____

SECTION III: PRACTICING FOR NCLEX

Activity F NCLEX-STYLE

Answer the following questions.

1. A patient with second-degree burns is admitted to a health care facility. Which of the following interventions should the nurse perform to improve the patient's treatment?
   a. Clean the surface of the skin
   b. Apply a half-inch layer of cream
   c. Apply the drug with bare hands
   d. Apply cream over debris on skin surface

2. A patient on sulfonamide therapy develops thrombocytopenia. Which of the following interventions should the nurse perform to alleviate the patient's condition?
   a. Prevent patient from being moved until therapy is over
   b. Instruct patient to avoid brushing teeth
   c. Palpate the patient's skin to assess for trauma
   d. Inspect the patient's skin daily

3. A nurse is educating a patient, who is being discharged, about the measures to combat the effects of photosensitivity. Which of the following precautions should the nurse instruct the patient to follow regarding the effects of photosensitivity while on sulfadiazine therapy?
   a. Stop using contact lenses during the treatment
   b. Apply sunscreen to exposed areas when outdoors
   c. Avoid lights while indoors
   d. Wear protective clothing while outdoors

4. A patient is admitted to a health care facility, and the primary health care provider has prescribed sulfonamide therapy. The patient has also been instructed to increase fluid intake by 2000 mL per day. Which of the following reasons should the nurse give to the patient for increasing fluid intake? Select all that apply.
   a. Removes microorganisms from urinary tract
   b. Allows for easy absorption of drug by GI system
   c. Prevents formation of crystals in urine
   d. Allows for easy excretion by kidneys
   e. Prevents stone formation in genitourinary tract

5. Which of the following adverse reactions should the nurse assess for in a patient during or after the application of mafenide?
   a. Orange-yellow urine
   b. Crystals in urine
   c. Edema
   d. Burning sensation in skin

6. A patient has been admitted to a health care facility and the primary health care provider has prescribed sulfasalazine. The patient is using soft contact lenses. Which of the following information should the nurse provide to the patient about the use of contact lenses during the treatment?

   a. Burning sensation in eyes

   b. Headache and dizziness

   c. Permanent yellow stain in lenses

   d. Impaired vision

7. A patient has been diagnosed with ulcerative colitis and is being administered sulfasalazine. Which of the following interventions should the nurse perform while caring for the patient? Select all that apply.

   a. Check the number and appearance of stool samples

   b. Administer drug during meals or immediately afterwards

   c. Check appearance of urine and measure output

   d. Assess for a loss of appetite or anorexia

   e. Monitor patient for relief or intensification of the symptoms

8. Sulfonamide therapy has been prescribed for a 30-year-old patient with a urinary tract infection. Which of the following information should the nurse give to the patient about the use of cranberries during the treatment?

   a. Prevents bacteria from attaching to walls of the urinary tract

   b. Prevents crystals from forming in the urine

   c. Prevents effect of photosensitivity

   d. Prevents formation of clots

9. A patient with a urinary tract infection is admitted to a health care facility. The physician has prescribed sulfonamide therapy. Which of the following is an advantage of sulfonamide therapy?

   a. Is easily absorbed by the GI system

   b. Kills bacteria cells to fight infection

   c. Decreases the number of white blood cells

   d. Does not have life-threatening adverse reactions

10. A 40-year-old patient is on sulfonamide therapy. Which of the following symptoms should the nurse assess for in the patient to detect Stevens-Johnson syndrome (SJS)?

    a. Inflammation of the mouth

    b. Lesions on mucous membranes

    c. Crystals in urine

    d. Diarrhea

11. The body is equipped with a natural defense system that includes which of the following? Select all that apply.

    a. Saliva

    b. Tears

    c. Skin

    d. Sweat

12. Which of the following are ways in which microbes enter the body? Select all that apply.

    a. Break in the skin

    b. Ingestion

    c. Breathing

    d. Mucous membrane contact

13. Sulfonamides are classified as which of the following?

    a. Antibacterial

    b. Antifungal

    c. Antiviral

    d. Antiprotozoal

14. Drugs that slow or retard the multiplication of bacteria are known as which of the following?

    a. Bacteriocidal

    b. Bacteriostatic

    c. Bacteriostationary

    d. Bacteriophage

15. Drugs that destroy bacteria are known as which of the following?

    a. Bacteriocidal

    b. Bacteriostatic

    c. Bacteriostationary

    d. Bacteriophage

Penicillins

Learning Objectives

- Identify the uses, general drug actions, and general adverse reactions, contraindications, precautions, and interactions of the penicillins
- Identify important preadministration and ongoing assessment activities the nurse should perform on the patient taking penicillin
- List nursing diagnoses particular to a patient taking penicillin
- Discuss hypersensitivity reactions and pseudomembranous colitis as they relate to antibiotic therapy
- Discuss ways to promote optimal response to therapy, nursing actions to minimize adverse effects, and important points to keep in mind when educating patients about the use of penicillins

SECTION I: ASSESSING YOUR UNDERSTANDING

Activity A MATCHING

1. Match the conditions caused by penicillins in Column A with their symptoms in Column B.

Column A	Column B
1. Pseudomembranous colitis	a. Lesions of the mouth or tongue, vaginal discharge, and anal or vaginal itching
2. Anaphylactic shock	b. Inflamed oral mucous membranes, swollen and red tongue, swollen gums, and pain in the mouth and throat
3. Candidiasis	c. Diarrhea or bloody diarrhea, rectal bleeding, fever, and abdominal cramping
4. Fungal superinfection (oral cavity)	d. Severe hypotension, loss of consciousness, and acute respiratory distress

2. *Match the groups of penicillins in Column A with their features in Column B.*

Column A

1. Natural penicillins
2. Penicillinase-resistant penicillins
3. Aminopenicillins
4. Extended-spectrum penicillins

Column B

a. Penicillin effective against a wide range of bacteria including pseudomonas

b. Combinations of penicillins with beta-lactamase inhibitors

c. First large-scale antibiotics used to combat infection

d. Antibiotic developed to combat penicillinase

Activity B FILL IN THE BLANKS

1. A patient may develop phlebitis, an administration route reaction, when penicillin is administered via the _____ route.

2. _____ - spectrum penicillins are a group of penicillins used to destroy bacteria such as *Pseudomonas*.

3. Adverse reactions associated with penicillin include _____ changes, such as anemia, leukopenia, and thrombocytopenia.

4. Treatment of minor hypersensitivity reactions caused by penicillins may include administration of _____ such as diphenhydramine (Benadryl) for a rash or itching.

5. An example of bacterial resistance is the ability of certain bacteria to produce _____, an enzyme that inactivates penicillin.

Activity C SHORT ANSWERS

A nurse's role in managing patients who are being administered penicillin involves monitoring them and implementing interventions that aid in their recovery. Answer the following questions, which involve the nurse's role in management of such situations.

1. A patient with pneumonia has been recommended penicillin. What should a nurse assess for in the patient before administering the first dose of penicillin?

2. A patient receiving penicillin is showing signs of impaired oral mucous membranes. What are the appropriate interventions a nurse should take to ensure the patient's well-being?

Activity D DOSAGE CALCULATION

1. A doctor prescribes 375 mg of ampicillin for a patient. The available solution contains 125 mg/5 cc. How many cc of the available solution will the nurse administer?

2. 1.5 million units of penicillin G (aqueous) have been prescribed for a patient. The available solution contains 500,000 units/cc. How many cc of the available solution are needed to meet the prescribed drug level?

3. A patient has been prescribed 500 mg of oxacillin sodium intramuscularly. After reconstitution, the vial contains 250 mg of active drug per 1.5 mL of solution. How much of the reconstituted solution will be administered to the patient?

4. A doctor prescribes 500 mg Nafcillin every 4 hours for a patient. After reconstitution, the concentration of the drug is 250 mg/mL. How many mL of the reconstituted solution should be administered to the patient?

_____

_____

5. A patient has been prescribed 1 g of penicillin V. The available penicillin V tablet is 500 mg. How many tablets will the nurse administer to the patient?

_____

_____

6. A doctor prescribes 1.5 g Unasyn (ampicillin/sulbactam) for a patient. After reconstitution, the concentration of Unasyn in the vial is 600mg/mL. How many mL of the reconstituted solution will be administered to the patient?

_____

_____

SECTION II: APPLYING YOUR KNOWLEDGE

Activity E CASE STUDY

Lori Jenkins is a Caucasian female 6 years of age. She presents to the physician's office today with bilateral ear pain, nasal congestion, cough, and a low-grade fever. Her mother reports she is not taking any medications and has no allergies that she is aware of at this point. The physician writes a prescription for amoxicillin 250 mg/5 mL, 2 teaspoonsful TID for 10 days.

Lori's mother is concerned that Lori may have an allergic reaction to the amoxicillin. What signs or symptoms should the nurse tell Lori's mother to look for that may indicate an allergic reaction has occurred?

_____

_____

_____

What should the nurse tell Lori's mother about oral suspensions?

_____

_____

SECTION III: PRACTICING FOR NCLEX

Activity F NCLEX-STYLE

Answer the following questions.

1. A patient has developed rashes after the administration of penicillin. The primary health care provider has diagnosed it as a mild hypersensitivity reaction. Which of the following interventions should the nurse perform to alleviate the patient's skin condition?
   a. Reduce the dosage to provide relief to the patient
   b. Instruct the patient to avoid taking baths
   c. Tell the patient to avoid contact of clothing with the affected areas
   d. Administer frequent skin care to the patient

2. A 27-year-old married woman is prescribed penicillin intramuscularly for an infection. Which of the following points should a nurse relay to the patient when educating her about penicillin therapy?
   a. Take the drug at the prescribed times of the day
   b. Discontinue dosage as soon as symptoms of affected condition disappear
   c. Stop taking birth control pills during the medical regimen
   d. Take the drug on an empty stomach, 1 hour before or 2 hours after meals

3. A nurse is caring for a patient who is receiving penicillin. Which of the following reactions to the drug is a cause for concern and should be reported immediately to the primary health care provider?
   a. Pain at injection site
   b. Redness/soreness at previous injection site
   c. Mild nausea
   d. Decrease in body temperature

4. Given below, in random order, are important interventions when caring for a patient receiving antibiotics for an infection. Arrange the interventions in the order they most likely occur in most situations.

   a. Identify the appropriate penicillin
   b. Order a culture and sensitivity test
   c. Record improvement on patient's chart
   d. Administer penicillin to patient
   e. Obtain general history of patient

5. A nurse is caring for a patient who is receiving penicillin. Which of the following assessments will a nurse perform as part of the ongoing assessment process? Select all that apply.

   a. Obtain patient's general health history
   b. Save sample of stool for tests
   c. Evaluate patient daily for response to therapy
   d. Record improvement on patient's chart
   e. Perform additional culture and sensitivity tests

6. A patient who is receiving penicillin complains of diarrhea. Arrange the interventions a nurse will perform in the most likely sequence.

   a. If the stool tests positive for blood, save sample
   b. Notify primary health care provider if diarrhea is confirmed
   c. Inspect all stools for signs of diarrhea
   d. Save a sample of the stool to test for occult blood

7. A nurse has just administered penicillin intramuscularly to a patient as prescribed. The nurse suspects that the patient is developing signs of anaphylactic shock. Which of the following reactions should a nurse monitor for in this patient? Select all that apply.

   a. Severe hypotension
   b. Nausea and vomiting
   c. Loss of consciousness
   d. Acute respiratory distress
   e. Pain at injection site

8. Which of the following interventions should a nurse perform in the event of impaired comfort or increased fever in a patient after he or she has been administered penicillin? Select all that apply.

   a. Discontinue administering the drug immediately
   b. Take vital signs every 4 hours or more
   c. Report any rise in temperature to the primary health care provider
   d. Change the patient's diet to a soft, non-irritating diet
   e. Administer antipyretic drug as per primary health provider's instructions

9. When caring for a patient who is receiving penicillin, a nurse is required to monitor for symptoms of a bacterial superinfection of the bowel. Which of the following symptoms should a nurse monitor for in the patient? Select all that apply.

   a. Diarrhea/bloody diarrhea
   b. Vomiting
   c. Abdominal cramping
   d. Lesions
   e. Rectal bleeding

10. Given below, in random order, are the steps for administering a crystalline drug intramuscularly. Arrange the steps in the correct order.

    a. Extract the penicillin from the vial
    b. Read manufacturer's directions on label
    c. Administer the drug to the patient
    d. Reconstitute the drug to a liquid form
    e. Obtain the appropriate diluent

11. Natural penicillins exert what types of effects on microorganisms?

    a. Bactericidal
    b. Bacteriostatic
    c. Fungicidal
    d. Fungistatic

12. Penicillinase causes bacterial resistance by which of the following mechanisms?
    a. Enzymatic inactivation of the penicillin
    b. Destruction of the beta-lactam ring of the penicillin
    c. Destruction of the penicillin cell wall
    d. Rupture of the penicillin membrane

13. Which of the following are ways that penicillins can be modified to broaden their spectrum of action? Select all that apply.
    a. Chemical modification of the penicillins to slow hepatic metabolism
    b. Addition of a chemical compound to inhibit beta-lactamase inhibitors
    c. Chemical modification of the penicillins to increase GI absorption
    d. Chemical modification to slow excretion of penicillins from the kidneys
    e. Chemical modification of the penicillin to increase tissue penetration

14. Which of the following classes of penicillins are used to treat *Pseudomonas*?
    a. Extended spectrum penicillins
    b. Natural penicillins
    c. Aminopenicillins
    d. Penicillinase-resistant penicillins

15. Penicillins are utilized in the treatment of which of the following bacterial infections? Select all that apply.
    a. Meningitis
    b. Syphilis
    c. Intra-abdominal infections
    d. Osteomyelitis

CHAPTER 8

Cephalosporins

Learning Objectives

- Explain the difference between the first-, second-, third-, and fourth-generation cephalosporins
- Discuss uses, general drug action, adverse reactions, contraindications, precautions, and interactions associated with cephalosporins
- Discuss important preadministration and ongoing assessment activities the nurse should perform on the patient taking cephalosporins
- List nursing diagnoses particular to a patient taking cephalosporins. Discuss ways to promote an optimal response to therapy, how to manage common adverse reactions, special considerations related to administration, and important points to keep in mind when educating patients about the use of the cephalosporins

SECTION I: ASSESSING YOUR UNDERSTANDING

Activity A MATCHING

1. *Match the cephalosporins group in Column A with its appropriate drug in Column B.*

Column A	Column B
1. First-generation	a. Cefepime (Maxipime)
2. Second-generation	b. Cefoperazone (Cefobid)
3. Third-generation	c. Cefoxitin (Mefoxin)
4. Fourth-generation	d. Cefazolin (Ancef)

2. *Match the nursing diagnoses in Column A with their appropriate causes in Column B.*

Column A	Column B
1. Risk for impaired skin integrity	a. Related to ineffectiveness of cephalosporin to the infection
2. Risk for impaired comfort	b. Related to superinfection
3. Impaired urinary elimination	c. Related to hypersensitivity to cephalosporin therapy
4. Diarrhea	d. Related to nephrotoxic effects on kidneys

Activity B FILL IN THE BLANKS

1. Administration route reactions to cephalosporins include pain, tenderness, and _____ at the injection site when given intramuscularly.

2. A_____ -like reaction may occur if alcohol is consumed within 72 hours after certain cephalosporin administration.

3. The needle insertion site and the area above the site are inspected several times a day for signs of redness, which may indicate_____.

4. The nurse should not administer cephalosporins if the patient has a history of allergies to cephalosporins or _____.

5. When cephalosporins are given IV, the nurse inspects the needle insertion site for signs of _____ or infiltration.

Activity C SHORT ANSWERS

A nurse's role in managing patients who are administered cephalosporins involves monitoring them and implementing interventions that lead to their recovery. Answer the following questions which involve the nurse's role in management of patients receiving cephalosporins therapy.

1. A patient diagnosed with a lung infection has been prescribed cephalosporins. What are the factors the nurse should consider before the first dose of the drug is administered?

   _____

   _____

   _____

2. An elderly patient has been prescribed cephalosporin.

   a. What nursing interventions are important when the patient is to be administered cephalosporin by IV?

   _____

   _____

   _____

   b. What nursing interventions are important when the patient is to be administered cephalosporin by IM?

   _____

   _____

   _____

Activity D DOSAGE CALCULATION

1. A middle-aged patient has been prescribed 500 mg of cefzil every 24 hrs. The available form of drug is a 250-mg tablet. To meet the recommended dose, how many tablets should the nurse administer each time?

   _____

   _____

2. A patient is undergoing the treatment of infections due to susceptible organisms. The patient has been prescribed 400 mg of loracarbef orally every 12 hours. For the first dosage, the nurse administers the patient four 100-mg capsules at 8 AM. For the next dosage, the drug is available only in the form of 200-mg capsules. To meet the recommended dose, how many capsules should the nurse administer at the next dosage and at what time?

   _____

   _____

3. A patient has been prescribed 250 mg of cefuroxime drug orally BID every day. The available drug is in the form of a 250-mg tablet. To meet the recommended dose, how many tablets should the nurse administer and how many times a day?

   _____

   _____

4. A patient undergoing hemodialysis has been prescribed a single 400-mg dose of ceftibuten orally 2 times weekly. After reconstitution, the vial contains 90 mg/5 mL of the drug. Approximately how many mL of the reconstituted solution should be administered to the patient for each dosage?

   _____

   _____

5. A patient has been prescribed 250 mg of velosef every 12 hours for infections due to susceptible microorganisms. The available drug is in the form of a 500-mg capsule. How many capsules should the nurse administer to the patient each time?

_____

_____

SECTION II: APPLYING YOUR KNOWLEDGE

Activity E CASE STUDY

Luis Labra is an Hispanic male, 65 years of age. He presents to the ED today with increased shortness of breath, cough, and a low-grade fever. His current medications are warfarin (Coumadin) 5 mg taken as directed and metoprolol 50 mg twice daily. He is admitted to the hospital and the physician writes an order for Mr. Labra to receive ceftriaxone (Rocephin) 1 g every 12 hours via IV infusion.

1. Prior to administering the ceftriaxone to Mr. Labra what information should the nurse obtain from the patient?

_____

_____

_____

2. He reports experiencing an upset stomach after having taken penicillin a long time ago. Is this a true allergy and should Mr. Labra not receive the ceftriaxone?

_____

_____

_____

SECTION III: PRACTICING FOR NCLEX

Activity F NCLEX-STYLE

Answer the following questions.

1. A patient with renal impairment is currently being administered cephalosporins. What are the nursing interventions the nurse should perform when caring for this patient?

a. Inspect each bowel movement

b. Administer antipyretic drugs

c. Record the fluid intake and output

d. Monitor for excessive perspiration

2. The nurse has administered a 32-year-old patient cephalosporin intravenously. What specific condition should the nurse monitor for when this drug is given intravenously?

a. Phlebitis

b. Angina

c. Fever

d. Tenderness

3. A patient has been administered oral anticoagulants while on cephalosporin therapy. What should the nurse identify as a maximized risk in this patient?

a. Increased risk for bleeding

b. Increased risk for nephrotoxicity

c. Increased risk of hypertension

d. Increase in the number of WBCs

4. A 45-year-old patient has been prescribed loracarbef by the physician. Which of the following instructions should the nurse give this patient?

a. Avoid direct sunlight for 1 hour after taking the drug

b. Take the drug with milk or fruit juice

c. Minimize consumption of alcohol while on therapy

d. Take the drug 1 hour before or 2 hours after meals

5. A patient is being administered cefdinir 300 mg orally q12h. However, the physician has prescribed a change in the dosage amount for each administration, where the amount of drug the patient receives per day is the same, but is administered with a 24-hour interval between each dose. Hence, the nurse should now administer _____ mg of the drug after every 24 hours.

6. A 72-year-old patient with paralysis has been prescribed cephalosporin intramuscularly for an infection. Why should the nurse monitor this patient carefully?

   a. The patient may experience a stinging or burning sensation

   b. There is an increased risk for hypersensitive reaction

   c. The large muscle may be atrophied

   d. There is an increased risk for thrombophlebitis

7. Which of the following are expected outcomes in a patient receiving cephalosporin? Choose all that apply.

   a. Complete recovery

   b. Optimal response to therapy

   c. Understanding the treatment

   d. Improved dietary patterns

   e. Compliance with treatment

8. The test reports of a patient on cephalosporin therapy show a deficient production of RBCs. Which of the following adverse effects has the patient developed?

   a. Nephrotoxicity

   b. Anorexia

   c. Aplastic anemia

   d. Toxic epidermal necrolysis

9. The patient on cephalosporin therapy has developed diarrhea. Which of the following is an ideal nursing intervention in this case? Select all that apply.

   a. Save samples of the stool

   b. Administer an antipyretic drug

   c. Discontinue the drug

   d. Immediately report to the physician

   e. Institute treatment for diarrhea

10. A patient has been prescribed cefditoven 200 mg orally TID. The available drug is in the form of a 100-mg tablet. To meet the recommended dose, the nurse will require _____ tablets each day.

11. Cephalosporins are structurally and chemically related to which classes of antibiotics?

    a. Fluoroquinolones

    b. Aminoglycosides

    c. Tetracyclines

    d. Penicillins

12. Which of the following is true of fourth-generation cephalosporins? Select all that apply.

    a. Fourth-generation cephalosporins have a broader spectrum of action

    b. Fourth-generation cephalosporins have a longer duration of resistance to beta-lactamase

    c. Fourth-generation cephalosporins have a narrower spectrum of action

    d. Fourth-generation cephalosporins have a shorter duration of resistance to beta-lactamase

    e. Fourth-generation cephalosporins have the ability to treat viral infections

13. Due to the close relationship cephalosporins have with penicillins, what percentage of clients who are allergic to penicillins are also allergic to cephalosporins?

    a. 10%

    b. 20%

    c. 30%

    d. 50%

14. A disulfiram-like reaction may occur if which of the following is consumed within 72 hours after administration of certain cephalosporins?

    a. Cheese

    b. Alcohol

    c. Meat

    d. Bananas

15. Which cephalosporins have been implicated in disulfiram-like reactions with alcohol? Select all that apply.

    a. Cefamandole

    b. Cefotetan

    c. Cefuroxime

    d. Cefoperazone

    e. Cephalexin

Tetracyclines, Aminoglycosides, Macrolides, and Lincosamides

Learning Objectives

- Discuss the uses, general drug action, adverse reactions, contraindications, precautions, and interactions of the tetracyclines, aminoglycosides, macrolides, and lincosamides
- Discuss important preadministration and ongoing assessment activities the nurse should perform on the patient taking a tetracycline, aminoglycoside, macrolide, or lincosamide
- List nursing diagnoses particular to a patient taking a tetracycline, aminoglycoside, macrolide, or lincosamide
- Discuss ways to promote an optimal response to therapy, how to manage adverse reactions, and important points to keep in mind when educating patients about the use of a tetracycline, aminoglycoside, macrolide, or lincosamide

SECTION I: ASSESSING YOUR UNDERSTANDING

Activity A MATCHING

1. *Match the drugs in Column A with the effect of their interaction with macrolides in Column B.*

Column A

1. Antacids
2. Digoxin
3. Anticoagulants
4. Lincomycin

Column B

a. Increased serum levels

b. Decreased therapeutic activity of macrolide

c. Decreased absorption and effectiveness of macrolide

d. Increased risk of bleeding

2. *Match the adverse reactions of aminoglycosides given in Column A with their signs and symptoms in Column B.*

Column A

1. Nephrotoxicity
2. Ototoxicity
3. Neurotoxicity

Column B

a. Numbness, skin tingling, circumoral paresthesia

b. Proteinuria, hematuria, increase in BUN level

c. Tinnitus, dizziness, roaring in the ears

3. *Match the drugs given in Column A with their adverse reactions given in Column B.*

Column A

1. Tetracyclines
2. Macrolides
3. Lincosamides

Column B

a. Blood dyscrasias
b. Epigastric distress
c. Abdominal pain or cramping

Activity B FILL IN THE BLANKS

1. _____ antibiotics are used for upper respiratory infections caused by *Haemophilus influenzae*.

2. Myasthenia gravis is a disease that affects the _____ junction in nerves and is manifested by extreme weakness and exhaustion of the muscles.

3. _____ act by inhibiting protein synthesis in susceptible bacteria, causing cell death.

4. _____ should not be ordered if a patient is taking cisapride or pimozide.

5. Food or drugs containing calcium, magnesium, aluminum, or iron prevent the absorption of the _____ if ingested concurrently.

6. _____ paralysis is a very serious adverse effect occurring due to the administration of aminoglycosides.

7. Kanamycin, neomycin, and paromomycin are used orally in the management of _____ coma.

Activity C SHORT ANSWERS

A nurse's role in managing patients involves assisting the patients in answering inquiries regarding the treatment being provided. The nurse also helps patients by educating them about precautions to take. Answer the following questions, which involve the nurse's role in management of such situations.

1. A patient with upper respiratory infections caused by *Haemophilus influenzae* is prescribed azithromycin. What is the role of the nurse in monitoring and managing the patient's needs?

_____

_____

_____

2. A patient is to be discharged from the health care facility. He has been prescribed to take demeclocycline for 4 days. What should the nurse include in her teaching plan to educate the patient regarding the medication?

_____

_____

_____

Activity D DOSAGE CALCULATION

1. A physician has prescribed 600 mg of demeclocycline per day for an adult patient. The physician has suggested 4 separate doses of 150 mg. Only 300-mg tablets are available. How many doses should the nurse administer per day?

_____

_____

2. Doxycycline is prescribed by the physician for a 7-year-old patient who weighs 75 lb. Two types of capsules are available, one containing 50 mg. How many capsules should the nurse administer per day if the child should be given 2 mg/lb per day for severe infection?

_____

_____

3. A patient has been prescribed 500 mg of clarithromycin, twice a day. The tablets contain 250 mg. How many tablets should the nurse administer to the patient each time?

_____

_____

4. The physician has prescribed 500 mg of erythromycin to be given every 12 hours for a patient. How many tablets should the nurse administer every 12 hours if they are available in tablets of 250 mg?

_____

_____

5. The physician has prescribed 2250 mg of clindamycin for a patient with severe infection. Each mL of Cleocin Phosphate Sterile Solution contains clindamycin phosphate equivalent to 150 mg of clindamycin. What amount of Cleocin Phosphate Sterile Solution should the nurse give to the patient?

_____

_____

6. The physician has prescribed 600 mg of lincomycin for a patient which is to be administered intramuscularly every 24 hours. Lincocin Sterile Solution is available which contains 300 mg of lincomycin per mL. What amount of the Lincocin Sterile Solution should the nurse give to the patient?

_____

_____

SECTION II: APPLYING YOUR KNOWLEDGE

Activity E CASE STUDY

Maria Lopez is an Hispanic female, 24 years of age. She presents to the physician's office today seeking treatment for her acne. Her only medication is Ortho Tri-Cyclen Lo. The physician writes Ms. Lopez a prescription for doxycycline (Doryx) 150 mg once daily.

1. What should the nurse tell Ms. Lopez about taking oral contraception with Doryx?

_____

_____

_____

2. What adverse reactions should the nurse discuss with Ms. Lopez?

_____

_____

_____

SECTION III: PRACTICING FOR NCLEX

Activity F NCLEX-STYLE

Answer the following questions.

1. Which of the following categories of patients are contraindicated for lincosamides?
   a. Patients with viral infections
   b. Patients less than 9 years of age
   c. Patients who are lactating
   d. Patients with liver disease

2. A patient being treated with lincosamides is to undergo an operation under anesthesia. If a neuromuscular-blocking drug is to be administered for anesthesia, what are the possible complications?
   a. Increased risk for bleeding
   b. Severe and profound respiratory depression
   c. Decreased absorption of the lincosamide
   d. Increased risk for digitalis toxicity

3. A nurse is assigned to take care of a patient with an infection. The nurse is required to identify and record signs and symptoms of the infection. For which of the following symptoms should the nurse closely monitor the patient? Select all that apply.

a. General malaise

b. Diabetes

c. Blood dyscrasias

d. Chills and fever

e. Redness

4. A patient with high fever has been prescribed doxycycline. Which of the following tests should be performed before the first dose of drug is given? Select all that apply.

a. Stress test

b. Sensitivity test

c. Glucose tolerance test

d. Renal function test

e. Urinalysis

5. A patient has been administered a tetracycline drug. Which of the following should the nurse immediately report to the primary health care provider during the ongoing assessment of the patient? Select all that apply.

a. Drop in blood pressure

b. Regular urine output

c. Increase in pulse rate

d. Normal blood sugar level

e. Increase in temperature

6. A patient has been administered Ketak as part of a dental treatment. Concerning which of the following adverse effects should the nurse inform the patient?

a. Esophagitis

b. Difficulty in focusing

c. Photosensitivity

d. Development of skin rashes

7. A patient has been prescribed oral preparations of tetracycline. Which of the following must the nurse include in the patient education plan?

a. Take the drug on an empty stomach

b. Take the drug just before a meal

c. Take the drug along with milk

d. Take the drug only at bedtime

8. A nurse is caring for a 12-year-old patient who has been prescribed dirithromycin. The patient's father inquires about the risks associated with the drug before it is administered. Which of these risks should the nurse include in her reply?

a. Anorexia, constipation, dry mouth, or electrolyte imbalance

b. Visual disturbance, headache, or dizziness

c. Abdominal pain, esophagitis, skin rash, or blood dyscrasias

d. Photosensitivity reactions, hematologic changes, or discoloration of teeth

9. A patient is admitted to a health care facility for diarrhea. The patient's stool tests positive for blood and mucus. What immediate nursing intervention should follow this observation?

a. Save urine sample for tests

b. Measure and record vital signs

c. Check patient's blood pressure

d. Save stool sample for occult blood test

10. A physician has prescribed lincomycin to a patient. How should the nurse administer this drug to the patient?

a. Administer the drug on empty stomach

b. Administer 1 to 2 hours before and after giving food

c. Administer the drug 4 hours after food in between meals.

d. Administer the drug with fruit juice

11. A patient is being administered cephalosporins with aminoglycosides. What is the possible effect of interaction of cephalosporins with aminoglycosides that the nurse should know?

a. Increased risk of ototoxicity

b. Increased risk of nephrotoxicity

c. Increased risk of neuromuscular blockage

d. Increased serum theophylline level

12. A nurse is caring for a patient with a gram-negative bacteria infection, who has been prescribed aminoglycosides. Which of the following interventions should the nurse perform as part of the preadministration assessment for the patient?

    a. Obtain patient's blood count

    b. Monitor vital signs every 4 hours

    c. Record findings in patient's chart

    d. Ensure that urinalysis is conducted

    e. Ensure that hepatic function tests are conducted

13. A nurse is assigned to care for a patient with hepatic coma who has been prescribed kanamycin. Which of the following observations is the nurse most likely to make when monitoring the patient's condition?

    a. Lethargy

    b. Abdominal pain

    c. Numbness

    d. Muscle twitching

14. A nurse is caring for a patient who is being administered aminoglycosides. When assessing the patient, the nurse understands that the patient has developed apnea. The nurse knows that the patient has developed a risk for which of the following conditions?

    a. Neuromuscular blockade

    b. Nephrotoxicity

    c. Pseudomembranous colitis

    d. Ototoxicity

15. Tetracyclines treat infection by which of the following effects?

    a. Inhibiting bacterial protein synthesis

    b. Inhibiting bacterial cell wall synthesis

    c. Inhibiting bacterial DNA gyrase

    d. Depolarizing the bacterial cell wall

CHAPTER 10

Fluoroquinolones and Miscellaneous Anti-Infectives

CHAPTER

Learning Objectives

- Discuss the uses, general drug action, contraindications, precautions, interactions, and adverse reactions of the fluoroquinolones and miscellaneous anti-infectives
- Discuss preadministration and ongoing assessment activities the nurse should perform on the patient taking the fluoroquinolones and miscellaneous anti-infectives
- List nursing diagnoses particular to a patient receiving a fluoroquinolone or miscellaneous anti-infectives
- Discuss ways to promote an optimal response to therapy, how to manage adverse reactions, and important points to keep in mind when educating patients about the use of a fluoroquinolone or miscellaneous anti-infectives

SECTION I: ASSESSING YOUR UNDERSTANDING

Activity A MATCHING

1. *Match the interacting drugs used along with fluoroquinolones given in Column A with their common uses in Column B.*

Column A

1. Theophylline
2. Cimetidine (Tagamet)
3. Oral anticoagulants
4. Non-steroidal anti-inflammatory drugs (NSAIDs)

Column B

a. Blood thinners
b. Relief of pain and inflammation
c. Management of respiratory problems
d. Management of GI upset

2. *Match the anti-infective drugs given in Column A with their uses in Column B.*

Column A

1. Spectinomycin
2. Fosfomycin tromethamine
3. Aztreonam
4. Quinupristin

Column B

a. Used for treating gonorrhea in patients who are allergic to penicillins, cephalosporins, or probenecid

b. Used in the treatment of vancomycin-resistant *Enterococcus faecium*

c. Used to treat urinary tract infections

d. Used to treat gram-negative microorganisms

3. *Match the anti-infective drugs in Column A with their most adverse reactions in Column B.*

Column A

1. Linezolid
2. Daptomycin
3. Spectinomycin
4. Vancomycin

Column B

a. Nephrotoxicity
b. Urticaria
c. Vein irritation
d. Pseudo membranous colitis and thrombocytopenia

Activity B **FILL IN THE BLANKS**

1. Linezolid is a _____ that acts by binding to a site on a specific ribosomal RNA.

2. Linezolid is contraindicated in patients with _____.

3. _____ is used to treat serious infections and community-acquired pneumonia caused by bacteria.

4. _____ are used cautiously in patients with central nervous system (CNS) disorders, seizure disorders, and in patients with renal or hepatic failure.

5. Nephrotoxicity and ototoxicity may be seen with the administration of _____.

6. _____ is a fluoroquinolone which is used in the management of respiratory problems, such as asthma.

7. Fluoroquinolones exert their _____ effect by interfering with the synthesis of bacterial DNA.

Activity C **SHORT ANSWERS**

A nurse's role in managing patients who are using fluoroquinolones involves monitoring and managing interventions that aid in their recovery. A patient with acute pain due to tissue injury is prescribed intravenous fluoroquinolones. What interventions should the nurse perform when caring for the patient who is administered fluoroquinolones?

A nurse's role in managing patients who are being administered anti-infective drugs involves monitoring the patients and implementing interventions that aid their recovery.

A nurse has been caring for a client with gonorrhea. Post-treatment, the nurse has to evaluate the effectiveness of the treatment plan. What factors should the nurse consider to determine the success of the treatment plan?

Activity D **DOSAGE CALCULATION**

1. A patient is prescribed 500 mg of aztreonam every 12 hours. The drug is available in the form of 125-mg tablets. How many tablets should the nurse administer per day to meet the recommended dose?

2. A patient is prescribed 400 mg of vancomycin per day. The drug is available in the form of 80-mg tablets. How many tablets should the nurse administer per day?

3. A patient with a bacterial infection is prescribed daptomycin to be administered intravenously. The normal dosage for daptomycin is 4 mg/kg. The patient weighs 65 kg. The normal dose of daptomycin available is 500 mg/10 mL. How much of the drug solution should the nurse prepare?

_____

_____

4. A patient with a rash on his hand is prescribed 500 mg of trobicin every 12 hours. The drug is available in the form of 100-mg tablets. How many tablets should the nurse administer in 2 days?

_____

_____

5. A pneumonia patient is prescribed 300 mg of ertapenem every 8 hours. The drug is available in the form of 150-mg tablets. How many tablets should the nurse administer per day to meet the recommended dose?

_____

_____

6. A patient with a bacterial infection is prescribed 700 mg of aztreonam to be taken intramuscularly. The drug is available in the form of 50 mL/g. How much of the drug solution should the nurse prepare for the intramuscular administration in the client?

_____

_____

SECTION II: APPLYING YOUR KNOWLEDGE

Activity E CASE STUDY

Darla Moore is an African American female, 54 years of age. She is hospitalized for pyelonephritis. The physician orders ciprofloxacin (Cipro), 400 mg every 12 hours for 2 days and then Cipro 500 mg by mouth every 12 hours for 12 more days.

1. What preadministration assessments should be completed prior to starting Mrs. Moore on Cipro?

_____

_____

2. Cipro is available in a 10 mg/mL vial. How many mL will the nurse need to prepare for one 400-mg dose?

_____

_____

_____

SECTION III: PRACTICING FOR NCLEX

Activity F NCLEX-STYLE

Answer the following questions.

1. A nurse is assigned to care for a patient who has developed a serious bacterial infection. The patient has been prescribed linezolid, which has to be administered orally. Which of the following most serious adverse reactions of linezolid should the nurse monitor for in the patient?
   a. Thrombocytopenia
   b. Nephrotoxicity
   c. Ototoxicity
   d. Phlebitis

2. A nurse has been caring for a patient who was treated for bacterial infection. The patient is now scheduled to receive treatment on an outpatient basis. Which of the following instructions should the nurse offer to the patient and patient's family under continuing care?
   a. Complete full course of treatment
   b. Always take the drug with food
   c. Avoid drinking alcoholic beverages
   d. Understand potential adverse reactions
   e. Monitor for adverse symptoms for 3 days

3. A nurse is caring for a 35-year-old patient with gonorrhea. The physician has prescribed a dosage of 4 g of spectinomycin to be given intravenously to the patient. The available dosage of this drug is 5 mL/2 g. How much of the drug in solution should the nurse prepare?
   a. 2 mL
   b. 10 mL
   c. 15 mL
   d. 4 mL

4. A nurse is caring for a patient with gonorrhea who is being prescribed spectinomycin. The nurse should monitor for which of the following adverse effects when caring for this patient?

   a. Sudden decrease in blood pressure

   b. Headache

   c. Urticaria

   d. Throbbing neck pain

5. A nurse is assigned to care for a patient who has to be administered quinupristin/dalfopristin. Which of the following precautions should the nurse take when administering quinupristin/dalfopristin to the patient?

   a. Monitor for cross-sensitivity if administered with cephalosporin

   b. Monitor for secondary bacterial or fungal infections

   c. Monitor for bone marrow depression

   d. Monitor for hearing or kidney problems

6. A nurse is caring for a patient with a bacterial infection. The nurse has to administer vancomycin to the patient through the parenteral route. The nurse ensures that every dose of vancomycin is administered over 60 minutes. The nurse should remain alert for which of the following conditions when caring for this patient?

   a. Shock

   b. Severe hypotension

   c. Sudden decrease in blood pressure

   d. Ringing in the ears

7. A patient with a urinary tract infection is administered fosfomycin tromethamine. The nurse is required to conduct an ongoing assessment for the patient. What are the required ongoing assessments for a patient that the nurse has to perform? Select all that apply.

   a. Monitor for sudden decrease in pulse and respiratory rate

   b. Monitor vital signs of the patient every 4 hours

   c. Observe for sudden increase in temperature in the patient

   d. Observe patient frequently during first 48 hours of therapy

   e. Determine signs of any infection in the patient

8. A nurse is caring for a patient with a gram-negative bacterial infection. The patient has to be administered aztreonam. The nurse has to assess the patient's medical history to determine the medications that the patient uses. The nurse knows aztreonam has to be administered cautiously in case the patient is taking which of the following drugs?

   a. Antiplatelet drugs

   b. Nephrotoxic drugs

   c. Warfarin

   d. Penicillin

9. A nurse is assigned to care for a patient who has to be administered an anti-infective drug intramuscularly. Which of the following nursing interventions should the nurse perform when caring for this patient receiving an intramuscular anti-infective?

   a. Check the infusion site every 12 hours

   b. Rotate the injection sites

   c. Inspect previous injection sites

   d. Assess for vein irritation

   e. Adjust rate of infusion every 30 minutes

10. A patient with a bacterial infection has been admitted to a health care facility. The patient has an infection caused by *Enterococcus faecium*, which is resistant to the effect of vancomycin. The nurse knows that which of the following drugs will help reduce the infection in the patient?

    a. Daptomycin

    b. Quinupristin/dalfopristin

    c. Fosfomycin tromethamine

    d. Spectinomycin

11. A nurse is required to care for a patient who is to be administered fluoroquinolones. The nurse knows that under which of the following conditions should fluoroquinolones be administered cautiously?

    a. Patients with a history of seizures

    b. Patients with renal failure

    c. Patients with neuromuscular disorders

    d. Patients who are elderly

12. A nurse is caring for a patient with a low respiratory rate. The patient is administered fluoroquinolones. The nurse is required to assess the client for which of the following adverse effects caused due to the administration of fluoroquinolones?

    a. Urticaria

    b. Anorexia

    c. Rash

    d. Dizziness

13. A nurse is caring for a patient who is receiving fluoroquinolones through the intravenous route. Which of the following nursing interventions should the nurse perform to avoid the occurrence of phlebitis or thrombophlebitis?

    a. Check the rate of infusion every 2 hours

    b. Inspect the vein used for infusion frequently

    c. Alternate the vein used for infusion

    d. Inform physicians of observations

    e. Perform assessment frequently

14. A nurse is caring for a patient with a sexually transmitted disease. The patient is to be administered fluoroquinolones. Which of the following should the nurse ensure to confirm that fluoroquinolone is not contraindicated in the patient?

    a. Patient is not younger than 18 years of age

    b. Patient does not have preexisting hearing loss

    c. Patient does not have myasthenia gravis

    d. Patient does not have Parkinsonism

15. A nurse is caring for a patient who is being administered fluoroquinolones. Which of the following instructions should the nurse offer to assist the patient to protect herself against photosensitive reactions?

    a. Wear brimmed hats

    b. Wear long-sleeve clothing

    c. Venture out preferably on hazy days

    d. Wear sunscreen

    e. Wear very light makeup

CHAPTER 11

Antitubercular Drugs

Learning Objectives

- Discuss the drugs used in the treatment of mycobacteria for tuberculosis and leprosy
- Discuss the uses, general drug actions, contraindications, precautions, interactions, and general adverse reactions associated with the administration of the antitubercular drugs
- Discuss important preadministration and ongoing assessment activities the nurse should perform on the patient taking an antitubercular drug
- List nursing diagnoses particular to a patient taking an antitubercular drug
- Describe directly observed therapy (DOT)
- Discuss ways to promote an optimal response to therapy, how to manage adverse reactions, and important points to keep in mind when educating patients about the use of the antitubercular drugs

SECTION I: ASSESSING YOUR UNDERSTANDING

Activity A MATCHING

1. *Match the drugs in Column A with the effects of their interaction with isoniazid in Column B.*

Column A	Column B
1. Aluminum salts	a. Increases serum levels
2. Anticoagulants	b. Exaggerated sympathetic-type response occurs
3. Phenytoin	
4. Tyramine	c. Increases risk for bleeding
	d. Reduces absorption of isoniazid

Activity B FILL IN THE BLANKS

1. Nephrotoxicity and ototoxicity may be seen with the administration of _____.

2. People with human _____ virus are at risk for tuberculosis because of their compromised immune systems.

3. _____ tuberculosis is the term used to distinguish TB affecting the lungs from infection with the *M. tuberculosis* bacillus in other organs of the body.

4. When isoniazid is taken with foods containing _____, an exaggerated sympathetic-type response can occur.

5. The recommended treatment regimen is for the administration of rifampin, isoniazid, pyrazinamide, and ethambutol for a minimum of _____ months.

Activity C SHORT ANSWERS

A nurse's role in managing patients who are diagnosed with tuberculosis and administered anti-tubercular drugs involves instructing the patients about adverse reactions and precautions to be taken during recovery. Answer the following questions regarding the nurse's role in the management of such situations.

1. The nurse is caring for a 24-year-old patient with tuberculosis. What interventions should the nurse perform as part of the preadministration assessment when providing care for this client?

   _____

   _____

2. A nurse has been caring for a patient with TB. Post-treatment, the nurse has to care for the patient on an outpatient basis. What instructions should the nurse offer the patient and patient's family to decrease the chances of non-compliance?

   _____

   _____

3. A nurse has been caring for a patient with TB. After the patient's treatment, the nurse has to evaluate the effectiveness of the treatment plan. What should the nurse keep in mind when evaluating the success of the treatment plan?

   _____

   _____

Activity D DOSAGE CALCULATION

1. A patient has been prescribed 150 mg of isoniazid per day. Each available tablet of isoniazid contains 100 mg of the drug. How many tablets will need to be administered to the patient in 2 days?

   _____

   _____

2. A physician prescribes 600 mg of rifampin per day for a patient. Rifampin is available as 300-mg tablets. How many tablets will need to be administered to the patient per day?

   _____

   _____

3. A patient has been prescribed 400 mg of pyrazinamide per day. If this antitubercular drug is available as splits of 25 mg each, then how many splits of the drug per day will have to be administered to the patient?

   _____

   _____

SECTION II APPLYING YOUR KNOWLEDGE

Activity E CASE STUDY

Charlie Price is a Caucasian male, 55 years of age, who presented to the physician's office 2 days ago with a 2-week history of coughing, sputum production, and night sweats. The nurse administered Mr. Price a PPD skin test. He presents today for the nurse to read the test, which is positive. The physician diagnoses Mr. Price with tuberculosis.

1. What assessment should be completed prior to starting Mr. Price on any antitubercular drugs?

   _____

   _____

2. What ongoing assessment should the nurse complete while Mr. Price is taking the antitubercular drugs?

   _____

   _____

SECTION IV: PRACTICING FOR NCLEX

Activity F NCLEX-STYLE

Answer the following questions.

1. A nurse is required to care for a patient who has been administered rifampin. Which of the following generalized adverse reactions should the nurse monitor for in the patient?

   a. Myalgia

   b. Jaundice

   c. Reddish-orange color of bodily fluids

   d. Dermatitis and pruritus

2. A nurse is assigned to care for a patient with TB, who has to be administered ethambutol. Which of the following conditions should the nurse ensure to confirm that ethambutol is not contraindicated in the patient? Select all that apply

   a. Patients is not younger than 13 years of age

   b. Patient does not have cataracts

   c. Patient does not have a hypersensitivity to drug

   d. Patient does not have diabetes mellitus

   e. Patient does not have acute gout

3. A nurse has been caring for a patient with TB in a health care facility. Posttreatment, the nurse now has to ensure that the patient follows his drug regimen regularly without missing a dose. The nurse suggests that the patient follow an alternative dosing regimen of twice weekly. How can this mode of taking the dosage help the client?

   a. Decreases gastric upset and promotes nutrition

   b. Promotes fluid balance in the patient's body

   c. Prevents the occurrence of neuropathy

   d. Prevents the occurrence of liver dysfunction

4. A nurse is assigned to care for a client with extrapulmonary tuberculosis in a health care facility. Which of the following organs can be affected by extrapulmonary tuberculosis? Select all that apply.

   a. Heart

   b. Liver

   c. Spleen

   d. Brain

   e. Kidneys

5. A nurse is assigned to care for a patient with TB. When conducting the preadministration assessment, the nurse should know that the patient is taking which of the following drugs so that she can closely monitor the patient when he is administered rifampin? Select all that apply.

   a. Oral anticoagulants

   b. Digoxin

   c. Oral contraceptives

   d. Colchicine

   e. Allopurinol

6. A nurse is caring for a patient with TB who has been administered isoniazid. The treatment has lasted for many months and ongoing assessment reveals that the patient is developing signs of a severe toxic reaction. The nurse should monitor for which of the following manifestations of a severe toxic reaction to isoniazid in the patient?

   a. Hepatotoxicity

   b. Anaphylactoid reactions

   c. Severe hepatitis

   d. Epigastric distress

7. A patient with tuberculosis is administered pyrazinamide as prescribed. The nurse caring for the patient suspects that the patient is developing signs of hepatotoxicity as an adverse reaction of pyrazinamide. Which of the following manifestations of a hepatotoxic reaction should the nurse look for in the patient?

   a. Severe jaundice

   b. Epigastric distress

   c. Severe hepatitis

   d. Hematologic changes

8. A nurse is required to care for a TB patient who has been administered antitubercular drugs. The nurse has to provide care to the patient on an outpatient basis. Which of the following interventions should the nurse perform to prevent the risk of hepatitis in the TB patient?

   a. Administer antitubercular drugs in combination

   b. Use DOT to administer drugs on outpatient basis

   c. Instruct patient to take pyridozine according to prescription

   d. Instruct the patient to minimize alcohol consumption

9. A nurse is assigned to care for a TB patient who is administered rifampin. The nurse knows that under which of the following conditions is the use of rifampin contraindicated?

   a. Patients who have tested positive for HIV

   b. Patients with hepatic or renal impairment

   c. Patients with diabetes mellitus

   d. Patients with diabetic retinopathy

10. Which of the following individuals are especially susceptible to tuberculosis? Select all that apply.

    a. Individuals living in crowded conditions

    b. Individuals with human immunodeficiency virus (HIV)

    c. Individuals less than 6 years of age

    d. Individuals more than 30 years of age

    e. Individuals with asthma

11. How is tuberculosis transmitted from person to person?

    a. Contact with infected blood

    b. Fecal oral transmission

    c. Inhalation of infected aerosolized droplets

    d. Contact with sweat

12. Tuberculosis can affect which of the following organs? Select all that apply.

    a. Lungs

    b. Liver

    c. Kidneys

    d. Spleen

    e. Uterus

13. Which of the following are true of antitubercular drugs? Select all that apply.

    a. Treat active cases of tuberculosis

    b. Prophylaxis to prevent the spread of tuberculosis

    c. Render the patient non-infectious to others

    d. Treat dormant cases of tuberculosis

    e. Cure tuberculosis infection

14. Active tuberculosis (TB) may be difficult to diagnose in patients infected with HIV because of their immune system deficiency. Which of the following can be used to determine if an HIV patient with a negative skin test has active TB? Select all that apply.

    a. X-ray studies

    b. Blood tests

    c. Sputum analyses

    d. Urinalysis

    e. Physical examinations

15. A client in the initial phase of tuberculosis treatment develops a decrease in visual acuity and changes in color perception. Which drug may be causing this reaction?

    a. Ethambutol

    b. Isoniazid

    c. Pyrazinamide

    d. Rifampin

CHAPTER 12

Antiviral Drugs

Learning Objectives

- Discuss the uses, general drug actions, adverse reactions, contraindications, precautions, and interactions of antiviral drugs
- Discuss important preadministration and ongoing assessment activities the nurse should perform on the patient receiving an antiviral/antiretroviral drug
- List nursing diagnoses particular to a patient taking an antiviral drug
- List possible goals for a patient taking an antiviral/antiretroviral drug
- Discuss ways to promote an optimal response to therapy and manage adverse reactions, and special considerations to keep in mind when educating the patient and the family about the antiviral/antiretroviral drugs

SECTION I: ASSESSING YOUR UNDERSTANDING

Activity A MATCHING

1. *Match the interactant drugs in Column A with their uses in Column B.*

Column A	Column B
1. Antifungals	a. Treat bacterial infection
2. Clarithromycin	b. Relieve pain
3. Sildenafil	c. Eliminate or manage fungal infections
4. Opioid analgesics	d. Treat erectile dysfunction

2. *Match the interactant drugs in Column A with their common uses in Column B.*

Column A	Column B
1. Probenecid	a. Gout treatment
2. Cimetidine	b. Pain relief
3. Ibuprofen	c. Anti-infective agent
4. Imipenem/cilastatin	d. Relief of gastric upset, heartburn

Activity B FILL IN THE BLANKS

1. _____ balm is a perennial herb with heart-shaped leaves that has been used for hundreds of years. Its scientific name is *Melissa officinalis*.

2. _____, also called Vistide, should not be given to patients who have renal impairment or in combination with medications that are nephrotoxic, such as aminoglycosides.

3. _____, also called Norvir, is contraindicated if the patient is taking bupropion (Wellbutrin), zolpidem (Ambien), or an antiarrhythmic drug.

4. The drug _____ has been known to cause kidney and/or bladder stones in patients.

5. _____ drugs are used in the treatment of human immunodeficiency virus (HIV) and acquired immune deficiency syndrome (AIDS).

Activity C SHORT ANSWERS

A nurse's role in managing patients who are being administered antiviral drugs includes observing and monitoring their progress and performing any necessary interventions. Answer the following questions which involve the nurse's role in management of such situations.

1. A patient is diagnosed with *Herpes simplex* virus (HSV) and the physician has prescribed antiviral drugs. What should the nurse assess for before administering the antiviral drug?

   _____

   _____

2. A patient has hepatitis B and the physician has prescribed an antiviral drug. What should nurse assess for while administerng the antiviral drug to the patient?

   _____

   _____

Activity D DOSAGE CALCULATION

1. A primary health care provider has prescribed 120 mg of Foscavir per day to be given intravenously. The strength of the drug in the available solution is 24 mg/mL. How many mL of the solution should the nurse administer to the patient in a day?

   _____

   _____

2. The primary health care provider has prescribed intravenous acyclovir to a patient. The standard dosage of the drug is 5 mg/kg to be given once a day. The patient weighs 50 kg. The drug available in solution is 10 mL/500 mg. How much of the drug dosage should the nurse prepare for the client to be administered for a week?

   _____

   _____

3. The primary health care provider has prescribed 100 mg of amantadine daily for a patient. The drug is available as syrup with a concentration of 50 mg/5 mL. How many mL of the given syrup should the nurse prepare for the patient to be administered for a week?

   _____

   _____

4. The primary health care provider has prescribed 500 mg of famciclovir per dose. The drug is available in 125-mg tablets. How many tablets should the nurse administer to the patient per dose?

   _____

   _____

5. The primary health care provider has prescribed 300 mg of cidofovir for a patient. The drug is available as syrup with a concentration of 375 mg/5 mL. How many mL of the given syrup should the nurse administer to the patient?

   _____

   _____

6. The primary health care provider has prescribed 1 mg of entecavir per dose. The drug is available in 0.05 mg/mL oral solution. How many mL for 6 such doses should the nurse prepare for the patient?

_____

_____

SECTION II: APPLYING YOUR KNOWLEDGE

Activity E CASE STUDY

John Jones is an African American male, 55 years of age, who has been HIV-positive for 5 years. He is currently taking Atripla one tablet by mouth daily. He presents to the physician's office complaining of pain in his mouth and white patches on his tongue and cheeks.

1. While triaging Mr. Jones, what information should the nurse obtain?

_____

_____

_____

2. Mr. Jones tells the nurse he has started taking St. John's wort because he heard it had antiviral effects and he was feeling a bit depressed lately. What should the nurse tell Mr. Jones about the St. John's wort?

_____

_____

_____

SECTION III: PRACTICING FOR NCLEX

Activity F NCLEX-STYLE

Answer the following questions.

1. A nurse is required to administer ribavirin to a patient. Which of the following points should the nurse keep in mind while administering the drug? Select all that apply.
   a. Discard and replace the solution every 24 hours
   b. The drug can worsen respiratory status
   c. The drug increases risk of nephrotoxicity
   d. Drug should be administered with a small-particle aerosol generator
   e. The drug induces anorexia and weight loss

2. A patient on antiretroviral drug is also taking clarithromycin. Which of the following are the effects of the antiretroviral therapy when it is combined with clarithromycin?
   a. Increased serum level of the antiretroviral
   b. Increased serum level of both drugs
   c. Risk of toxicity
   d. Decreased effectiveness of the antiretroviral

3. A patient with HSV 1 has been prescribed antiretroviral therapy. Before beginning the treatment, which of the following interventions should the nurse perform that is most appropriate considering the patient's infection?
   a. Save a sample of patient's urine
   b. Record patient's temperature
   c. Inspect areas with lesions
   d. Check patient's blood pressure

4. A nurse is caring for a patient who is on antiretroviral therapy for HIV. The patient has developed anorexia and nausea due to the therapy. Which of the following interventions should the nurse perform in the given situation? Select all that apply.
   a. Reduce frequency of meals but increase quantity of meals
   b. Ensure that client's diet includes soft, non-irritating foods
   c. Keep the atmosphere clean and free of odors
   d. Eliminate carbonated beverages or hot tea from diet
   e. Provide good oral care before and after meals

5. In which of the following cases should a nurse monitor for phlebitis in a patient?
   a. Patient is given drugs orally
   b. Patient is given drugs intramuscularly
   c. Patient is given drugs intravenously
   d. Patient is given drugs transdermally

6. In which of the following cases should the nurse exercise caution while caring for clients who have been administered indinavir?
   a. Patients with renal impairment
   b. Patients with cardiac disorders
   c. Patients with sulfonamide allergy
   d. Patients with history of bladder stone formation

7. A nurse is required to administer didanosine to an HIV patient. Which of the following points should the nurse keep in mind while administering the drug?
   a. Administer drug with meals
   b. Administer with 2 oz of water
   c. Avoid generating dust
   d. Refrigerate solution

8. A primary health care provider has prescribed 5400 mg of foscavir per day to be administered intravenously. The strength of the drug in the available solution is 24 mg/mL. How many mL of the solution should the nurse administer to the patient in a day?
   a. 250 mL
   b. 225 mL
   c. 275 mL
   d. 200 mL

9. The primary health care provider has prescribed 800 mg of acyclovir per dose. The drug is available in 200-mg tablets. How many tablets should the nurse administer to the patient per dose?
   a. 1
   b. 2
   c. 4
   d. 8

10. The primary health care provider has prescribed 200 mg of amantadine daily. The drug is available as syrup with a concentration of 50 mg/5mL. How many mL of the given syrup should the nurse administer to the patient?
    a. 10 mL
    b. 15 mL
    c. 20 mL
    d. 25 mL

11. Which of the following represents a route of entry for viruses into the body? Select all that apply.
    a. Insect bite
    b Blood on intact skin
    c. Needle stick
    d. Inhalation
    e. Ingestion

12. Which of the following can be caused by a virus? Select all that apply.
    a. Common cold
    b. Impetigo
    c. Wart
    d. Influenza
    e. Hepatitis C

13. Why are viruses so difficult to treat even with the use of antiviral medications? Select all that apply.
    a. Viruses are tiny
    b. Viruses can develop resistance to antiviral drugs
    c. Viruses have a hard-to-penetrate outer layer
    d. Viruses are large
    e. Viruses replicate inside human cells

14. Highly active antiretroviral therapy (HAART) is used to treat which of the following infections?
    a. Human immunodeficiency virus (HIV)
    b. *Herpes simplex* virus (HSV)
    c. Cytomegalovirus (CMV)
    d. Rotavirus
    e. Rhinovirus

15. How are retroviruses different from viruses? Select all that apply.
    a. Human immunodeficiency virus is an example of a retrovirus.
    b. Retroviruses contain an enzyme called reverse transcriptase.
    c. RNA is the primary component of the retrovirus instead of DNA.
    d. DNA is the primary component of the retrovirus instead of RNA.
    e. Cytomegalovirus is an example of a retrovirus.

Antifungal and Antiparasitic Drugs

- Distinguish between superficial and systemic fungal infections
- Distinguish between helminthic infections, protozoal infections, and amebiasis
- Discuss the uses, general drug action, adverse reactions, contraindications, precautions, and interactions of antifungal and antiparasitic drugs
- Discuss important preadministration and ongoing assessment activities the nurse should perform on the patient receiving an antifungal and antiparasitics drug
- List nursing diagnoses particular to a patient taking an antifungal and antiparasitic drug
- List possible goals for a patient taking an antifungal and antiparasitic drug
- Discuss ways to promote an optimal response to therapy, how to manage adverse reactions, and important points to keep in mind when educating the patient and the family about the antifungal and antiparasitic drugs

SECTION I: ASSESSING YOUR UNDERSTANDING

Activity A MATCHING

1. *Match the antifungal drugs in Column A with their uses in Column B.*

Column A

1. Flucytosine
2. Ketoconazole
3. Griseofulvin
4. Miconazole
5. Micafungin sodium

Column B

a. Treat infections of the skin, hair, or nails

b. Inhibit DNA and RNA synthesis in the fungi

c. Prevention in stem cell transplantation

d. Treat systemic fungal infections

e. Treat vaginal infections

2. *Match the anthelmintics in Column A with their effect on helminthic infections in Column B.*

Column A

1. Albendazole
2. Mebendazole
3. Pyrantel
4. Thiabendazole

Column B

a. Interrupts the life cycle of the helminth

b. Interferes with the synthesis of helminth microtubules

c. Blocks uptake of glucose by the helminth

d. Paralyzes the helminth

Activity B FILL IN THE BLANKS

1. _____ fungal infections are serious infections that occur when fungi gain entrance into the interior of the body.

2. _____ mycotic infections occur on the surface of, or just below, the skin or nails.

3. _____ clearance tests are done before administering fluconazole to an elderly patient or a patient with renal impairment.

4. The use of griseofulvin is contraindicated for patients having severe _____ disease.

5. The systemic agent itraconazole should not be used to treat fungal nail infections in patients with a history of _____ problems.

6. Use of amphotericin B for patients who have _____ imbalances can cause severe bone marrow suppression.

7. _____ due to fungal infections may cause anxiety for a patient undergoing antifungal treatment.

8. _____ or Vermox blocks the uptake of glucose by the helminth, resulting in a depletion of the helminth's own glycogen.

9. Parenteral injection of the antimalarial drug _____ is avoided because the drug can cause cardiovascular collapse when given intramuscularly (IM) or intravenously (IV).

10. _____ is an aminoglycoside with amebicidal activity and is used to treat intestinal amebiasis.

11. _____ interferes with the results of thyroid function tests up to 6 months after therapy.

12. Irreversible_____ damage has occurred in patients on long-term therapy with antimalarial drugs.

Activity C SHORT ANSWERS

A nurse's role in managing a patient who is prescribed an antifungal drug involves preadministration assessment. The nurse also monitors patients who are administered with an antifungal drug. Answer the following questions, which involve the nurse's role in management of patients on antifungal therapy.

1. A patient with vaginal fungus is prescribed an antifungal drug. What preadministration assessments should the nurse conduct before administering an antifungal drug?

_____

_____

2. After the preadministration assessment, the patient is administered an antifungal drug for the vaginal infection. What is the nurse's role when caring for the patient administered a topical antifungal infection preparation?

_____

_____

A nurse's role in managing patients who are administered anthelmintic drugs involves monitoring the patients and implementing interventions that aid in their recovery. Answer the following questions, which involve the nurse's role in the management of such situations.

3. A patient with a pinworm infection has been recommended an anthelmintic drug. What should a nurse assess for in the patient before administering the drug?

_____

_____

4. A patient receiving an anthelmintic drug is showing signs of nausea, vomiting, and abdominal pain. What are the appropriate interventions a nurse should take to ensure the patient's well-being?

_____

_____

Activity D DOSAGE CALCULATIONS

1. A patient has been prescribed 400 mg of fluconazole every 24 hours. The available drug is in the form of a 200-mg tablet. To meet the prescribed dose, how many tablets should the nurse administer each day?

_____

_____

2. A patient has been prescribed 200 mg of fluconazole every 12 hours. The available drug is in the form of a 50-mg tablet. To meet the prescribed dose, how many tablets should the nurse administer each time?

_____

_____

3. A patient has been prescribed 100 mg of flucytosine every 6 hours. The available drug is in the form of a 50-mg tablet. To meet the prescribed dose, how many tablets should the nurse administer each day?

_____

_____

4. An athletic patient has been prescribed 500 mg of griseofulvin in 4 doses every day. The available drug is in the form of 125 mg/5 mL suspension. To meet the prescribed dose, how many mL should the nurse administer for each dose?

_____

_____

5. A patient with a nail infection has been prescribed 200 mg of itraconazole twice daily. The drug is available in the form of 100-mg capsules at the local pharmacy. The patient would like to know the total number of capsules he should buy for a 3-day course to meet the prescribed dose. What is the total number of capsules required for this patient?

_____

_____

6. A patient with a fungal infection has been prescribed 400 mg of ketoconazole in 2 doses every day. The available drug is in the form of 200-mg capsules. To meet the prescribed dose, how many capsules should the nurse administer each time?

_____

_____

7. A doctor prescribes 500 mg per day of chloroquine. The available chloroquine tablet is 250 mg. How many tablets should the patient consume daily?

_____

_____

8. A patient has been prescribed 780 mg of quinine sulfate per day (divided into 3 equal doses). The available quinine sulfate tablet is 260 mg. How many tablets should the nurse administer to the patient every day?

_____

_____

SECTION II: APPLYING YOUR KNOWLEDGE

Activity E CASE STUDY

Jessica Landry is a Caucasian female, 24 years of age, who is a 2 years status post-kidney transplant. Her current medications include: prednisone 5 mg QD, Prograf 1 mg BID, Cellcept 500mg 2 capsules BID, warfarin 5 mg QD, enalapril 10 mg QD, simvastatin 10 mg QD, Ortho Novum 7/7/7 QD, Advair 250/50 1 inhalation BID, and Proventil HFA 2 puffs Q 4–6 hours PRN wheezing and shortness of breath. She presents today complaining of irritation and soreness in her mouth and throat.

1. Which of Ms. Landry's medications or medical conditions put her at risk for a fungal infection?

   _____

   _____

   _____

2. The physician diagnoses Ms. Landry with oral candidiasis and prescribes nystatin suspension 1 teaspoonful QID for 7 days. As part of the nurse's teaching plan, how should she counsel Ms. Landry to use the suspension?

   _____

   _____

   _____

SECTION III: PRACTICING FOR NCLEX

Activity F NCLEX-STYLE

Answer the following questions.

1. A nurse is required to assess a patient for symptoms of deep myotic infection. Which parts of the body should the nurse check for deep myotic infections?
   a. Liver
   a. Lungs
   b. Mouth
   c. Heart

2. A patient with a fungal infection is admitted to the health care facility. The physician prescribes topical administration of an antifungal drug. What kinds of reactions should the nurse monitor for in the patient?
   a. Dehydration
   b. Nausea
   c. Stinging
   d. Diarrhea

3. The nurse is documenting the history of a patient who is to be started on itraconazole therapy. In which of the conditions is itraconazole contraindicated?
   a. Bone marrow suppression
   b. Severe liver disease
   c. History of heart failure
   d. History of asthma

4. What care should the nurse take when administering an IV solution of amphotericin B?
   a. Ensure that the IV solution is protected from light
   b. Freeze the unused IV solution
   c. Ensure that the IV solution is used within 24 hours
   d. Store the drug in a heated environment

5. A patient has been prescribed intravenous administration of amphotericin B to cure a fungal infection. What adverse reactions should a nurse monitor for in the patient?
   a. Vomiting
   b. Abdominal pain
   c. Muscle pain
   d. Anorexia

6. A patient is undergoing antifungal treatment. The patient has lesions due to fungal infections, and the reaction to the treatment is slow. As a result, the patient is anxious. What should the nurse do to help reduce the anxiety of the patient undergoing antifungal treatment?
   a. Check the patient's blood pressure
   b. Encourage the patient to verbalize feelings
   c. Provide the patient with a warm blanket
   d. Keep the patient away from light

7. A patient who is being treated for a fungal infection has recovered and is to be discharged. The nurse needs to instruct the patient how to take care of the infection after the discharge. What are the important instructions that the nurse should include in the patient's teaching plan?

   a. There should be no sexual contact while lesions are present

   b. Precautions to avoid sunlight should be taken when going out of doors

   c. Physical activities should be avoided

   d. Towels should be kept separate from those of other family members

8. A patient undergoing treatment with ketoconazole is soon to be discharged. What reactions for the ketoconazole drug should a nurse instruct the patient to expect?

   a. Unusual fatigue, yellow skin, and darkened urine

   b. Fever, sore throat, or skin rash

   c. Headache, dizziness, and drowsiness

   d. Nausea, vomiting, or diarrhea

9. A nurse is required to care for a malaria patient who is acutely ill. Which of the following interventions should the nurse perform?

   a. Record vital signs of the patient every 12 hours

   b. Observe the patient every 4 hours for malaria symptoms

   c. Collect urine samples of the patient and send for testing

   d. Carefully measure and record the fluid intake and output

10. For which of the following patients is the antimalarial drug quinine contraindicated?

   a. Patients with myasthenia gravis

   b. Patients with thyroid disease

   c. Patients with blood dyscrasias

   d. Patients with diabetes

11. Which of the following are adverse effects associated with anthelmintic drugs? Select all that apply.

   a. Drowsiness, dizziness

   b. Nausea, vomiting

   c. Visual disturbances

   d. Abdominal pain, cramps

   e. Tinnitus (ringing sound in ears)

12. A nurse is caring for a patient with a helminthic infection. Which of the following interventions should the nurse perform?

   a. Save stool samples during the first day of treatment only

   b. Follow hospital procedure for transporting stool to the laboratory

   c. Visually inspect stools only if patient reports anything unusual

   d. Use any container to save a sample of the stool

13. A nurse is caring for a patient who has been administered chloroquine. Which of the following patient conditions is a cause for concern that the nurse should report immediately to the primary health care provider?

   a. Unusual muscle weakness

   b. Peripheral neuropathy

   c. Yellow or brown urine

   d. Ringing in the ears

   e. Visual changes

14. Which of the following information should be given to women of child-bearing age regarding the possible effects of Albendazole?

   a. Albendazole can cause serious harm to a developing fetus

   b. Albendazole increases the risk of miscarriage

   c. Albendazole may decrease the chances of conception

   d. Albendazole may adversely affect the estrogen hormone

15. A female patient is prescribed pyrantel for roundworms. Which of the following should a nurse tell the patient when educating her about taking an anthelmintic drug?
    a. Use birth control pills instead of the barrier method for contraception
    b. Discontinue dosage as soon as symptoms of the affected condition disappear
    c. Use chlorine bleach to disinfect toilet facilities or shower stall after bathing
    d. Take the drug with milk and not water, unless the patient is lactose intolerant

16. Which of the following adverse effects associated with Paromomycin should a nurse monitor for in a patient?
    a. Vertigo, hypotension
    b. Nephrotoxicity and ototoxicity
    c. Thrombocytopenia
    d. Peripheral neuropathy

17. Which of the following pieces of information should a nurse give to a patient who has been prescribed Metronidazole?
    a. Take the drug with meals or immediately afterward
    b. Avoid alcohol for the first week of treatment
    c. Take cimetidine for gastric upset or other stomach problems
    d. Wear protective clothing to guard against photosensitivity

18. A patient has been prescribed doxycycline for malaria. Which of the following side effects should the nurse inform the patient about regarding the drug?
    a. Photosensitivity
    b. Skin eruptions
    c. Cinchonism
    d. Thrombocytopenia

Nonopioid Analgesics: Salicylates and Nonsalicylates

Learning Objectives

- Discuss the types, uses, general drug actions, common adverse reactions, contraindications, precautions, and interactions of the salicylates and acetaminophen
- Discuss important preadministration and ongoing assessment activities the nurse should perform for the patient taking salicylates or acetaminophen
- List nursing diagnoses particular to a patient taking salicylates or acetaminophen
- Discuss the ways to promote an optimal response to therapy, how to manage common adverse reactions, and important points to keep in mind when educating patients about the use of salicylates or acetaminophen

SECTION I: ASSESSING YOUR UNDERSTANDING

Activity A MATCHING

1. *Match the interactant drug in Column A with the likely effect it may have when taken with a salicylate from Column B.*

Column A

1. Anticoagulant b
2. Activated charcoal d
3. Antacid a
4. Carbonic anhydrase inhibitor c

Column B

a. Decreased effects of the salicylates

b. Increased risk of bleeding

c. Increased risk for salicylism

d. Decreased absorption of the salicylates

2. *Match the nursing diagnosis checklist options in Column A with their nursing diagnoses in Column B.*

Column A

1. Impaired comfort C

2. Chronic or acute a pain

3. Impaired physical d mobility

4. Disturbed sensory b perception

Column B

a. Peripheral nerve damage and/or tissue inflammation due to the aspirin therapy

b. Auditory related to adverse drug reactions

c. Fever of the disease process (e.g., infection or surgery)

d. Muscle and joint stiffness

Activity B FILL IN THE BLANKS

1. The analgesic action of the salicylates is due to the inhibition of prostaglandins which are fatty acid derivatives found in almost every tissue of the body and bodily fluid.

2. Aspirin prolongs bleeding time by inhibiting the aggregation (clumping) of platelets

3. Pancytopenia a reduction in all cellular components of the blood.

4. The use of aspirin may be involved in the development of Reye syndrome in children who have chickenpox or influenza.

5. Tinnitus, a ringing sound in the ear, is one of the symptoms of salicylism.

Activity C SHORT ANSWERS

A nurse's role in managing discomfort of patients involves assisting them with relieving their pain. The nurse also helps administer drugs and provide physical comfort. Briefly answer the following questions, which involve the nurse's role in the management of such situations.

1. What are the different ways in which a nurse can assess patients' pain?

Different ways to assess pain would be a scale, either a color scales, faces or numeric # scale 0-10. 0 being no pain and 10 the most.

2. A patient had been prescribed salicylates. How can the nurse monitor and manage this patient's discomfort?

Nurse can monitor and manage pts comfort from relief of pain, any inflammation or bleeding, color or odor of stool and by decreasing of pain and distress.

Activity D DOSAGE CALCULATION

1. A patient has been prescribed 650 mg of aspirin every 4 hours. The available tablets are 325 mg. How many tablets will the nurse administer to the patient daily?

12 tablets

2. The physician prescribes 500 mg of Dolobid orally, every 8 hours, for a patient. The available tablets are 250 mg. How many tablets will the nurse administer to the patient daily?

6 tablets

3. Salsalate, 3000 mg daily, has been prescribed for a patient. The available tablet contains 500 mg of salsalate. How many tablets are needed daily to meet the prescribed drug level?

6 tablets

4. A patient has been prescribed 600 mg of acetaminophen every day. The available drug is in the form of a 300-mg tablet, which is to be administered every 6 hours. To meet the recommended dose, how many tablets should the nurse administer each time?

1/2 tablet

5. A patient can be given 650 mg of buffered aspirin every 4 hours. The available tablets are 325 mg. How many tablets will the nurse administer to the patient each time if the tablets are to be administered every 8 hours?

4 tablets

6. A patient is prescribed 650 mg of Ecotrin every 4 hours. The nurse has 325-mg tablets. How many tablets should the nurse administer every 4 hours?

2 tablets

SECTION II: APPLYING YOUR KNOWLEDGE

Activity E CASE STUDY

Martha Matthews is an African American female, 34 years of age, who was admitted to the hospital 2 days ago with a VTE. She is being discharged from the hospital today on Coumadin (warfarin) 5 mg QD. She tells the nurse she often takes Ecotrin for headaches.

1. What should the nurse tell Mrs. Matthews about the use of Ecotrin with Coumadin (warfarin)?

The nurse should indicate that the use of Ecotrin with warfarin will increase bleeding and increases the the time of clotting.

2. What should the nurse recommend Mrs. Matthews take for her headaches?

The nurse should recommend Mrs. Matthew to take acetaminophen tylenol for headaches because it won't cause clotting problems.

SECTION III: PRACTICING FOR NCLEX

Activity F NCLEX-STYLE

Answer the following questions.

1. A patient has been prescribed salicylates as an analgesic agent. Which of the following adverse reactions caused by salicylates should the nurse monitor for?
   a. Skin eruptions
   b. GI bleeding
   c. Jaundice
   d. Bleeding disorders

2. For which of the following patients are salicylates contraindicated? Select all that apply.
   a. Patients with hypersensitivity to the drug
   b. Patients with a history of heart failure
   c. Patients with influenza or viral illness
   d. Patients with bleeding disorders
   e. Patients with hepatic disorders

3. In which of the following patients is acetaminophen preferred over aspirin?
   a. Patients with severe pain
   b. Patients with high fever
   c. Patients with bleeding tendencies
   d. Patients with inflammatory disorders

4. A patient has been administered acetaminophen. Which of the following interventions should the nurse perform as part of the ongoing assessment?
   a. Reassess patient's pain rating 3 hours after administration
   b. Monitor the patient's vital signs every 8 hours
   c. If stools are dark, send a sample for testing immediately
   d. Assess for decrease in inflammation and greater mobility

5. Which of the following symptoms can be observed in a patient with salicylate levels between 150 and 250 micrograms/mL?
   a. Nausea
   b. Respiratory alkalosis
   c. Hemorrhage
   d. Asterixis

6. Which of the following is an effect of combining loop diuretics with acetaminophen?
   a. Increased possibility of toxicity
   b. Decreased effect of acetaminophen
   c. Increased risk for bleeding
   d. Decreased effectiveness of the diuretic

7. Which of the following information should a nurse provide to a patient who has been prescribed salicylates regarding their purchase and storage?
   a. Do not use OTC drugs containing aspirin
   b. Include paprika, licorice, prunes, and raisins in diet
   c. Store the drug in a cool, ventilated area
   d. Purchase salicylates in small amounts
   e. Notify the physician before surgery or a dental procedure

8. Which of the following adverse reactions should a nurse monitor for in a patient who has been administered salsalate?
   a. GI bleeding
   b. Hypoglycemia
   c. Pancytopenia
   d. Hemolytic anemia

9. In which of the following instances can aspirin be used to treat patients?
   a. Patients with hemophilia
   b. Patients with rheumatoid arthritis
   c. Patients with postoperative pain
   d. Patients taking anticoagulants

10. A patient has been prescribed acetaminophen. Which of the following are signs of acetaminophen toxicity that the nurse should monitor for in the patient?
    a. Malaise
    b. Increased anxiety
    c. Hyperglycemia
    d. Bradycardia

11. Which body system is the agent involved in the recognition and perception of pain?
    a. Nervous system
    b. Cardiovascular system
    c. Integumentary system
    d. Endocrine system

12. Pain is classified into which of the following basic types? Select all that apply.
    a. Acute
    b. Traumatic
    c. Chronic
    d. Postoperative
    e. Neuropathic

13. Which of the following are classified as acute pain? Select all that apply.
    a. Postoperative pain
    b. Procedural pain
    c. Osteoarthritis pain
    d. Fibromyalgia pain
    e. Diabetic neuropathic pain

14. Chronic pain is classified as pain that lasts for more than how long?
    a. 1 week
    b. 1 month
    c. 6 weeks
    d. 6 months

15. Which of the following are examples of chronic pain? Select all that apply.
    a. Fibromyalgia pain
    b. Postoperative pain
    c. Traumatic pain
    d. Rheumatoid arthritis pain
    e. Osteoarthritis pain

Nonopioid Analgesics: Nonsteroidal Anti-Inflammatory Drugs (NSAIDs) and Migraine Headache Medications

Learning Objectives

- Discuss the types, uses, general drug actions, common adverse reactions, contraindications, precautions, and interactions of the NSAIDs
- Describe the types, general drug actions, common adverse reactions, contraindications, precautions, and interactions of drugs used to treat migraine headaches
- Discuss important preadministration and ongoing assessment activities the nurse should perform on the patient taking the NSAIDs
- List nursing diagnoses particular to a patient taking an NSAID
- Discuss the ways to promote an optimal response to therapy, how to manage common adverse reactions, and important points to keep in mind when educating patients about the use of NSAIDs

SECTION I: ASSESSING YOUR UNDERSTANDING

Activity A MATCHING

1. *Match the discomforts faced by patients in Column A with their NANDA nursing diagnoses in Column B.*

Column A	Column B
1. Impaired physical mobility _C_	a. Visual disturbance
2. Disturbed sensory perception _A_	b. Peripheral tissue damage
3. Acute or chronic pain _B_	c. Muscle and joint stiffness

2. *Match the drugs that interact with NSAIDs in Column A with their interacting effects in Column B.*

Column A

1. Anticoagulants _d_
2. Hydantoins _c_
3. Acetaminophen _a_
4. Diuretics _b_

Column B

a. Increased risk of renal impairment
b. Increased excretion of extracellular fluid
c. Increased effectiveness of the anticonvulsant
d. Increased risk of bleeding

Activity B FILL IN THE BLANKS

1. NSAIDs act by inhibiting prostaglandin synthesis by inhibiting the action of the enzyme _cyclooxygenase_

2. _Celecoxib_ is associated with an increased risk of serious cardiovascular thrombosis, myocardial infarction (MI), and stroke.

3. _Ibuprofen_ a drug for pain relief, is available over-the-counter without a prescription.

4. _Reye_ syndrome is an adverse effect of aspirin.

5. NSAIDs are prescribed for the pain and _inflammation_ associated with arthritis.

Activity C SHORT ANSWERS

A nurse's role in managing patients who are being administered NSAIDs involves monitoring the patients and implementing interventions that aid in their recovery. Answer the following questions, which involve the nurse's role in the management of such situations.

1. What are NSAIDs used for?

   NSAIDs are used for fever reduction, mild to moderate pain and pain related to musculoskeletal disorders such as arthritis and osteoarthritis.

2. A nurse is caring for a patient receiving an NSAID drug for moderate pain. For which adverse reactions of NSAIDs on the sensory organs should the nurse monitor the patient?

   Adverse reactions to be monitored would be changes in taste, runny nose, tinnitus, blurry vision, swollen eyes and visual disturbances.

Activity D DOSAGE CALCULATION

1. A patient has been prescribed 150 mg of Cataflam orally per day. Cataflam is available as 50-mg tablets. How many tablets will the nurse administer to the patient per day?

   3 tablets

2. A patient has been prescribed 1 g of Lodine orally per day. The drug is available in 200-mg tablets. How many tablets will the nurse administer to the patient per day?

   5 tablets

3. A patient has been prescribed 1.2 g of Nalfon orally in 4 doses a day. The drug is available in 200-mg tablets. How many tablets will the nurse administer to the patient each time?

   1 1/2 tablets

4. A patient has been prescribed 200 mg of Ansaid orally in 2 equally divided doses. The drug is available in 100-mg tablets. How many tablets will the nurse administer to the patient daily?

   2 tablets

5. A patient has been prescribed 400 mg of meclofenamate sodium orally in 4 divided doses. The drug is available as 100-mg tablets. How many tablets will the nurse administer to the patient per day?

   4 tablets

SECTION II: APPLYING YOUR KNOWLEDGE

Activity E CASE STUDY

James Smith is a Caucasian male, 55 years of age, who presents to the physician's office today complaining of knee and hip pain. He has hypertension, diabetes, and generalized anxiety disorder. His medications include lisinopril 20 mg QD, metformin ER 500 mg BID, and aspirin 81 mg QD. He has tried acetaminophen in the past to treat his joint pain, but with little relief. The physician diagnoses him with osteoarthritis and writes a prescription for ibuprofen 800 mg q8h PRN Pain. The physician has asked the nurse to bring Mr. Smith the prescription.

1. What should the nurse tell Mr. Smith about taking the ibuprofen with his other medications?

   The nurse should indicate that Ibuprofen can cause bleeding, bruising, increase in BP, weakness w/ his other medications.

2. How should the nurse advise Mr. Smith to take his ibuprofen?

   The nurse should advise Mr. Smith to take his medicine with fluids either milk or water, don't take more than needed and follow directions on the bottle when to take pills, how many hours in between.

SECTION III: PRACTICING FOR NCLEX

Activity F NCLEX-STYLE

Answer the following questions.

1. A patient with rheumatoid arthritis has been administered an NSAID. For which of the following adverse reactions of NSAIDs on the gastrointestinal system should the nurse monitor the patient? Select all that apply.
   a. **Epigastric pain**
   b. Appendicitis
   c. **Abdominal distress**
   d. Indigestion
   e. **Intestinal ulceration**

2. Why is celecoxib not used to relieve postoperative pain for a patient who has undergone coronary artery bypass graft (CABG) surgery?
   a. Increased risk of duodenal ulcer
   b. Increased risk of gastric bleeding
   c. **Increased risk of myocardial infarction**
   d. Increased risk of diarrhea

3. A nurse is documenting the history of a patient who is to be initiated on NSAID therapy. In which of the following conditions is ibuprofen contraindicated?
   a. Patients with sulfonamide allergy
   b. **Patients with peptic ulceration**
   c. Patients with cardiac disease
   d. Patients with history of stroke

4. A nurse is assigned to care for a patient who has to be administered an NSAID. Which of the following precautions should the nurse take before administering NSAID to the patient?
   a. Monitor for visual disturbances
   b. Monitor for skin reactions
   c. Monitor for dizziness
   d. **Monitor for bleeding disorders**

5. A patient is prescribed an NSAID for osteoarthritis. What assessments should the nurse perform before the administration of NSAIDs?
   a. **Document limitations in mobility**
   b. Examine the level of consciousness in the patient
   c. Check the level of mental stability of the patient
   d. Determine the patient's body temperature

6. A nurse is caring for a patient undergoing NSAID treatment. Which of the following should the nurse suggest to the patient to promote an optimal response to therapy?
   a. Avoid exercise
   b. Restrict to a liquid diet
   c. **Take medication with food**
   d. Restrict mobility

7. A patient has been prescribed indomethacin for rheumatoid disorders. Which of the following adverse conditions should the nurse monitor the patient for?

    a. Tinnitus

    b. Diarrhea

    c. Rash

    d. GI bleeding

8. A 68-year-old patient is prescribed an NSAID for arthritis. Why should treatment for the elderly begin with a reduced dosage that is increased slowly?

    a. Increased risk of inflammation

    b. Increased risk of erythema

    c. Increased RBC count

    d. Increased risk of serious ulcer diseases

9. A patient has been prescribed 1 g of oral nabumetone in 2 equal doses per day. The drug is available in 500-mg tablets. How many tablet(s) should the nurse administer the patient per day?

    a. 2

    b. 1

    c. 2.5

    d. 1.5

10. A patient being treated for arthritis is to be discharged. Which of the following instructions should the nurse include in the patient's teaching plan? Select all that apply.

    a. Avoid physical activities during drug therapy

    b. Do not use the drugs on a regular basis unless the PHCP is notified

    c. Keep towels separate from those of other family members

    d. Avoid use of aspirin

    e. Take the drug with a full glass of water or with food

11. Blocking of which of the following is responsible for the pain-relieving effects of NSAIDs?

    a. Cyclooxygenase-2

    b. Cyclooxygenase-1

    c. Cyclooxygenase-3

    d. Cyclooxygenase-4

12. Blocking of which of the following is responsible for the gastrointestinal side effects caused by NSAIDs?

    a. Cyclooxygenase-2

    b. Cyclooxygenase-3

    c. Cyclooxygenase-1

    d. Cyclooxygenase-4

13. The most common side effects caused by NSAIDs involve which of the following?

    a. Stomach

    b. Lungs

    c. Liver

    d. Peripheral nerves

14. A hypersensitivity to which of the following medications is a contraindication for all NSAIDs?

    a. Acetaminophen

    b. Hydrochlorothiazide

    c. Aspirin

    d. Lisinopril

15. Which of the following NSAIDs appears to work by specifically inhibiting cyclooxygenase-2, without inhibiting cyclooxygenase-1?

    a. Celecoxib (Celebrex)

    b. Ibuprofen (Motrin)

    c. Naproxen (Naprosyn)

    d. Meloxicam (Mobic)

CHAPTER 16

Opioid Analgesics

Learning Objectives

- Discuss the uses, general drug action, general adverse reactions, contraindications, precautions, and interactions of the opioid analgesics
- Discuss important preadministration and ongoing assessment activities the nurse should perform on the patient taking the opioid analgesics
- List nursing diagnoses particular to a patient taking an opioid analgesic
- Discuss ways to promote optimal response to therapy, how to manage adverse reactions, and important points to keep in mind when educating patients about the use of opioid analgesics

SECTION I: ASSESSING YOUR UNDERSTANDING

Activity A MATCHING

1. *Match the adverse reaction in Column A with the associated drug name in Column B.*

Column A	Column B
1. Vertigo b	a. Demerol
2. Dry mouth d	b. Dilaudid
3. Constipation a	c. Ultiva
4. Skeletal muscle rigidity c	d. Levo-Dromoran

2. *Match the discomforts faced by patients in Column A with their nursing diagnoses in Column B.*

Column A	Column B
c 1. Effects on breathing B	a. Decreased gastrointestinal motility caused by opioids
a 2. Constipation d	b. Anorexia caused by opioids
d 3. Risk for injury a	c. Ineffective breathing pattern
b 4. Imbalanced nutrition c	d. Dizziness or lightheadedness from opioid administration

Activity B FILL IN THE BLANKS

1. The most widely used opioid, _morphine_ sulfate, is an effective drug for moderately severe to severe pain.

2. All opioid analgesics are contraindicated in patients with _hypersensitivity to_ the drugs.

3. Opioid analgesics are the analgesics obtained from the _opium_ plant.

4. _Heroin_ is an illegal narcotic substance in the United States and is not used in medicine.

5. Elderly, _cachectic,_ or debilitated patients may have a reduced initial opioid dose until their response to the drug is known.

Activity C SHORT ANSWERS

A nurse's role in managing patients who are prescribed opioid analgesics involves helping the patients deal with chronic pain. The nurse also assists patients in coping with their drug regimens and helps them in the event of opiate addiction. Answer the following questions, which involve the nurse's role in managing such situations.

1. A patient who has cancer is prescribed morphine through an IV infusion pump. What information should the nurse offer the patient with regard to the use of the PCA infusion pump?

   The location of the control button and button that activates the drug, The difference between the control button and the call light button. Call the nurse if the pain med is not wearing.

2. What factors should the nurse evaluate to determine the success of an opioid treatment plan?

   The nurse shall evaluate the therapeutic effects occur and when pain is relieved. Adverse reactions are identified and reported to the primary health care provider and nursing interventions.

Activity D DOSAGE CALCULATION

1. A physician prescribes 30 mg of aspirin-codeine orally 4 times a day for a patient. The available tablets are 60 mg. How many tablets will the nurse need to administer to the patient daily?

   2 tablets

2. A physician prescribes 60 mg of methadone for a patient, to be spread over 6 doses per day. Each available tablet contains 10 mg of the drug. How many tablets will the nurse need to administer to the patient in each dose?

   1 tablet

3. A physician prescribes butorphanol to a patient. The standard dose is 4 mg/70 kg. The patient weighs 110 kg. The drug has to be taken 3 times a day. How much of butorphanol has the physician prescribed, and how much should the nurse administer to the patient in one day?

   6.3 mg of butorphanol will be prescribed and pt should take 18.9 mg a day

4. A patient is prescribed Fentanyl 50 mcg IM 30 minutes before surgery. The available vial has dosage strength of 0.05 mg/1 mL. How much fentanyl will the nurse need to administer to the patient?

   _1 mL_

5. A physician prescribes 250 mg of morphine sulfate daily to a patient. Each 5 mL of Roxanol 100TM contains 100 mg of morphine sulfate. How much Roxanol 100TM will the nurse need to administer to the patient daily?

   _12.5 mL_

6. A physician prescribes 100 mg of tramadol hydrochloride daily to a patient. Tramadol hydrochloride is available in the form of Ultram tablets, each tablet containing 50 mg of tramadol hydrochloride. How many Ultram tablets will the nurse need to administer to the patient daily?

   2 tablets

SECTION II: APPLYING YOUR KNOWLEDGE

Activity E CASE STUDY

Janice Wiggins is an African American female, 45 years of age, who is in the hospital for an elective hysterectomy. She is to receive morphine via a PCA pump postop.

1. How should the nurse instruct Mrs. Wiggins to use the pump during preoperative teaching?

   How the pump works the location of the control button that activates the administration of the morphine.

2. After the surgery, what information should be included in the nurse's ongoing assessment and how often should the assessments be completed?

   BP, Pulse, R pain rate 5-10 mins be morphine given which will include location, type and intensity.

SECTION III: PRACTICING FOR NCLEX

Activity F NCLEX-STYLE

Answer the following questions.

1. A nurse is caring for a patient who is prescribed opioid analgesics. Which of the following allergic reactions of opioid analgesics should the nurse monitor for in the patient?
   a. Constipation
   b. Urticaria
   c. Palpitations
   d. Facial flushing

2. A patient is prescribed an opioid analgesic for the treatment of pain. What preadministration assessments should the nurse conduct before the administration of an opioid analgesic?
   a. Obtain patient's blood pressure
   b. Assess the intensity and location of pain
   c. Monitor patient's pulse rate
   d. Assess patient's respiratory rate

3. A nurse is caring for a patient who would like to use herbal doses of passion flower. Which of the following should the nurse confirm to ensure that the use of passion flower is not contraindicated in the patient?
   a. Patient is not taking monoamine oxidase inhibitors
   b. Patient is not taking opioid analgesics
   c. Patient does not have acute ulcerative colitis
   d. Patient does not have a history of asthma

4. A patient is prescribed an opioid analgesic for pain relief caused by terminal illness. The nurse notices that the patient has developed severe anorexia due to the opioid treatment. What interventions should the nurse perform for a patient with imbalanced nutrition due to prolonged administration of an opioid?
   a. Ensure an increase in patient's fluid intake
   b. Assess the patient's food intake after each meal
   c. Complement patient's meal with protein supplements
   d. Record patient's bowel movements daily

5. A nurse is caring for a patient who has delivered a baby. The patient was opioid-dependent during her pregnancy. Which of the following withdrawal symptoms should the nurse monitor for in the newborn?
   a. Excessive crying
   b. Vomiting
   c. Yawning
   d. Coughing
   e. Sneezing

6. Which of the following enforces a cautious use of naloxone to a patient experiencing a decrease in respiratory rate?
   a. Naloxone leads to withdrawal symptoms
   b. Naloxone leads to vomiting
   c. Naloxone leads to dizziness
   d. Naloxone leads to headache

7. A patient is being prescribed opioid analgesics in a local health care facility. Which of the following is the nurse most likely to observe in this patient that would require immediate attention by the physician?
   a. Decrease in respiratory rate
   b. Change in pulse quality
   c. Decrease in blood pressure
   d. Increase in body weight
   e. Increase in body temperature

8. A nurse is assigned to care for a patient who has to be prescribed opioid therapy. Which of the following statements in the patient's health history will require cautious use of opioid analgesics by the nurse? Select all that apply.
   a. Patient has undiagnosed abdominal pain
   b. Patient is 13 years old
   c. Patient has hepatic or renal impairment
   d. Patient has hypoxia
   e. Patient has fungal infections

9. A nurse is caring for a patient on opioid therapy. The patient is also prescribed barbiturates, under close supervision. Which of the following risks is likely to occur in this patient?
   a. Bacterial infections
   b. Hypertension
   c. Respiratory depression
   d. Hypoxia

10. A patient who was being treated for severe diarrhea with opioid analgesics has recovered and is to be discharged. Which of the following instructions should the nurse include in the patient's teaching plan?
   a. Avoid traveling
   b. Avoid alcohol
   c. Avoid exercising
   d. Avoid starchy food

11. Which of the following is considered the gold standard in pain management?
   a. Morphine sulfate
   b. Codeine
   c. Oxymorphone
   d. Hydromorphone

12. Which of the body systems does not adapt and compensate for the secondary effects of opioids?
   a. GI system
   b. Respiratory system
   c. Cardiovascular system
   d. Nervous system

13. Lactating females may use opioid analgesics, but should wait how long after taking an opioid analgesic to breastfeed the infant?
   a. 2 to 4 hours
   b. 4 to 6 hours
   c. 6 to 8 hours
   d. 8 to 10 hours

14. Which of the following herbs has been used to treat pain?
   a. Passion flower
   b. Ginger
   c. Garlic
   d. Ginseng

15. Patient taking which of the following medications should not use the passion flower herb?
   a. Ibuprofen (Motrin)
   b. Lisinopril (Prinivil)
   c. Warfarin (Coumadin)
   d. Amoxicillin (Amoxil)

Opioid Antagonists

Learning Objectives

- Discuss the uses, general drug action, general adverse reactions, contraindications, precautions, and interactions of the opioid antagonists
- Discuss important preadministration and ongoing assessment activities the nurse should perform on the patient receiving the opioid antagonists
- List nursing diagnoses particular to a patient taking an opioid antagonist
- Discuss ways to promote optimal response to therapy, how to manage adverse reactions, and important points to keep in mind when educating patients about the use of opioid antagonists

SECTION I: ASSESSING YOUR UNDERSTANDING

Activity A MATCHING

1. *Match the opioid antagonists in Column A with their uses in column B.*

Column A *a , b*

1. Naloxone (Narcan)

2. Nalmefene (Revex)

    a , b

Column B

a. Complete or partial reversal of opioid effects after overdose

b. Postoperative acute respiratory depression

Activity B FILL IN THE BLANKS

1. A drug that is a(n) _Antagonist_ has a greater affinity for a cell receptor than an opioid drug, and by binding to the cell it prevents a response to the opioid.

2. _Opioid_ antagonists reverse the actions of an opioid.

3. _Naloxone_ is capable of restoring respiratory function within 1 to 2 minutes of administration.

4. Antagonists are contraindicated in patients with _hypersensitivity to_ opioid antagonists.

5. Naloxone is used within the controlled settings of the _postanesthesia_ recovery unit.

6. Opioid antagonists are used for the treatment of postoperative acute _respiratory_ depression.

7. The trade name for naloxone is _Narcan_

Activity C SHORT ANSWERS

A nurse's role in managing respiratory depression in patients involves assisting the patients with the administration of opioid antagonists. The nurse is also expected to monitor and assess the patients' needs. Answer the following questions, which involve the nurse's role in managing such situations.

1. A patient with respiratory depression is administered an opioid antagonist in a health care facility. What preadministration assessments should a nurse perform when caring for the patient?

   Wake the pt, instruct deep breathing patterns, take vitals and review history, allergy history and current treatment provided.

2. What circumstances that enforce the use of opioid antagonists should a nurse be aware of?

   Postop acute respiratory depression, reverse of opioids and adverse effects and acute opioid overdosage suspected.

Activity D DOSAGE CALCULATION

1. A patient is prescribed naloxone for a narcotic overdose. A total of 3 mg has to be given to the patient, and the available dosage is in the form of 0.5-mg tablets. Considering that one tablet has already been administered, how many more tablets should the patient take to complete the dosage?

   5 tablets

2. A patient is prescribed 15 mg of intramuscular nalmefene. The available drug concentration is 2.5 mg/mL. How much drug will the nurse have to administer to the patient?

   6mL

3. A patient has been prescribed 10 mg of buprenorphine intravenously. How much buprenorphine should the nurse administer to the patient when the available dose is 2 mg/mL?

   5mL of Buprenorphine

SECTION II: APPLYING YOUR KNOWLEDGE

Activity E CASE STUDY

Jeffrey Smith is a Caucasian male, 17 years of age, who is driven to the ED after collapsing at a party. After examining the patient and talking to others at the party, the physician suspects Mr. Smith has overdosed on oxycodone.

1. Prior to administering naloxone (Narcan) to Mr. Smith, what should be included in the nurse's preadministration assessment?

   Preadministration assessment should be monitoring BP, pulse and Respiratory rate.

2. During the third dose, Mr. Smith vomits. How should the nurse handle this situation?

   After Mr. Smith vomits the nurse should maintain a patent airway repositioning him on his side and suction prn.

SECTION III: PRACTICING FOR NCLEX

Activity F NCLEX-STYLE

Answer the following questions.

1. A patient is administered a postoperative opioid antagonist for pain management. Which of the following should the nurse identify as the action of the opioid antagonist in the patient's body?

   a. Opioid antagonist instantly relieves pain

   b. Opioid antagonist reverses the effect of pain medication

   c. Opioid antagonist neutralizes the effect of opioid drug

   d. Opioid antagonist decreases pain

2. A nurse has been caring for a patient with respiratory depression. Which of the following critical factors are used to evaluate the treatment of a patient receiving an opioid antagonist for respiratory depression? Select all that apply.

    a. Positive response to therapeutic treatment
    b. Normal blood pressure
    c. Normal respiratory rate
    d. Resumption of pain relief
    e. Normal heart rate

3. A patient has been prescribed naloxone for respiratory depression. Which of the following interventions should the nurse perform to promote an optimal response in the patient?

    a. Monitor for an increase in the patient's body temperature
    b. Monitor for any signs of dehydration and water loss in the patient
    c. Balance need for continued pain relief with patient's ability to breathe
    d. Administer the drug through a rapid IV push in the patient

4. A patient in a health care facility is prescribed a postoperative dose of naloxone. Which of the following interventions should the nurse perform during and after naloxone administration when caring for this patient? Select all that apply.

    a. Monitor the patient for symptoms of hypotension
    b. Make the suction equipment available
    c. Turn and suction the patient when needed
    d. Provide artificial ventilation
    e. Monitor hematologic changes

5. A patient in a health care facility is prescribed an opioid antagonist. Which of the following statements in the patient's health records will require a cautious use of the opioid antagonist in this patient?

    a. Patient has liver impairment
    b. Patient is lactating
    c. Patient has renal failure
    d. Patient is hypersensitive to the drug

6. Which of the following interventions should a nurse perform when caring for patients with respiratory depression to ensure an expected outcome from the treatment?

    a. Provide adequate ventilation of body
    b. Provide patients with controlled analgesic pumps
    c. Administer prescribed sedatives through IV route
    d. Ensure that patients' rooms are odor free

7. Which of the following is defined as a substance that counteracts the action of something else?

    a. Antagonist
    b. Agonist
    c. Analgesic
    d. Anti-inflammatory

8. A nurse working in an alcohol detoxification clinic may use which of the following to treat patients with alcohol dependence?

    a. Naloxone (Narcan)
    b. Nalmefene (Revex)
    c. Naltrexone (Depade)
    d. Nifedipine (Procardia)

9. How quickly does naloxone (Narcan) work to reverse opioid-induced respiratory depression?

    a. 1 to 2 minutes
    b. 10 to 15 minutes
    c. 15 to 30 minutes
    d. 30 to 60 minutes

10. A patient presents to the ED with symptoms of an acute opioid overdose. The physician orders the patient naloxone (Narcan) for the patient. Several minutes after the nurse administers the naloxone (Narcan), the patient's respiratory depression and other symptoms have not changed. This is most likely due to which of the following?

    a. The patient was not administered a large enough dose of naloxone (Narcan)
    b. The patient is not experiencing an opioid overdose
    c. The patient overdosed on multiple opioids
    d. The naloxone (Narcan) has not been given enough time to work

11. Naloxone (Narcan) will reverse the effects of which of the following drugs?
    a. Fentanyl (Duragesic)
    b. Lorazepam (Ativan)
    c. Valproic Acid (Depakote)
    d. Warfarin (Coumadin)

12. A nurse should not administer nalmefene (Revex) to which of the following patients?
    a. Patients with a hypersensitivity to nalmefene (Revex)
    b. Patients with uncontrolled type 2 diabetes
    c. Patients with a history of opioid abuse
    d. Patients with a history of alcohol abuse

13. Opioid antagonists may produce withdrawal symptoms in patients physically dependent on which of the following?
    a. Alcohol
    b. NSAIDs
    c. Opioids
    d. Benzodiazepines

14. Opioid naïve patients are defined as which of the following?
    a. Patients who do not routinely take opioids
    b. Patients who routinely take opioids
    c. Patients who are physically dependent on opioids
    d. Patients who are psychologically dependent on opioids

15. Opioid naïve patients are most at risk for which of the following?
    a. Hypertension
    b. Respiratory depression
    c. Diarrhea
    d. Physical dependence

CHAPTER 18

Anesthetic Drugs

Learning Objectives

- State the uses of local anesthesia, methods of administration, and nursing responsibilities when administering a local anesthetic
- Describe the purpose of a preanesthetic drug and the nursing responsibilities associated with the administration of a preanesthetic drug
- Identify several drugs used for local and general anesthesia
- List and briefly describe the four stages of general anesthesia
- Discuss important nursing responsibilities associated with caring for a patient receiving a preanesthetic drug and during the postanesthesia care (recovery room) period

SECTION I: ASSESSING YOUR UNDERSTANDING

Activity A MATCHING

1. **Match the various types of local anesthesia in Column A with their application in Column B.**

Column A

1. Spinal anesthesia C
2. Local infiltration d anesthesia
3. Regional anesthesia a
4. Topical anesthesia b

Column B

a. Injection of anesthetic around nerves

b. Application of the anesthetic to the surface of the skin

c. Injection of local anesthetic drug into the subarachnoid space

d. Injection of a local anesthetic drug into tissues

2. *Match the drugs used for general anesthesia in Column A with their uses in Column B.*

Column A	Column B
1. Methohexital *d*	a. Used for surgical procedures that do not require the relaxation of skeletal muscles
2. Midazolam *c*	
3. Propofol *b*	b. Used for continuous sedation of intubated or respiratory-controlled patients in intensive care units
4. Ketamine *a*	
	c. Used for conscious sedation before minor procedures
	d. Used for short surgical procedures with minimal painful stimuli

Activity B FILL IN THE BLANKS

1. A ~~Conduction~~ block is a type of regional anesthesia produced by injection of a local anesthetic drug into or near a nerve trunk.

2. ~~general~~ anesthesia is the provision of a pain-free state for the entire body.

3. ~~Anesthesia~~ is a loss of feeling or sensation.

4. A nurse ~~anesthetist~~ is a nurse with a master's degree and special training who is qualified to administer anesthetics.

5. A ~~anesthesiologist~~ a physician with special training in administering anesthesia.

6. ~~Volatile~~ *Cholinergic* preanesthetic blocking drug decreases secretions of the upper respiratory tract.

7. ~~Volatile~~ liquid anesthetics produce anesthesia when their vapors are inhaled.

Activity C SHORT ANSWERS

A nurse is required to care for patients who are to be administered anesthesia. A number of nursing interventions are associated with the administration of anesthesia. Answer the following questions, which involve the nurse's role in managing such situations.

1. A nurse observes that an abnormal laboratory test finding was included in the patient's chart shortly before surgery. What should be the nurse's immediate reaction?

The nurse should make sure the surgeon and anesthesiologist know about the abnormal lab findings and look over the pts chart and have the chart noted about the abnormal finding

2. What are the postoperative nursing interventions that a nurse has to perform when caring for a patient?

Admit the pt for procedure, check vitals, check airway so theres no risk of aspiration, and review pts records w/ previous surgeries and use of anesthesia.

3. What factors should a nurse be aware of that influence the choice of anesthetic drug?

The anticipated time of the surgery length, the area, organ for operation and pts general physical condition.

Activity D DOSAGE CALCULATION

1. A patient is to be administered 0.6 mg of robinul. The dose is available as 0.2 mg/mL and is to be administered intramuscularly. How much robinul should the nurse prepare to be administered as a preanesthetic to the patient?

3mL

2. A patient is to be administered 30-mg chlordiazepoxide a day. Chlordiazepoxide is available as 15-mg tablets. How many tablets should the nurse administer to the patient?

2 tablets

3. A patient is to be administered 25 mL of marcaine HCl over 5 days. Each dose of marcaine HCl contains 5 mL. How many doses should the nurse administer if one dose is to be administered each day?

5 doses in 5 days and take 1 dose each day

4. A patient is to be administered 240 mg of fentanyl. Fentanyl is available as 80-mg tablets. How many tablets should be administered to the patient?

3 tablets

5. A patient is prescribed Ultiva. The normal dosage of this drug is 0.5 mcg/kg, and the patient weighs 90 kg. If the rate of infusion of the drug is 0.5 mcg/30 seconds, calculate the time taken (in minutes) for the infusion of the entire dose of the drug.

It will take 45 mins

SECTION II: APPLYING YOUR KNOWLEDGE

Activity E CASE STUDY

James Jones is a Caucasian male, 29 years of age, admitted to the hospital to undergo surgery to repair a torn ACL on his left knee. He has no chronic medical conditions and is in good health. His only medication is Lortab 5/500 mg, and he is allergic to penicillin.

1. As the preoperative nurse, what are your responsibilities to Mr. Jones?

Preparation of surgery, physician, physical status of pt, describe post op care and activities during post op as well as working the PCA pump.

2. As part of preanesthesia, the physician has ordered Mr. Jones to receive midazolam (Versed) 5 mg, 45 minutes prior to surgery. Midazolam is available in a 1 mg/mL vial. How much would the nurse need to prepare to administer to the patient?

The nurse needs to prepare 5mL to the pt.

SECTION III: PRACTICING FOR NCLEX

Activity F NCLEX-STYLE

Answer the following questions.

1. A patient is prescribed the drug methohexital by the physician. The nurse knows that which of the following are the effects of methohexital?
   a. Produces mild stimulation of respiratory and bronchial secretions
   b. Brings about moderate muscle relaxation
   c. Depresses CNS to produce hypnosis and anesthesia
   d. Decreases secretions in the upper respiratory tract

2. Which of the following stages of general anesthesia begins with a loss of consciousness?
   a. Analgesia
   b. Delirium
   c. Surgical analgesia
   d. Respiratory paralysis

3. Which of the following are effects of topical anesthesia of which a nurse should be aware?
   a. Decreased anxiety and apprehension
   b. Desensitized skin or mucous membrane
   c. Loss of feeling in the lower extremities
   d. Cardiovascular stimulation

4. Which of the following should the nurse perform as postoperative interventions after the administration of anesthesia?

   a. Review patient's laboratory test records

   b. Administer a hypnotic agent to the patient

   c. Position the patient to prevent aspiration of vomitus

   d. Monitor patient's blood pressure every 12 hours

5. A patient who was administered a preanesthetic drug is experiencing an increase in his respiratory secretions. The nurse knows that which of the following has occurred during the administration of the preanesthetic drug?

   a. Patient's anesthesia records were not reviewed

   b. The drug was not administered on time

   c. Patient's respiratory status was not assessed

   d. Patient's IV lines were not well assessed

6. A nurse is caring for a patient who is to receive local anesthesia for the suturing of a wound. Which of the following interventions should the nurse perform when caring for this client? Select all that apply.

   a. Observe if there is any oozing

   b. Apply dressing to the surgical areas

   c. Observe the patient for any signs of bleeding

   d. Assess the patient's pulse every 5 to 15 minutes

   e. Exercise caution in administering opioids

7. A nurse is assigned to care for a patient who is to receive anesthesia. Which of the following should the nurse confirm to ensure that the use of preanesthetic drugs is not contraindicated in this patient?

   a. Patient is not over 60 years of age

   b. Patient does not need anesthesia on his or her extremities

   c. Patient is not younger than 13 years of age

   d. Patient does not have a low body weight

8. A patient is admitted to a local health care facility for a kidney operation. Which of the following preanesthetic drugs should be administered to reduce the incidence of upper respiratory tract secretions in the patient?

   a. Cholinergic-blocking drug

   b. Scopolamine and glycopyrrolate

   c. Opioid or antianxiety drug

   d. Diazepam or Valium

9. A pregnant patient is admitted to a local health care facility for a C-section delivery. The primary health care provider decides to administer a transsacral block as anesthesia. Where is the transsacral block injected in a patient?

   a. Epidural space at level of sacrococcygeal notch

   b. Space surrounding the dura of spinal cord

   c. Subarachnoid space of the spinal cord

   d. Injection into the brachial plexus

10. A nurse is assigned to care for a patient who is to be administered local anesthesia. Which of the following should the nurse confirm to ensure that the use of epinephrine along with the local anesthesia is not contraindicated in the patient?

    a. Patient does not have anemia

    a. Patient does not have low blood pressure

    b. Patient is not older than 60 years of age

    c. Patient does not need anesthesia for his or her extremities

11. Which of the following is an example of regional anesthesia?

    a. Spinal anesthesia

    b. Topical anesthesia

    c. Local infiltration anesthesia

    d. General anesthesia

12. Which type of anesthesia may be applied by the nurse with a cotton swab or sprayed on the area to be desensitized?

    a. Local infiltration anesthesia

    b. General anesthesia

    c. Topical anesthesia

    d. Conduction block anesthesia

13. Which type of anesthesia is commonly used for the suturing of small wounds?
    a. Local infiltration anesthesia
    b. General anesthesia
    c. Conduction block anesthesia
    d. Topical anesthesia

14. Which of the following can be mixed in certain situations with an injectable local anesthetic to cause local vasoconstriction?
    a. Epinephrine
    b. Phenylephrine
    c. Oxymetazoline
    d. Diphenhydramine

15. A nurse may be asked to administer which of the following drugs prior to a colonoscopy in order to help the patient relax?
    a. Midazolam (Versed)
    b. Meperidine (Demerol)
    c. Lidocaine (Xylocaine)
    d. Fentanyl (Sublimaze)

CHAPTER 19

Central Nervous System Stimulants

Learning Objectives

- List the three types of central nervous system (CNS) stimulants
- Discuss the uses, general drug actions, general adverse reactions, contraindications, precautions, and interactions of the CNS stimulants
- Discuss important preadministration and ongoing assessment activities the nurse should perform on the patient taking a CNS stimulant
- List nursing diagnoses particular to a patient taking a CNS stimulant
- Discuss ways to promote an optimal response to drug therapy, how to manage common adverse drug reactions, and important points to keep in mind when educating patients about the use of CNS stimulants

SECTION I: ASSESSING YOUR UNDERSTANDING

Activity A MATCHING

1. *Match the interactant drug in Column A with the likely interaction effect when combined with a CNS stimulant in Column B.*

Column A	Column B
1. Anesthetics	a. Decreased effect of the oral contraceptive
2. Theophylline	b. Increased risk of cardiac arrhythmias
3. Modafinil	c. Increased risk of hyperactive behaviors

Activity B FILL IN THE BLANKS

1. Analeptics increase the depth of respirations by stimulating special receptors located in the _____ arteries and upper aorta.

2. Modafinil analeptic is used to treat _____.

3. Amphetamines are _____ drugs that stimulate the CNS.

4. The doxapram drugs increase the respiratory rate by stimulating the _____.

5. When a CNS stimulant is administered with anesthetics there is an increased risk of cardiac _____.

Activity C SHORT ANSWERS

A nurse's role in managing patients who are administered CNS stimulants involves understanding the effects of the drug and performing appropriate interventions depending on the type of drug administered. Answer the following questions, which involve the nurse's role in managing such situations.

1. A nurse is caring for a patient undergoing CNS stimulant treatment. What are the nursing interventions while caring for a patient with an ineffective breathing pattern who is being administered CNS stimulants?

   _____

   _____

   _____

2. A nurse is caring for a patient undergoing CNS stimulant treatment. What are the nursing interventions for a patient experiencing nausea and vomiting from an analeptic?

   _____

   _____

   _____

Activity D DOSAGE CALCULATION

1. A patient has been prescribed 400 mg of modafinil per day. The available tablets are 100 mg each. How many tablets will the nurse administer to the patient daily?

   _____

   _____

2. A patient has been prescribed 80 mg of Doxapram HCl to be administered intravenously. The drug is available in 20-mL vials containing 400 mg of the drug. How many mL of the available solution should be administered to the patient?

   _____

   _____

3. A patient has been prescribed 20 mg of Focalin twice a day. The available tablets are 10 mg each. How many tablets will the nurse administer to the patient daily?

   _____

   _____

4. A patient has been prescribed 15 mg of Meridia once daily. The available tablets are 5 mg each. How many tablets will the nurse administer to the patient daily?

   _____

   _____

5. A patient has been prescribed 90 mg of Meridia, to be taken over a period of 6 days. The available tablets are 15 mg each. How many tablets will the nurse administer to the patient each day?

   _____

   _____

SECTION II: APPLYING YOUR KNOWLEDGE

Activity E CASE STUDY

Amanda Johnson is a Caucasian female, 29 years of age, who presents to the physician's office for her yearly physical. She is 65 in tall and weighs 220 lb. She is prehypertensive with a blood pressure of 125/85 mm Hg. She has no other medical conditions and takes only a daily multivitamin. The physician writes a prescription for sibutramine (Meridia) 10 mg daily for weight loss.

1. What preadministration and ongoing assessments should the nurse make?

   _____

   _____

2. What side effects should the nurse advise Ms. Johnson about?

_____

_____

_____

SECTION III: PRACTICING FOR NCLEX

Activity F NCLEX-STYLE

Answer the following questions.

1. A nurse is caring for a patient who is receiving CNS stimulants. Which of the following adverse reactions should the nurse monitor for in this patient?

   a. Bradycardia

   b. Hyperactivity

   c. High blood pressure

   d. Elevated temperature

2. Which of the following points should the nurse include in the teaching plan for patients who are being administered CNS stimulants for attention deficit hyperactivity disorder (ADHD)?

   a. Administer drug half an hour before breakfast

   b. Administer drug in the late afternoon

   c. Administer drug with milk, not water

   d. Dissolve drug in milk or water before consuming

3. In which of the following patients is the use of CNS stimulants contraindicated?

   a. Liver disorders

   b. Acute ulcerative colitis

   c. Ventilation mechanism disorder

   d. Bone marrow suppression

4. Which of the following reactions could occur if theophylline is combined with CNS stimulants?

   a. Decreased effectiveness of the CNS stimulant

   b. Increased risk of cardiac arrhythmias

   c. Increased risk of hyperactive behaviors

   d. Decreased effectiveness of theophylline

5. Which of the following interventions should the nurse perform as part of the ongoing assessment after administering an analeptic?

   a. Send blood sample for a platelet count test

   b. Check pulse rate and blood pressure every hour

   c. Monitor consciousness levels every 5 to 15 minutes

   d. Monitor respiratory rate for 5 minutes after administration

6. A nurse is caring for a patient on CNS stimulant therapy. The patient complains of insomnia. Which of the following interventions should the nurse perform to diminish sleep disturbances?

   a. Encourage patient to avoid napping during daytime

   b. Administer the drug in the evening, if possible

   c. Take stimulants such as coffee or tea

   d. Administer any OTC sleeping pills

7. CNS stimulants have been prescribed for a child with ADHD. Which of the following points should the nurse include in the teaching plan? Select all that apply.

   a. Monitor the child's eating patterns

   b. Teach the parents the importance of preparing nutritious meals

   c. Provide a light breakfast so that the child stays alert

   d. Advise parents to give OTC sleeping pills in case of insomnia

   e. Check the child's height and weight measurements to monitor growth

8. A patient is prescribed amphetamines as part of obesity treatment. Which of the following interventions should the nurse perform as part of the preadministration process? Select all that apply.

   a. Record blood pressure

   b. Observe urinary output

   c. Record blood pressure

   d. Measure blood glucose

   e. Record weight

9. Which of the following represent the parts of the central nervous system (CNS)? Select all that apply.
   a. Brain
   b. Spinal cord
   c. Afferent nerves
   d. Efferent nerves
   e. Autonomic nerves

10. The analeptics are CNS stimulants that do which of the following? Select all that apply.
    a. Stimulate the cardiovascular system
    b. Stimulate the limbic system of the brain
    c. Stimulate the digestive system
    d. Stimulate the respiratory center of the brain
    e. Stimulate endocrine system

11. Anorexiants are primarily used for which purposes?
    a. Treat ADHD
    b. Suppress the appetite
    c. Suppress the cardiovascular system
    d. Stimulate the respiratory system

12. Which of the following medications is used to treat narcolepsy and does not cause cardiac and other systemic stimulatory effects like other CNS stimulants?
    a. Provigil
    b. Caffeine
    c. Dopram
    d. Focalin

13. Most anorexiants are classified in which pregnancy category?
    a. Category A
    b. Category B
    c. Category C
    d. Category X

14. Pediatric patients given atomoxetine (Strattera) should be monitored closely for which of the following?
    a. Suicidal ideation
    b. Hypertension
    c. Dyspnea
    d. Hyperglycemia

15. Children taking CNS stimulants for the long-term treatment of ADHD should be monitored closely for which of the following?
    a. Hyperglycemia
    b. Growth
    c. Hypotension
    d. Weight loss
    e. Respiratory depression

Antianxiety Drugs

Learning Objectives

- Discuss the uses, general drug actions, general adverse reactions, contraindications, precautions, and interactions associated with the administration of the antianxiety drugs
- Discuss important preadministration and ongoing assessment activities the nurse should perform on the patient taking antianxiety drugs
- List nursing diagnoses particular to a patient taking antianxiety drugs
- Discuss ways to promote an optimal response to therapy, how to manage common adverse reactions, and important points to keep in mind when educating patients about the use of antianxiety drugs

SECTION I: ASSESSING YOUR UNDERSTANDING

Activity A MATCHING

1. *Match the drug interacting with an anxiolytic in Column A with its interacting effect in Column B.*

Column A	Column B
1. Alcohol	a. Increased risk for central nervous system (CNS) depression
2. Digoxin	b. Increased risk for convulsions
3. Antipsychotic	c. Increased risk for digitalis toxicity
4. Analgesic	d. Increased risk for sedation and respiratory depression

2. *Match the generic drugs (trade names in parentheses) in Column A with their actions in Column B.*

Column A

1. Buspirone (BuSpar)
2. Hydroxyzine (Atarax, Vistaril)
3. Chlordiazepoxide (Librium)

Column B

a. Acts on the hypothalamus and brainstem reticular formation
b. Acts by enhancing the actions of a natural brain chemical GABA (gamma-aminobutyric acid)
c. Acts on the brain's serotonin receptors

Activity B FILL IN THE BLANKS

1. Drugs used to treat anxiety are called _____.

2. _____ drugs are used for the management of cardiac problems.

3. Antianxiety drugs are used in the management of _____ sedatives and muscle relaxants.

4. _____ administration is indicated primarily in acute states when it is difficult to have the patient take the medication by mouth.

5. _____ symptoms occur if benzodiazepines are taken for more than three months and discontinued abruptly.

Activity C SHORT ANSWERS

A nurse's role in managing patients who are being administered antianxiety drugs involves monitoring the patients and implementing interventions that aid in their recovery. Answer the following questions, which involve the nurse's role in managing such situations.

1. A patient with anxiety has been prescribed alprazolam. What should a nurse assess for in this patient before administering the first dose of alprazolam?

_____

_____

2. A patient receiving alprazolam complains of constipation. What effective interventions should the nurse perform to ensure the patient's well-being?

_____

_____

Activity D DOSAGE CALCULATION

1. A patient is prescribed 0.25 mg of alprazolam orally 3 times a day. The drug is available in 0.5-mg tablets. How many tablets should the nurse administer to the patient daily?

_____

_____

2. A patient is prescribed 30 mg of oxazepam orally 4 times a day. At what interval should the nurse administer the drug, which is available in 15-mg tablets?

_____

_____

3. A patient is prescribed 15 mg of BuSpar daily. The tablet is available in 5-mg doses. How many tablets are needed daily to meet the prescribed drug level?

_____

_____

4. A physician prescribes 25 mg of chlordiazepoxide orally 4 times a day for a patient. The drug is available in 10-mg tablets. How many tablets will the nurse administer to the patient daily?

_____

_____

5. A physician prescribes 0.25 mg of clonazepam every 12 hours for the first 3 days. How many milligrams of the drug would the nurse administer to the patient over 3 days?

_____

_____

6. A patient has been prescribed 150 mg of doxepin HCl daily. The drug is available in 25-mg tablets. How many tablets are needed daily to meet the prescribed drug level?

_____

_____

SECTION II: APPLYING YOUR KNOWLEDGE

Activity E **CASE STUDY**

Ruby Hinton is an African American female, 87 years of age. Due to worsening dementia, she is often agitated. The physician has written an order for Mrs. Hinton to receive lorazepam (Ativan) 0.5 mg TID PRN.

1. What are some things to consider as the nurse caring for Mrs. Hinton with regards to the lorazepam?

    _____

    _____

    _____

2. What should the nurse's ongoing assessment consist of for Mrs. Hinton?

    _____

    _____

    _____

SECTION III: PRACTICING FOR NCLEX

Activity F **NCLEX-STYLE**

Answer the following questions.

1. A nurse is caring for a patient who is receiving antianxiety drugs. Which of the following is an adverse reaction for which the nurse should monitor the patient?
    a. Seizures
    b. Diarrhea
    c. Abdominal cramps
    d. Bradycardia

2. A patient who was on benzodiazepine therapy for 4 weeks visits a health care facility. The patient exhibits benzodiazepine withdrawal symptoms. Which of the following should the nurse assess for in the patient?
    a. Increased RBC count
    b. Decreased pulse rate
    c. Increased anxiety
    d. Increased appetite

3. A patient undergoing digoxin therapy for cardiac problems is prescribed diazepam for anxiety disorders. Which of the following effects is a result of a drug interaction for which the nurse should monitor the patient?
    a. Increased risk for central nervous system depression
    b. Increased risk for respiratory depression
    c. Increased risk for sedation
    d. Increased risk for digitalis toxicity

4. A patient visits a health care facility with symptoms of anxiety. The primary health care provider has prescribed hydroxyzine. For which of the following patients should the nurse take precautions when administering the hydroxyzine drug? Select all that apply.
    a. Patients with impaired liver function
    b. Patients with impaired pancreas function
    c. Patients with impaired kidney function
    d. Patients with bone marrow depression
    e. Patients with debilitation

5. The primary health care provider has diagnosed a patient with anxiety due to withdrawal from alcohol. Which of the following should the nurse relate to alcohol withdrawal?
    a. Diarrhea
    b. Acute panic
    c. Dry mouth
    d. Lightheadedness

6. A nurse is caring for a patient with anxiety. The patient is to be administered lorazepam. Which of the following should the nurse ensure to confirm that lorazepam is not contraindicated in the patient?
    a. Patient is not younger than 18 years of age
    b. Patient is not hypersensitive
    c. Patient does not have myasthenia gravis
    d. Patient does not have Parkinsonism

7. A patient is prescribed a chlordiazepoxide drug for anxiety. Which of the following interventions should the nurse perform to prevent the occurrence of constipation in the patient?
    a. Provide vitamin supplements
    b. Restrict patient's diet to fluids only
    c. Provide patient with a fiber-rich diet and plenty of fluids
    d. Restrict patient to a strict vegetarian diet

8. A patient being treated for anxiety is to be discharged. Which of the following instructions should the nurse include in the patient's teaching plan?
   a. Avoid sunlight
   b. Avoid alcohol
   c. Avoid yogurt
   d. Avoid sour cream

9. A nurse is assigned to care for an elderly patient who has to be administered doxepin. Which of the following safety measures should the nurse take while administering doxepin?
   a. Administer the drug intramuscularly on the gluteus muscle
   b. Monitor for hearing or kidney problems
   c. Administer the drug intramuscularly on the arms
   d. Monitor for secondary bacterial or fungal infections

10. A patient on alprazolam therapy for has discontinued treatment for a week. Which of the following is a withdrawal symptom for which the nurse should monitor the patient?
    a. Diarrhea
    b. Dizziness
    c. Metallic taste
    d. Dry mouth

11. Antianxiety drugs are also referred to as which of the following?
    a. Anxiolytics
    b. Opioids
    c. NSAIDs
    d. Anesthetics

12. Which of the following is classified as a controlled substance by DEA regulations?
    a. Lorazepam (Ativan)
    b. Buspirone (BuSpar)
    c. Doxepin (Sinequan)
    d. Hydroxyzine (Atarax)

13. Which of the following exerts its anxiolytic effect by acting on the brains serotonin receptors?
    a. Buspirone (BuSpar)
    b. Lorazepam (Ativan)
    c. Doxepin (Sinequan)
    d. Hydroxyzine (Atarax)

14. Which of the following exerts its anxiolytic effect by acting on the hypothalamus and brainstem reticular formation?
    a. Buspirone (BuSpar)
    b. Doxepin (Sinequan)
    c. Hydroxyzine (Atarax)
    d. Diazepam (Valium)

15. How early can benzodiazepine withdrawal occur in a patient?
    a. 7 days
    b. 12 hours
    c. 1 day
    d. 1 month

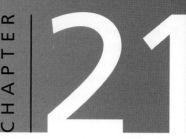

Sedatives and Hypnotics

- Differentiate between a sedative and a hypnotic.
- Discuss the uses, general drug actions, adverse reactions, contraindications, precautions, and interactions of sedatives and hypnotics
- Discuss important preadministration and ongoing assessment activities the nurse should perform with the patient taking a sedative or hypnotic
- List nursing diagnoses particular to a patient taking a sedative or hypnotic
- Discuss ways to promote an optimal response to therapy, how to manage common adverse reactions, and important points to keep in mind when educating patients about the use of a sedative or hypnotic

SECTION I: ASSESSING YOUR UNDERSTANDING

Activity A MATCHING

1. *Match the types of drugs in Column A with their common uses in Column B.*

Column A	Column B
1. Antidepressants	a. Pain relief
2. Opioid analgesics	b. Management of gastric upset
3. Antihistamines	c. Management of depression
4. Phenothiazines	d. Relief of allergy symptoms
5. Cimetadine	e. Management of agitation and psychotic symptoms

2. *Match the key terms in Column A with their definitions in Column B.*

Column A	Column B
1. Ataxia	a. Produce a relaxing, calming effect
2. Hypnotics	b. Unsteady gait
3. Sedatives	c. Induce drowsiness or sleep

Activity B FILL IN THE BLANKS

1. Sleep deprivation may interfere with the _____ process of a patient.

2. Sedatives and hypnotics are primarily used to treat _____ and convulsions or seizures.

3. The herb _____ was originally used in Europe for its sedating effects in conditions of mild anxiety or restlessness.

4. Drinking beverages containing caffeine contributes to _____.

5. _____ is a hormone produced by the pineal gland in the brain.

6. _____, when given in the presence of pain, may cause restlessness, excitement, and delirium.

Activity C SHORT ANSWERS

A nurse's role in managing patients who are being administered sedatives and hypnotic drugs involves monitoring the patients and implementing interventions that aid in their recovery. Answer the following questions, which involve the nurse's role in managing such situations.

1. A patient is prescribed a sedative. What assessments should the nurse perform before administering the drug?

   _____

   _____

2. List nursing diagnoses specific to a patient taking a sedative or hypnotic.

   _____

   _____

Activity D DOSAGE CALCULATION

1. A patient is prescribed 2 mg of estazolam twice a day. Estazolam is available in 1-mg tablets. How many tablets will the nurse have to administer to the patient in a day?

   _____

   _____

2. A patient is prescribed 15 mg of temazepam per day. The available tablet of temazepam contains 5 mg of the drug. How many tablets will the nurse have to administer to the patient at one time?

   _____

   _____

3. A patient is prescribed 10 mg of zaleplon at bedtime. The available zaleplon tablet contains 5 mg of the drug. How many tablets of zaleplon will the nurse have to administer to the patient?

   _____

   _____

4. A patient is prescribed 0.25 mg of triazolam (Halcion) orally at bedtime. Triazolam is available in the form of 0.125-mg tablets. How many tablets will the nurse have to administer to the patient?

   _____

   _____

5. A patient is prescribed 10 mg of zolpidem tartrate orally at bedtime. Zolpidem tartrate is available in 5-mg tablets. How many tablets of the drug will the nurse have to administer to the patient?

   _____

   _____

SECTION II: APPLYING YOUR KNOWLEDGE

Activity E CASE STUDY

Richard Howard is an African American male, 34 years of age He presents to the physician's office with a chief complaint of insomnia. The physician writes Mr. Howard a prescription for temazepam (Restoril) 15 mg at bedtime as needed for sleep.

1. Is temazepam (Restoril) a sedative or hypnotic?

   _____

   _____

1. What is the difference between a sedative and a hypnotic?

_____

_____

_____

SECTION III: PRACTICING FOR NCLEX

Activity F **NCLEX-STYLE**

Answer the following questions.

1. A nurse is caring for a patient who is prescribed a sedative. Which of the following measures can ensure an optimal response to sedative therapy? Select all that apply.
   a. Back rubs
   b. Alcohol intake
   c. Night lights
   d. Darkened room
   e. Bedtime coffee

2. A nurse is caring for a patient who has been administered sedatives for insomnia. Which of the following is a criterion for evaluating the effectiveness of the treatment?
   a. Decreased level of consciousness
   b. Normal respiration rate
   c. Improved sleep pattern
   d. Decrease in restlessness

3. A patient is admitted to a health care facility with convulsions and is prescribed a sedative. Which of the following should the nurse record before administration of the drug?
   a. Platelet count
   b. Blood pressure
   c. Hematocrit
   d. Blood sugar

4. A nurse is caring for a patient who is to undergo surgery. The patient is prescribed a preoperative sedation. For which adverse reactions should the nurse monitor this patient?
   a. Nausea
   b. Headache
   c. Restlessness
   d. Anxiety

5. Which of the following types of patients should a nurse identify as candidates for cautious use of sedatives and hypnotics?
   a. Patients with hearing impairment
   b. Patients with hyperglycemia
   c. Patients with glucose intolerance
   d. Patients with renal impairment

6. A patient undergoing treatment for allergy is prescribed sedatives for anxiety. Which of the following should the nurse monitor the patient for as a possible effect of the interaction between antihistamines and sedatives?
   a. Restlessness
   b. Increased sedation
   c. Headache
   d. Chronic pain

7. A nurse is caring for a patient who has been prescribed barbiturates. Which of the following is a symptom of acute drug toxicity?
   a. Increased blood pressure
   b. Respiratory depression
   c. Lowered blood sugar
   d. Frequent micturition

8. A patient is admitted to the local health care facility for the treatment of insomnia caused by pain. Why would the primary health care provider not prescribe barbiturates for the patient?
   a. They cause allergic reaction
   b. They cause an increase in temperature
   c. They cause delirium
   d. They cause an increase in blood sugar

9. A patient who was prescribed a barbiturate has abruptly discontinued use of the drug. The nurse expects withdrawal symptoms. Which of the following are withdrawal symptoms of barbiturates? Select all that apply.
   a. Restlessness
   b. Euphoria
   c. Seizures
   d. Confusion
   e. Convulsions

10. A patient is admitted to the health care facility with insomnia related to chronic headache. The patient is prescribed a sedative. Which of the following are benefits of sedatives? Select all that apply.

   a. Relaxing effect

   b. Nausea

   c. Calming effect

   d. Dizziness

   E. Drowsiness

11. Sedatives and hypnotics are used to primarily treat which of the following? (Choose one)

   a. Insomnia

   b. Anxiety

   c. Hypertension

   d. Depression

12. Which of the following is defined as a drug that induces drowsiness?

   a. Anxiolytic

   b. Sedative

   c. Hypnotic

   d. Opioid

13. Which of the following hypnotics produces the most respiratory depression? (Choose one)

   a. Secobarbital (Seconal)

   b. Temazepam (Restoril)

   c. Zolpidem (Ambien)

   d. Ramelteon (Rozerem)

14. The nonbenzodiazepines have diminished hypnotic effects after how long?

   a. 1 day

   b. 7 days

   c. 10 days

   d. 14 days

15. Benzodiazepines are classified in which pregnancy category?

   a. Category A

   b. Category X

   c. Category B

   d. Category C

CHAPTER 22

Antidepressant Drugs

Learning Objectives

■ Define depression and identify symptoms of a major depressive episode

■ Name the different types of antidepressant drugs

■ Discuss the uses, general drug actions, general adverse reactions, contraindications, precautions, and interactions of the antidepressant drugs

■ Discuss important preadministration and ongoing assessment activities that the nurse should perform on the patient taking antidepressant drugs

■ List nursing diagnoses particular to a patient taking antidepressant drugs

■ Discuss ways to promote an optimal response to therapy, how to manage common adverse reactions, and important points to keep in mind when educating patients about the use of antidepressant drugs

SECTION I: ASSESSING YOUR UNDERSTANDING

Activity A MATCHING

1. **Match the key terms in Column A with their meanings in Column B.**

Column A

1. Depression
2. Dysphoric mood
3. Priapism
4. Tardive dyskinesia

Column B

a. Syndrome of involuntary movement that may be irreversible

b. A persistent erection of the penis

c. Extreme sadness, anxiety, or unhappiness that interferes with daily functioning

d. Feeling sad, unhappy, or "down in the dumps"

2. *Match the key terms in Column A with their meanings in Column B.*

Column A

1. Endogenous
2. Hypertensive crisis
3. Tyramine
4. Strokes

Column B

a. Extremely high blood pressure
b. An amino acid present in some foods
c. Cerebrovascular accidents
d. Produced within the body

FILL IN THE BLANKS

1. _____ is used with antidepressants in treating major depressive episodes.

2. Patients receiving MAOIs should not eat foods containing _____.

3. Injection of alpha-adrenergic stimulants may be helpful in treating _____.

4. Older men with prostatic enlargement are at increased risk for urinary retention when they take _____ antidepressants.

5. Parenteral administration of antidepressants is given intramuscularly in a large muscle mass, such as the _____ muscle.

Activity C **SHORT ANSWERS**

A nurse's role in administering antidepressant drugs involves assisting patients in managing the common adverse reactions of the drugs. The nurse also educates patients about the use of these drugs. Answer the following questions, which involve the nurse's role in managing such situations.

1. How is clinical depression treated?

_____

_____

_____

2. What are the different types of antidepressants?

_____

_____

_____

3. What are the effects of antidepressants?

_____

_____

_____

4. What are the uses of tricyclic antidepressants?

_____

_____

_____

Activity D **DOSAGE CALCULATION**

1. A physician prescribes 150 mg of amitriptyline (Sinequan) per day for a patient. The available tablets are 50 mg. How many tablets should the nurse administer to the patient daily?

_____

_____

2. A patient is prescribed 50 mg of amoxapine 3 times a day. The drug is available in 25-mg tablets. How many tablets should the nurse administer to the patient daily?

_____

_____

3. A patient is prescribed 25 mg of clomipramine (Anafranil) daily. The available tablet contains 10 mg of clomipramine. How many tablets are needed each day to meet the prescribed drug level?

_____

_____

4. A patient is prescribed 25 mg of nortriptyline 4 times a day. The drug is available in 25-mg tablets. To give the drug equally, what should be the time interval between consecutive administrations?

_____

_____

5. A physician has prescribed 90 mg of phenelzine (Nardil) per day for a patient. The available tablets are 15 mg. How many tablets should the nurse administer to the patient daily?

_____

_____

6. A patient has been prescribed 80 mg of fluox-etine (Prozac) per day to be administered in two equal doses, once in the morning and once at noon. The drug is available in 20-mg tablets. How many tablets should the nurse administer to the patient each time?

_____

_____

SECTION II: APPLYING YOUR KNOWLEDGE

Activity E CASE STUDY

Jane Smith is a Caucasian female, 27 years of age. She presents to the physician's office for follow-up after giving birth to her first child 6 weeks ago. The triage nurse notices that Mrs. Smith has a monotonous speech pattern and is slow to answer questions.

1. The nurse suspects Mrs. Smith might be depressed. What are other symptoms of depression that the nurse should attempt to identify?

_____

_____

2. The physician diagnoses Mrs. Smith with depression and gives her a prescription for escitalopram (Lexapro) 10 mg QD. What information should be included in the nurse's teaching plan for educating Mrs. Smith about her medication?

_____

_____

SECTION III: PRACTICING FOR NCLEX

Activity F NCLEX-STYLE

Answer the following questions.

1. A nurse is caring for a patient who is pre-scribed a tricyclic antidepressant drug for depression. Which of the following is an adverse reaction to the drug?
   a. Photosensitivity
   b. Hypertensive episodes
   c. Severe convulsions
   d. Nervous system depression

2. A patient undergoing psychotherapy in a local health care facility is prescribed monoamine oxidase inhibitors. Which of the following contraindications should the nurse screen the patient for when administering the MAOIs?
   a. Urinary retention
   b. Seizure disorder
   c. Myocardial infarction
   d. Cerebrovascular disease

3. A nurse is caring for a patient undergoing antidepressant therapy. The patient is also prescribed warfarin for circulatory disorders. For which of the following risks should the nurse monitor the patient?
   a. Increased risk for bleeding
   b. Increased risk for hypotension
   c. Increased anticholinergic symptoms
   d. Increased risk for nervous system depression

4. A nurse is caring for a patient with bulimia nervosa. The patient is prescribed fluoxetine, an SSRI. Which of the following is an adverse reaction of this type of drug for which the nurse should monitor the patient?
   a. Vertigo
   b. Blurred vision
   c. Somnolence
   d. Tremor

5. A patient under treatment with MAOI antidepressants shows symptoms including a headache followed by a sore neck, nausea, vomiting, sweating, fever, chest pain, dilated pupils, and bradycardia indicative of hypertensive crisis. Which of the following factors needs immediate attention?

   a. Blood pressure
   b. Blood sugar
   c. Temperature
   d. Respiration rate

6. A nurse is caring for a patient under treatment with trazodone. Which of the following is a major adverse reaction that the nurse should ask the patient to report immediately?

   a. Priapism
   b. Orthostatic hypotension
   c. Insomnia
   d. Diarrhea

7. A nurse is required to administer antidepressant therapy to an outpatient. Which of the following activities should the nurse perform as a part of the preadministration assessment? Select all that apply.

   a. Obtain a complete medical history
   b. Obtain blood pressure measurements
   c. Obtain a complete blood count
   d. Obtain blood sugar levels
   e. Obtain pulse and respiratory rate

8. A nurse is caring for a patient receiving MAOI antidepressants. The nurse instructs the patient to avoid foods containing tyramine. Which of the following is the result of tyramine interacting with an MAOI antidepressant?

   a. Blurred vision
   b. Hypertensive crisis
   c. Orthostatic hypotension
   d. Photosensitivity

9. A nurse is caring for a patient undergoing antidepressant therapy. The nurse observes the patient showing signs of orthostatic hypotension. What intervention should the nurse perform in this case?

   a. Instruct the patient to change positions slowly
   b. Instruct the patient to drink plenty of fluids
   c. Monitor the patient for hyperglycemia
   d. Monitor the patient's vital signs frequently

10. A nurse is caring for a patient with bulimia nervosa who has been prescribed fluoxetine. Which of the following should the nurse identify as the best time to administer an SSRI?

    a. At bedtime
    b. With dinner
    c. In the morning
    d. With lunch

11. Anticholinergic effects such as dry mouth, sedation, and urinary retention are common adverse events occurring with the use of which of the following classes of antidepressants?

    a. Tricyclic antidepressants
    b. Selective serotonin reuptake inhibitors
    c. Monoamine oxidase inhibitors
    d. Atypical antidepressants

12. Which of the following class of antidepressants exert their effects by inhibiting reuptake of norepinephrine and serotonin?

    a. Selective serotonin reuptake inhibitors
    b. Tricyclic antidepressants
    c. Monoamine oxidase inhibitors
    d. Atypical antidepressants

13. Which of the following class of antidepressants exert their effects by inhibiting reuptake serotonin?

    a. Selective serotonin reuptake inhibitors
    b. Tricyclic antidepressants
    c. Monoamine oxidase inhibitors
    d. Atypical antidepressants

14. Which of the following drugs exerts its effect by inhibiting the activity of monoamine oxidase leading to increases in epinephrine, norepinephrine, dopamine, and serotonin?

    a. Sertraline (Zoloft)

    b. Amitriptyline (Elavil)

    c. Bupropion (Wellbutrin)

    d. Phenelzine (Nardil)

15. Which of the following antidepressants exert its effects by affecting the neurotransmission of norepinephrine, serotonin, and dopamine?

    a. Bupropion (Wellbutrin)

    b. Sertraline (Zoloft)

    c. Phenelzine (Nardil)

    d. Amitriptyline (Elavil)

23

Antipsychotic Drugs

Learning Objectives

- List the uses, general drug actions, general adverse reactions, contraindications, precautions, and interactions associated with the administration of the antipsychotic drugs
- Discuss important preadministration and ongoing assessment activities the nurse should perform on the patient taking an antipsychotic drug
- List nursing diagnoses particular to a patient taking an antipsychotic drug
- Discuss ways to promote an optimal response to therapy, how to manage common adverse reactions, and important points to keep in mind when educating patients about the use of antipsychotic drugs

SECTION I: ASSESSING YOUR UNDERSTANDING

Activity A MATCHING

1. **Match the drug in Column A with their interactions to antipsychotic drugs in Column B.**

Column A

1. Anticholinergic drugs
2. Immunologic drugs
3. Antacids
4. Loop diuretics

Column B

a. Decreased effectiveness of lithium
b. Increased risk for TD and psychotic symptoms
c. Increased risk for lithium toxicity
d. Increased severity of bone marrow suppression

2. *Match the conditions in Column A with their manifestations in Column B.*

Column A

1. Hallucinations
2. Delusions
3. Flattened affect
4. Anhedonia

Column B

a. False beliefs that cannot be changed with reason

b. Finding no pleasure in activities that are normally pleasurable

c. False perceptions having no basis in reality

d. Absence of an emotional response to any situation or condition

Activity B FILL IN THE BLANKS

1. _____ disorder is a psychiatric disorder characterized by severe mood swings from extreme hyperactivity to depression.

2. Antipsychotic drugs are thought to act by inhibiting or blocking the release of the neurotransmitter _____ in the brain.

3. Atypical antipsychotics act upon _____ receptors as well as the dopamine receptors in the brain.

4. _____ affect is the absence of an emotional response to any situation or condition.

5. The term _____ syndrome refers to a group of adverse reactions occurring in the extrapyramidal portion of the nervous system as a result of antipsychotic drugs.

Activity C SHORT ANSWERS

A nurse's role in managing patients being administered antipsychotic drugs involves monitoring and performing interventions for serious manifestations of acute psychosis. Answer the following questions, which involve the nurse's role in managing such situations.

1. What should a nurse assess for in the patient before administering the first dose of an antipsychotic drug?

_____

_____

_____

2. A patient receiving Risperdal is showing signs of hallucinations. What should the nurse closely monitor for in the patient who is showing signs of hallucinations?

_____

_____

_____

Activity D DOSAGE CALCULATION

1. A physician prescribes 400 mg of Thorazine daily for a patient with psychiatric disorders. The available Thorazine tablet is 100 mg. How many tablets will the nurse administer to the patient?

_____

_____

2. A physician prescribes 5 mg of haloperidol daily to be administered intramuscularly. After reconstitution, the concentration of the drug is 2 mg/mL. How many mL should the nurse administer to the patient?

_____

_____

3. A physician prescribes 1200 mg of lithium per day in divided doses for a patient having manic episodes of bipolar disorder. The available lithium tablet is 300 mg. How many total tablets will the nurse administer to the patient?

_____

_____

4. A physician prescribes 100 mg of Moban in 2 doses to a patient with schizophrenia. Moban is available as a syrup in 120-mL bottles with a concentration of 20 mg/mL. How many milliliters should the nurse administer the patient in a single dose?

_____

_____

5. A physician prescribes 5 mg of Compazine 3 times a day for a patient with anxiety. Compazine is available as 120 mL syrup. Five mL of Compazine is equivalent to 5 mg. How many milliliters should the nurse administer to the patient?

_____

_____

SECTION II: APPLYING YOUR KNOWLEDGE

Activity E CASE STUDY

Joe Jenkins is a 45-year-old African American male with a diagnosis of bipolar disorder. He is admitted to a psychiatric facility after he stopped taking his medications and suffered a manic episode. His prior medications consisted of quetiapine (Seroquel) 300 mg QHS and olanzapine (Zyprexa) 10 mg QD. The physician decides to restart Mr. Jenkins' quetiapine (Seroquel) but instead of restarting the olanzapine (Zyprexa), the physician starts Mr. Jenkins on lithium (Eskalith) 300 mg TID.

1. What should you as the nurse discuss with Mr. Jenkins regarding his new medication lithium (Eskalith)?

2. What labs would need to be obtained, and how frequently, now that Mr. Jenkins is taking lithium (Eskalith)?

SECTION III: PRACTICING FOR NCLEX

Activity F NCLEX-STYLE

Answer the following questions.

1. A patient administered Haldol has developed photosensitivity. What should the nurse include in patient teaching?
   a. Ask the patient to minimize alcohol use
   b. Ask the patient to avoid natural sunlight
   c. Suggest the patient use tanning beds
   d. Suggest the patient drink at least 5 glasses of water per day

2. A nurse has administered lithium carbonate to a patient. Which of the following adverse reactions should the nurse monitor in the patient?
   a. Rashes
   b. Polyuria
   c. Dystonia
   d. Insomnia

3. Before beginning antipsychotic drug therapy, a nurse is required to assess a patient. Which of the following should the nurse record as deviations from normal behavior?
   a. Shy or timid behavior
   b. Brief replies to questions
   c. Frequent laughter
   d. Poor eye contact

4. A patient is displaying violent behavior, and antipsychotic drugs have to be given parenterally. Which of the following interventions should the nurse perform while administering the drug?
   a. Administer the drug intravenously to the patient
   b. Ensure the injection site has minimal muscle mass
   c. Ensure the patient remains upright after the injection
   d. Ensure that assistance is available for securing the patient

5. A nurse is required to give antipsychotic drugs to a patient orally. Which of the following interventions should the nurse perform during the drug regimen?
   a. Give the drugs in one single daily dose only, not divided doses
   b. Confirm whether the drug has been swallowed by asking the patient
   c. Mix the drug in liquids such as fruit juices, tomato juice, or milk
   d. Compel the patient to swallow drug if he or she refuses to do so

6. Which of the following are symptoms of tardive dyskinesia (TD) that the nurse should report immediately?
   a. Dry feeling in mouth
   b. Rhythmic face movements
   c. Orthostatic hypotension
   d. Lethargy or drowsiness

7. A schizophrenic patient has been prescribed clozapine. Which of the following points should the nurse include in the teaching program?

   a. Purchase a month's supply of the drug

   b. Schedule WBC count tests every 2 weeks

   c. Continue WBC test for 1 week after end of therapy

   d. Monitor the patient for bone marrow suppression

8. A nurse is required to obtain a blood sample from a patient in the acute phase to test serum lithium levels. Which of the following interventions should the nurse perform?

   a. Obtain sample at least 5 hours after last dose

   b. Monitor patient for muscular weakness

   c. Monitor serum lithium levels every 2 weeks

   d. Obtain sample 1 hour before next dose

9. A patient with schizophrenia has been prescribed chlorpromazine. If symptoms of hypotension and sedation are observed after administration of the drug, which of the following interventions should the nurse perform to minimize the risk of injury to the patient?

   a. Administer the drug with food

   b. Administer the drug with calcium supplement

   c. Administer the drug every 8 hours

   d. Administer the drug at bedtime

10. A patient who has undergone antipsychotic drug therapy is being discharged from a health care facility. Which of the following points should the nurse include in the teaching plan? Select all that apply.

    a. Report any unusual changes or physical effects

    b. Inform the patient about the risks of EPS and TD

    c. Decrease dosage if the symptoms increase

    d. Take the drug on an empty stomach

    e. Avoid exposure to the sun

11. Which of the following is a symptom of psychosis that is defined as finding no pleasure in activities that are normally pleasurable?

    a. Anhedonia

    b. Delusions

    c. Hallucinations

    d. Flattened affect

12. Lithium is not a true antipsychotic medication but is used to treat which of the following antipsychotic disorders?

    a. Bipolar mania

    b. Bipolar depression

    c. Schizophrenia

    d. Personality disorder

13. Typical antipsychotic medications are thought to exert their effects in which of the following ways?

    a. Stimulating the release of dopamine in the brain

    b. Inhibiting the release of dopamine in the brain

    c. Inhibiting the release of serotonin in the brain

    d. Stimulating GABA receptors in the brain

14. Which of the following antipsychotics can be administered rectally to a patient?

    a. Chlorpromazine (Thorazine)

    b. Aripiprazole (Abilify)

    c. Clozapine (Clozaril)

    d. Haloperidol (Haldol))

15. Monitoring of patients taking lithium (Eskalith) includes periodically obtaining a serum lithium level; at what level may toxic reactions occur?

    a. Greater than 0.5 mEq/mL

    b. Greater than 1 mEq/mL

    c. Greater than 1.5 mEq/mL

    d. Greater than 1.25 mEq/mL

CHAPTER 24

Adrenergic Drugs

Learning Objectives

- Discuss the activity of the autonomic nervous system, specifically the sympathetic branch
- Discuss the types of shock, physiologic responses of shock, and the use of adrenergic drugs in the treatment of shock
- Discuss the uses, general drug actions, contraindications, precautions, interactions, and adverse reactions associated with the administration of adrenergic vasopressor drugs
- Discuss important preadministration and ongoing assessment activities the nurse should perform on the patient taking adrenergic drugs
- List nursing diagnoses particular to a patient taking adrenergic drugs
- Discuss ways to promote an optimal response to therapy, how to manage common adverse reactions, and important points to keep in mind when educating patients about the use of adrenergic drugs

SECTION I: ASSESSING YOUR UNDERSTANDING

Activity A MATCHING

1. *Match the drug names in Column A with their corresponding contraindications in Column B.*

Column A	Column B
1. Isoproterenol	a. Narrow-angle glaucoma
2. Dopamine	b. Tachyarrhythmias
3. Midodrine	c. Ventricular fibrillation
4. Epinephrine	d. Severe hypertension

2. *Match the drugs in Column A with the effect of the drug when mixed with an adrenergic in Column B.*

Column A	Column B
1. Antidepressants	a. Increased risk of hypertension
2. Oxytocin	b. Increased risk of bradycardia
3. Bretylium	c. Increased sympathomimetic effect
4. Dilantin	d. Increased risk of arrhythmias

Activity B FILL IN THE BLANKS

1. Adrenergic drugs are useful in improving hemodynamic status by improving _____ contractility and increasing heart rate.

2. The autonomic nervous system is divided into the sympathetic and the _____ nervous branches.

3. Supine _____ is a potentially dangerous adverse reaction that can occur when a patient is taking midodrine.

4. Adrenergic drugs are classified as Pregnancy Category _____ and are used with extreme caution during pregnancy.

5. _____ are drugs that raise the blood pressure because of their ability to constrict blood vessels.

Activity C SHORT ANSWERS

A nurse's role in managing patients who are being administered adrenergic drugs involves monitoring and interventions. Answer the following questions, which involve the nurse's role in managing such situations.

1. A patient is admitted to a health care facility after receiving a shock. The primary care provider has recommended an adrenergic drug. What should a nurse assess for in the patient before administering the first dose?

_____

_____

2. A nurse is monitoring a patient receiving metaraminol. What are the appropriate nursing interventions involved during the ongoing administration of metaraminol?

_____

_____

Activity D DOSAGE CALCULATION

1. A patient is prescribed 20 mg of Midodrine HCl per day. The available tablet contains 10 mg of Midodrine HCl. How many tablets are needed daily to meet the prescribed drug level?

_____

_____

2. A primary health care provider has prescribed 15 mg of ProAmatine to be taken orally 3 times a day. The available tablets contain ProAmatine equivalent to 5 mg. The nurse should administer how many tablets in a day?

_____

_____

3. A primary health care provider prescribes 2.5 mg of Requip, a dopamine agonist, orally 4 times a day for a patient. The available tablets are of 5 mg. How many tablets will the nurse administer to the patient daily?

_____

_____

4. A patient is prescribed 10 mg of Aramine to be administered intramuscularly. Aramine is available as a solution in 10-mL vials with a concentration of 100 mg of the drug. How many milliliters of Aramine should the nurse administer to the patient?

_____

_____

5. A primary health care provider prescribes 2 mg of Requip, a dopamine agonist, orally 4 times a day for a patient. The available tablets are 4 mg. How many tablets will the nurse administer to the patient daily?

_____

_____

SECTION II: APPLYING YOUR KNOWLEDGE

Activity E CASE STUDY

Kim Lacy is a 25-year-old African American female who was involved in a motor vehicle accident and has just arrived in the ED. She is in shock and preliminary exam shows significant head trauma, a spinal cord injury, and several lacerations and contusions. Her blood pressure is 85/60 mm Hg.

1. Based on her current condition from which type of shock is Ms. Lacy likely suffering?

_____

_____

2. Besides hypotension what other symptoms of shock might the ED nurse observe in Ms. Lacy?

_____

_____

SECTION III: PRACTICING FOR NCLEX

Activity F NCLEX-STYLE

Answer the following questions.

1. A nurse is required to administer metaraminol for a patient who is taking digoxin. The patient is at an increased risk for which of the following adverse reactions?

a. Epigastric distress

b. Pheochromocytoma

c. Cardiac arrhythmias

d. Decrease in blood pressure

2. For which of the following patients is isoproterenol contraindicated?

a. Patients with narrow-angle glaucoma

b. Patients with tachycardia

c. Patients with hypotension

d. Patients with pheochromocytoma

3. A 65-year-old patient has been prescribed isoproterenol. Which of the following should the nurse report immediately to the primary care provider?

a. Feeling of nausea

b. Changes in pulse rate

c. Severe headache

d. Urinary urgency

4. A patient has been prescribed midodrine. Which of the following is an adverse effect of Midodrine that the nurse should monitor for?

a. Supine hypertension

b. Tachycardia

c. Orthostatic hypotension

d. Respiratory distress

5. A nurse is required to administer dopamine to a patient. Which of the following nursing interventions should the nurse perform when caring for the client? Select all that apply.

a. Administer dopamine only via intravenous route

b. Mix dopamine with alkaline solutions before administering

c. Use an electronic infusion pump to administer these drugs

d. Monitor blood pressure every 30 minutes

e. Inspect needle site and surrounding tissues at frequent intervals

6. A nurse is caring for a patient who has been administered metaraminol. Which of the following changes should the nurse report to the primary care provider immediately?

a. Consistent fall in blood pressure

b. Rise in blood glucose levels

c. Decrease in gastric motility

d. Increase in the heart rate

7. A patient is experiencing insomnia during epinephrine therapy. Which of the following interventions should the nurse perform while caring for the client? Select all that apply.

a. Identify circumstances that disturb sleep

b. Draw curtains over windows

c. Provide bedtime snacks to the patient

d. Give frequent sips of tea and coffee

e. Administer drugs only during daytime

8. A nurse observes leakage of norepinephrine from the IV line. Which of the following interventions should the nurse perform to minimize tissue perfusion?

a. Discontinue old IV line immediately

b. Do not add another IV line unless instructed

c. Move the head of the bed to an elevated position

d. Mix alkaline solutions with norepinephrine

9. The adrenergic branch of the autonomic nervous system is also known by which of the following names?

a. Parasympathetic nervous system

b. Sympathetic nervous system

c. Central nervous system

d. Somatic nervous system

10. Which of the following is stimulated during the body's fight-or-flight response to a stressful condition?
    a. Sympathetic nervous system
    b. Parasympathetic nervous system
    c. Central nervous system
    d. Somatic nervous system

11. Which of the following is the primary neurotransmitter of the sympathetic nervous system?
    a. Norepinephrine
    b. Dopamine
    c. Serotonin
    d. Acetylcholine

12. Drugs that produce activity similar to the neurotransmitter norepinephrine are known as which of the following?
    a. Sympatholytics
    b. Antiadrenergic drugs
    c. Sympathomimetics
    d. Anticholinergic drugs

13. Which of following adrenergic receptors is responsible for the vasoconstriction of peripheral blood vessels?
    a. α_1 receptors
    b. α_2 receptors
    c. β_1 receptors
    d. β_2 receptors

14. Which of following adrenergic receptors is responsible for increased heart rate and increased force of myocardial contraction?
    a. α_1 receptors
    b. α_2 receptors
    c. β_2 receptors
    d. β_1 receptors

15. Which of following adrenergic receptors is responsible for decreased tone, motility, and secretions of the GI tract?
    a. α_2 receptors
    b. β_1 receptors
    c. α_1 receptors
    d. β_2 receptors

Adrenergic Blocking Drugs

Learning Objectives

- List the four types of adrenergic blocking drugs
- Discuss the uses, general drug actions, general adverse reactions, contraindications, precautions, and interactions of the adrenergic blocking drugs
- Discuss important preadministration and ongoing assessment activities the nurse should perform on the patient taking adrenergic blocking drugs
- List nursing diagnoses particular to a patient taking adrenergic blocking drugs
- Discuss ways to promote an optimal response to therapy, how to manage common adverse reactions, nursing actions that may be taken to minimize orthostatic or postural hypotension, and important points to keep in mind when educating patients about the use of adrenergic blocking drugs

SECTION I: ASSESSING YOUR UNDERSTANDING

Activity A MATCHING

1. **Match the drugs in Column A with the effect of their interaction with beta-adrenergic blockers in Column B.**

Column A

1. Clonidine
2. Lidocaine
3. Antidepressants (MAOI, SSRI)
4. Loop diuretics

Column B

a. Increased effect of the beta-blocker, bradycardia

b. Increased risk of paradoxical hypertensive effect

c. Increased risk of hypotension

d. Increased serum level of the beta-blocker

2. *Match the drugs in Column A with their common uses in Column B.*

Column A

1. Adrenergics
2. Levodopa
3. Lithium
4. Anesthetic agents

Column B

a. Surgery
b. Treatment of psychosis
c. Management of cardio-vascular problems
d. Management of Parkin-son's disease

Activity B FILL IN THE BLANKS

1. _____ is the substance that transmits nerve impulses across the sympathetic branch of the autonomic nervous system.

2. _____ drugs block the transmission of norepinephrine in the sympathetic system.

3. When _____ is administered with epi-nephrine, there is decreased vasoconstrictor and hypertensive action.

4. Beta-adrenergic blocking drugs are also called beta _____.

5. _____ is a narrowing or blockage of the drainage channels between the anterior and posterior chambers of the eye.

6. _____ is given on an empty stomach because food may reduce absorption of the drug.

Activity C SHORT ANSWERS

A nurse's role in managing a patient who is prescribed adrenergic blocking drugs involves assisting the patient for preadministration assessment and monitoring. Answer the following questions, which involve the nurse's role in the management of patients on adrenergic blocking drug therapy.

1. A patient is prescribed an adrenergic blocking drug. What preadministration assessments should the nurse follow for the patient receiving an adrenergic blocking drug?

2. After the preadministration assessment, the patient is administered an antifungal drug for a vaginal infection. What are the nursing interventions for a patient receiving adrener-gic blocking drug therapy for hypertension?

Activity D DOSAGE CALCULATION

1. A patient has been prescribed 20 mg of biso-prolol every 24 hours. The available drug is in the form of a 5-mg tablet. To meet the pre-scribed dose, how many tablets should the nurse administer each day?

2. A patient with hypertension has been pre-scribed 30 mg of pindolol twice daily. The drug is available in the form of 10-mg tablets at the local pharmacy. The patient would like to know the total number of tablets he should buy for a 3-day course to meet the prescribed dose. What is the total number of tablets required for this patient?

3. A patient has been prescribed 10 mg of alfu-zosin daily. The available drug is in the form of a 10-mg tablet. The patient would like to know the total number of tablets he should buy for a 9-day course to meet the prescribed dose. What is the total number of tablets required for this patient?

4. A patient with hypertension has been pre-scribed 5 mg of doxazosin daily. The drug is available in the form of 1-mg tablets at the local pharmacy. The patient would like to know the total number of tablets he should buy for a 10-day course to meet the pre-scribed dose. What is the total number of tablets required for this patient?

5. A patient has been prescribed 10 mg of prazosin every 24 hours. The available drug is in the form of a 5-mg tablet. To meet the prescribed dose, how many tablets should the nurse administer each day?

_____

_____

SECTION II: APPLYING YOUR KNOWLEDGE

Activity E CASE STUDY

Lori Anderson is a Caucasian female, 66 years of age. She presents to the ED via ambulance with nausea and substernal chest pain. After being assessed by the ED physician, it is determined Mrs. Anderson is having an acute MI. The physician orders metoprolol (Lopressor) 3 bolus doses of 5 mg IV.

1. Prior to administering the 3 bolus doses of metoprolol (Lopressor) to Mrs. Anderson, what should the nurse's preadministration include?

_____

_____

2. What ongoing assessment should the nurse conduct with Mrs. Anderson?

_____

_____

SECTION III: PRACTICING FOR NCLEX

Activity F NCLEX-STYLE

Answer the following questions.

1. A patient with pheochromocytoma is admitted to a health care facility. The physician prescribes Phentolamine, an alpha-adrenergic blocking drug, to the patient. Which of the following reactions should the nurse monitor for in the patient?
   a. Diarrhea
   b. Orthostatic hypotension
   c. Bradycardia
   d. Bronchospasm

2. The nurse is documenting the history of a patient who is to be initiated in alpha-adrenergic blocking drug therapy. In which of these conditions are alpha-adrenergic blocking drugs contraindicated?
   a. Sinus bradycardia
   b. Heart failure
   c. Coronary artery disease
   d. Emphysema

3. A nurse is caring for a patient receiving adrenergic blocking drugs. Which of the following actions should the nurse perform when the patient receiving adrenergic blocking drugs shows a decrease in blood pressure?
   a. Monitor for excessive perspiration
   b. Monitor for confusion
   c. Adjust into a more conducive position
   d. Discontinue the drug

4. A nurse is caring for an elderly patient. The physician has prescribed a beta-adrenergic blocking drug to the patient. What should the nurse monitor for in the elderly patient when administering a beta-adrenergic blocking drug?
   a. Monitor vascular insufficiency
   b. Monitor occipital headache
   c. Monitor dizziness
   d. Monitor CNS depression

5. A nurse is caring for a patient on beta-adrenergic blocker therapy. The patient is also to be administered lidocaine. Which of the following risks will this maximize?
   a. Increased risk of hypotension
   b. Increased serum level of the beta-blocker
   c. Increase risk of paradoxical hypertensive effect
   d. Increased effect of the beta-blocker

6. A nurse is caring for a patient who has been administered prazosin. For which of the following adverse reactions should the nurse monitor the patient who is administered peripherally acting anti-adrenergic drugs?
   a. Dry mouth
   b. Drowsiness
   c. Malaise
   d. Light-headedness

7. A nurse is caring for a patient who has been prescribed the sympatholytic drug propranolol by the physician. What nursing interventions should the nurse perform when the patient is administered the sympatholytic drug?
   a. Measure the apical pulse rate
   b. Measure the body temperature
   c. Measure the heart rate
   d. Measure the respiration rate

8. A nurse at a health care center is assigned to prepare a teaching plan for a patient undergoing adrenergic blocking drug therapy for glaucoma. Which of the following should the nurse include in the teaching plan of the patient?
   a. Inform the patient to monitor his/her own pulse and blood pressure
   b. Take drugs as directed with food or on an empty stomach
   c. Contact primary health care provider if change in vision occurs
   d. Ask the patient to keep ambulating often

9. A nurse is caring for a patient with glaucoma. The patient is administered a beta-adrenergic blocking ophthalmic preparation, such as timolol. What is the role of the nurse in determining the effect of drug therapy?
   a. Measure intraocular pressure of the patient
   b. Monitor blood pressure of the patient
   c. Monitor respiratory rate of the patient
   d. Measure pulse rate of the patient

10. A patient has been administered an antiadrenergic drug. The patient has also been taking haloperidol for the treatment of psychosis. Which of the following interactions should the nurse monitor in the patient?
   a. Increased risk of lithium toxicity
   b. Increased risk of psychotic behavior
   c. Increase risk of hypertension
   d. Increased effect of anesthetic

11. The use of an alpha-adrenergic blocker will result in which of the following patient outcomes?
   a. Vasoconstriction
   b. Vasodilation
   c. Tachypnea
   d. Bradycardia

12. Which of the following medications is an alpha-adrenergic blocker?
   a. Phentolamine (Regitine)
   b. Metoprolol (Lopressor)
   c. Losartan (Cozaar)
   d. Lisinopril (Prinivil)

13. In which organ are the majority of beta-adrenergic receptors found?
   a. Heart
   b. Kidney
   c. Brain
   d. Liver

14. Which of the following ethnic groups would benefit from atenolol/chlorthalidone (Tenoretic) over lisinopril (Prinivil) for the treatment of hypertension?
   a. Caucasians
   b. Latinos
   c. African Americans
   d. Asians

15. Which of following is an example of an alpha/beta-adrenergic blocking drug?
   a. Metoprolol (Lopressor)
   b. Losartan (Cozaar)
   c. Lisinopril (Prinivil)
   d. Carvedilol (Coreg)

CHAPTER 26

Cholinergic Drugs

Learning Objectives

- Discuss important aspects of the parasympathetic nervous system
- Discuss the uses, drug actions, general adverse reactions, contraindications, precautions, and interactions of the cholinergic drugs
- Identify important preadministration and ongoing assessment activities the nurse should perform on the patient taking cholinergic drugs
- List nursing diagnoses particular to a patient taking cholinergic drugs
- Discuss ways to promote an optimal response to therapy, how to manage common adverse reactions, and important points to keep in mind when educating the patient about the use of cholinergic drugs

SECTION I: ASSESSING YOUR UNDERSTANDING

Activity A MATCHING

1. *Match the disorders in Column A with the effect of treatment with cholinergic drugs in Column B.*

Column A	Column B
1. Myasthenia gravis	a. Produces constriction of the iris
2. Urinary retention	b. Inhibits the activity of AChE
3. Glaucoma	c. Contracts the bladder's smooth muscles

2. *Match the cholinergic drugs in Column A with their uses in Column B.*

Column A	Column B
1. Edrophonium	a. Glaucoma
2. Bethanechol chloride	b. Diagnosis of myasthenia gravis
3. Carbachol	c. Acute nonobstructive urinary retention

Activity B FILL IN THE BLANKS

1. _____ receptors stimulate the smooth muscle.

2. Cholinergic drugs mimic the activity of the _____ nervous system.

3. _____ is the substance that transmits nerve impulses across the parasympathetic branch of the autonomic nervous system.

4. Drugs that inhibit the enzyme acetyl-cholinesterase are called _____.

5. _____ receptors stimulate the skeletal muscles in the parasympathetic nerve branch of the autonomic nervous system.

Activity C SHORT ANSWERS

A nurse's role in managing patients with myasthenia gravis involves monitoring them and implementing interventions that aid in their recovery. Answer the following questions which involve the nurse's role in the management of such situations.

1. A patient with myasthenia gravis has been recommended ambenonium. What should a nurse assess for in the patient before administering the first dose?

   _____

   _____

2. A patient is undergoing the treatment of myasthenia gravis. What should the nurse explain to the patient about the disorder and the drug to be administered for myasthenia gravis?

   _____

   _____

Activity D DOSAGE CALCULATION

1. A physician prescribes 70 mg of Mytelase 4 times a day for the treatment of myasthenia gravis. Mytelase is available as 10-mg tablets. How many tablets should the nurse administer to the patient for the whole day?

   _____

   _____

2. A patient has been prescribed 30 mg of bethanechol chloride 3 times a day for the treatment of urinary retention. Bethanechol chloride is available as 5-mg tablets. How many tablets should the nurse administer the patient in a single dose?

   _____

   _____

3. A patient has been prescribed 0.2 mL of carbachol 5 times a day. Carbachol is available as 1.0-mL sterile glass vials. How many vials should the patient be administered in a single day?

   _____

   _____

4. A physician has prescribed 240 mg of Mestinon over 2 doses for myasthenia gravis. Mestinon is available as 60-mg tablets. How many tablets should the nurse administer to the patient for each dose?

   _____

   _____

5. A patient has been prescribed 5 mg of edrophonium intravenously. Edrophonium is available as 15-mL vials. One mL of edrophonium is equivalent to 10 mg. How many mL should the nurse administer to the patient?

   _____

   _____

SECTION II: APPLYING YOUR KNOWLEDGE

Activity E CASE STUDY

Jeffrey Simms is a 36-year-old Caucasian male who has recently been diagnosed with myasthenia gravis. The physician has given him a prescription for ambenonium (Mytelase) 5 mg TID. He has no other medical conditions and takes no medications at this time.

1. Prior to administering ambenonium (Mytelase) to Mr. Simms, what should the nurse's preadministration assessment include?

   _____

   _____

2. What adverse effects may occur with the use of ambenonium (Mytelase)?

_____

_____

SECTION III: PRACTICING FOR NCLEX

Activity F **NCLEX-STYLE**

Answer the following questions.

1. A nurse is caring for a patient with urinary retention. Which of the following adverse effects should the nurse monitor during the topical administration of cholinergic drugs?

a. Temporary reduction of visual acuity

b. Increased ocular tension

c. Decreased sweat production

d. Anaphylactic shock

2. A patient has been prescribed the pilocarpine ocular system. What should the nurse instruct the patient about the system?

a. Remove and replace the system every 7 days

b. Instruct the patient that replacement is best during daytime

c. Change the system every day if eye secretions are excessive

d. Instruct the patient to carry identification about the disorder

3. A physician has prescribed bethanecol to a patient for acute nonobstructive urinary retention. What should the nurse check in the patient before the administration of bethanecol?

a. Tachyarrhythmias

b. Myocardial infarction

c. Coronary occlusion

d. Mechanical obstruction of the GI

4. A patient with myasthenia gravis has been prescribed ambenonium. The patient informs the nurse that he has respiratory problems and is taking corticosteroids. Which of the following effects of interactions between the two drugs should the nurse anticipate in the patient?

a. Increased neuromuscular blocking effect

b. Decreased effect of the cholinergic

c. Increased absorption of the cholinergic

d. Decreased serum level of corticosteroids

5. A nurse is caring for a patient undergoing Pilopine drug therapy for glaucoma. Which of the following should be the ongoing assessments for the patient after instilling the drug?

a. Assess for signs of muscle weakness in the patient

b. Dry the upper respiratory and oral secretions

c. Remove excessive secretions with a cotton ball soaked in normal saline solution

d. Measure and record the fluid intake and output

6. A patient is undergoing cholinergic drug therapy. The nurse knows that which other drug needs cautious use if it has to be administered along with cholinergic drugs?

a. Salicylates

b. Analgesics

c. Aminoglycoside antibiotics

d. Antidiabetics

7. What interventions should the nurse perform when caring for a patient who has been prescribed Miostat? Select all that apply.

a. Instill drug in lower conjunctival sac

b. Avoid tip of dropper touching the eye

c. Support hand by holding dropper against patient's forehead

d. Allow patient to instill his or her own eye drops

e. Instruct the patient to wear or carry identification

8. A nurse is caring for a patient with myasthenia gravis. The patient has been administered pyridostigmine bromide. What symptoms of drug overdose should the nurse monitor in the patient to make frequent dosage adjustments? Select all that apply.

   a. Drooping of the eyelids

   b. Rapid fatigability of the muscles

   c. Salivation

   d. Clenching of the jaw

   e. Muscle rigidity and spasm

9. A patient has been admitted for urinary retention. What is the role of the nurse when caring for the patient administered cholinergic therapy?

   a. Instruct the patient to void before the drug is administered

   b. Encourage the patient to take the drug with milk to enhance absorption

   c. Place call light and items that patient might need within easy reach

   d. Encourage the patient to have 5 to 7 glasses of water after drug administration

10. Which of the following interventions should the nurse perform if the patient develops diarrhea after administering the urecholine drug orally? Select all that apply.

   a. Ensure that bedpan or bathroom is readily available

   b. Check for blood stains in the stool

   c. Encourage the patient to ambulate to assist the passing of flatus

   d. Encourage the patient to increase their fibrous food intake

   e. Keep record of the number, consistency, and frequency of stools

11. Which of the following is the substance responsible for transmission of nerve impulses across the parasympathetic nervous system?

   a. Acetylcholine

   b. Norepinephrine

   c. Dopamine

   d. Serotonin

12. The stimulation of which of the following receptors in the parasympathetic nervous system stimulates smooth muscle?

   a. Muscarinic receptors

   b. Nicotinic receptors

   c. Alpha-adrenergic receptors

   d. Beta-adrenergic receptors

13. The stimulation of which of the following receptors in the parasympathetic nervous system stimulates skeletal muscle?

   a. Muscarinic receptors

   b. Nicotinic receptors

   c. Alpha-adrenergic receptors

   d. Beta-adrenergic receptors

14. Which of the following is the enzyme responsible for activating acetylcholine, the primary neurotransmitter in the parasympathetic nervous system?

   a. Acetylcholinesterase

   b. DNA gyrase

   c. Protease

   d. Lipase

15. Which of the following is an example of a direct-acting cholinergic that acts like the neurotransmitter acetylcholine?

   a. Bethanechol (Urecholine)

   b. Pyridostigmine (Regonol)

   c. Pilocarpine (Pilopine)

   d. Ambenonium (Mytelase)

CHAPTER 27

Cholinergic Blocking Drugs

Learning Objectives

- Discuss the uses, general drug actions, general adverse reactions, contraindications, precautions, and interactions of the cholinergic blocking drugs (also called anticholinergic drugs and cholinergic blockers.
- Discuss important preadministration and ongoing assessment activities the nurse should perform on the patient taking cholinergic blocking drugs
- List nursing diagnoses particular to the patient taking cholinergic blocking drugs
- Discuss ways to promote an optimal response to therapy, how to manage common adverse reactions, and important points to keep in mind when educating patients taking a cholinergic blocking drug.

SECTION I: ASSESSING YOUR UNDERSTANDING

Activity A MATCHING

1. *Match the cholinergic blocking drugs in Column A with their uses in Column B.*

Column A	Column B
1. Atropine	a. Treatment of irritable bowel syndrome
2. Belladonna alkaloids	b. Adjunctive treatment of peptic ulcer
3. Dicyclomine HCl	c. Adjunctive therapy for diverticulitis
4. Mepenzolate bromide	d. Treatment of pylorospasm

2. *Match the adverse reactions associated with cholinergic blocking drugs in Column A with the measures to lessen their intensity in Column B.*

Column A	Column B
1. Photophobia	a. Chew gum or dissolve hard candy in mouth
2. Dry mouth	
3. Constipation	b. Schedule tasks requiring alertness before the first dose of the drug is taken
4. Drowsiness	
	c. Schedule outdoor activities before first dose of drug is taken
	d. Eat foods high in fiber

Activity B FILL IN THE BLANKS

1. _____ is the primary neurotransmitter in the parasympathetic branch of the autonomic nervous system.

2. Cholinergic blocking drugs inhibit the activity of acetylcholine at the _____ nerve synapse.

3. _____ is a type of visual impairment occurring due to the use of cholinergic blocking drugs, characterized by a difficulty in focusing resulting from paralysis of the ciliary muscle.

4. The nurse should use _____ with caution in patients with asthma.

5. An unexpected or unusual effect to cholinergic blocking drugs is known as drug _____.

Activity C SHORT ANSWERS

A nurse's role in caring for patients receiving cholinergic blocking drugs involves monitoring and managing the patients' needs and helping them in their recovery. Answer the following questions which involve the nurse's role in the management of such situations.

1. A nurse has been caring for a patient with a peptic ulcer. Which points should the nurse include when evaluating the patient's treatment plan?

_____

_____

_____

2. What instructions should the nurse offer an elderly patient's family when monitoring the patient receiving cholinergic blocking drugs?

_____

_____

_____

Activity D DOSAGE CALCULATION

1. A patient with an overactive bladder is prescribed 60 mg of trospium per day. The drug is available in the form of 20-mg tablets. How many tablets should the nurse administer per day to meet the recommended dose?

_____

_____

2. The physician has prescribed 800 mg of flavoxate for a patient to be administered 4 times a day. The available drug is in the form of 100 mg tablets. How many tablets should the nurse administer each time to meet the recommended dose?

_____

_____

3. A patient with peptic ulcers is prescribed 0.25 mg of glycopyrrolate to be injected in a patient intramuscularly. The available drug is in the form of a 0.2 mg/mL solution. How much glycopyrrolate should the nurse prepare to be administered to the patient?

_____

_____

4. A patient with irritable bowel syndrome is prescribed 120 mg of dicyclomine HCl, to be administered 4 times per day. The available drug is in the form of 10-mg tablets. How many tablets should the nurse administer the patient each time?

_____

_____

SECTION II: APPLYING YOUR KNOWLEDGE

Activity E CASE STUDY

Janet Mason is an African American female, 74 years of age. She presents to the clinic complaining of symptoms of overactive bladder. The physician writes Mrs. Mason a prescription for tolterodine (Detrol LA) 4 mg QD.

1. Discuss the adverse reactions that should be included in the nurse's teaching plan for Mrs. Mason?

_____

_____

2. What should the nurse observe Mrs. Mason for as an elderly patient taking a cholinergic blocking drug?

_____

_____

SECTION III: PRACTICING FOR NCLEX

Activity F NCLEX-STYLE

Answer the following questions.

1. In which of the following patients should a nurse use atropine cautiously?
   a. Patients with tachyarrhythmias
   b. Patients with myasthenia gravis
   c. Patients with glaucoma
   d. Patients with asthma

2. A patient is being administered propantheline bromide for the treatment of a peptic ulcer. After receiving the drug, the patient complains of constipation. Which of the following instructions should the nurse provide this patient to help relieve constipation?
   a. Consume an antacid after meals for severe constipation
   b. Increase the consumption of food rich in fiber
   c. Increase the consumption of citrus fruits
   d. Restrict fluid consumption to prevent urinary fequency

3. Which of the following interventions should a nurse perform when caring for a patient receiving atropine for third-degree heart block?
   a. Place the patient on a cardiac monitor before drug administration
   b. Provide oxygen support to the patient every hour
   c. Monitor for symptoms of mydriasis and cycloplegia
   d. Monitor for a change in pulse rate or rhythm

4. A patient with bladder overactivity is admitted to a health care facility. The nurse administers a cholinergic blocking drug to the patient as prescribed by the physician. The drug is known to cause heat prostration. What instructions should the nurse offer the patient to help lessen the intensity of heat prostration? Select all that apply.
   a. Wear loose-fitting clothes
   b. Sponge the skin with cool water
   c. Apply sunscreen when outside
   d. Use fans to cool the body
   e. Wear sunglasses when outdoors

5. A patient with excessive vagal-induced bradycardia has been prescribed atropine. The patient informs the nurse that he is receiving tricyclic antidepressants for the treatment of depression. What drug interactions should the nurse assess for in the patient?
   a. Decreased effectiveness of the antidepressant
   b. Increased respiratory rate
   c. Increased effect of the atropine drug
   d. Decreased blood pressure

6. A nurse is administering glycopyrrolate to a patient through the parenteral route to reduce bronchial and oral secretions. Which of the following adverse reactions of the drug should the nurse monitor for in this patient? Select all that apply.

   a. Nausea

   b. Altered taste perception

   c. Tachycardia

   d. Mydriasis

   e. Dysphagia

7. A nurse is caring for a 65-year-old patient with pylorospasm. Which of the following interventions should the nurse perform when caring for this patient as a part of preoperative interventions?

   a. Ensure that a cholinergic drug is not administered preoperatively

   b. Monitor for changes in the patient's pulse rate or rhythm

   c. Ensure that the patient has not received antibiotics recently

   d. Place the patient in the Fowler position

8. A nurse needs to administer a cholinergic blocking drug preoperatively to a patient. Why should the nurse administer the drug to the patient at the exact time as prescribed by the physician?

   a. To avoid abdominal cramping in the patient after the drug administration

   b. To ensure effectiveness of the drug after administration of the anesthetic

   c. To allow the drug to produce the greatest effect before administration of anesthetic

   d. To avoid excessive salivation and make the patient feel comfortable

9. A nurse is caring for a patient with bladder overactivity. The patient has been prescribed oxybutynin by the physician. Which of the following conditions should the nurse monitor for in the patient if the drug is administered on a daily basis?

   a. Mydriasis

   b. Mouth dryness

   c. Blurred vision

   d. Hesitancy

10. A nurse is caring for a patient who has been administered atropine preoperatively to reduce the production of secretions in the respiratory tract. Which of the following drug reactions should the nurse identify as a part of the desired response?

    a. Vomiting

    b. Elevated temperature

    c. Low pulse rate

    d. Drowsiness

11. Which of the following is an example of a parasympatholytic drug?

    a. Oxybutynin (Ditropan)

    b. Bethanechol (Urecholine)

    c. Ambenonium (Mytelase)

    d. Pyridostigmine (Regonol)

12. Oxybutynin (Ditropan), used for the treatment of overactive bladder, exerts its effect by inhibiting the action of which of the following receptors?

    a. Nicotinic receptors

    b. Alpha-adrenergic receptors

    c. Muscarinic receptors

    d. Beta-adrenergic receptors

13. The antispasmodic dicyclomine (Bentyl) used for the treatment of irritable bowel syndrome exerts its effect by inhibiting the action of which of the following receptors?

    a. Muscarinic receptors

    b. Nicotinic receptors

    c. Alpha-adrenergic receptors

    d. Beta-adrenergic receptors

14. The cholinergic blocking drug glycopyrrolate (Robinul) is used in conjunction with anesthesia for which of the following reasons?

    a. Increase muscle rigidity

    b. Relaxation

    c. Prolongation of anesthesia

    d. Reduction of oral secretions

15. The nurse should observe patients receiving a cholinergic blocking drug during the hot summer months because these patients are at increased risk of which of the following?

    a. Sunburn

    b. Heart attack

    c. Heat prostration

    d. Dehydration

CHAPTER 28

Cholinesterase Inhibitors

Learning Objectives

- Discuss the clinical manifestations of Alzheimer's disease
- List the uses, general drug actions, general adverse reactions, contraindications, precautions, and interactions associated with the administration of the cholinesterase inhibitors
- Discuss important preadministration and ongoing assessment activities the nurse should perform with the patient taking a cholinesterase inhibitor
- List nursing diagnoses particular to a patient taking a cholinesterase inhibitor
- Discuss ways to promote an optimal response to therapy, how to manage common adverse reactions, and important points to keep in mind when educating patients about the use of the cholinesterase inhibitors

SECTION I: ASSESSING YOUR UNDERSTANDING

Activity A MATCHING

1. *Match the cholinesterase inhibitor drugs given in Column A with their corresponding adverse reactions given in Column B.*

Column A		Column B
1. Donepezil	d	**a.** Vomiting
2. Memantin	C	**b.** Dyspepsia
3. Rivastigmine	b	**c.** Confusion
4. Tacrine	a	**d.** Muscle cramps

2. *Match the interactant drugs given in Column A with their corresponding uses given in Column B.*

	Column A	Column B
b	**1.** Anticholinergics	**a.** Breathing problems
C	**2.** Non-steroidal anti-inflammatory drugs	**b.** Decrease of bodily secretions
a	**3.** Theophylline	**c.** Pain relief

Activity B   FILL IN THE BLANKS

1. _Alzheimer's_ disease is a progressive deterioration of emotional, physical, and cognitive abilities.

2. Acetylcholine is a transmitter in the _cholinergic_ neuropathway.

3. Disease or injury to the _Liver_ causes alanine aminotransferase (ALT) enzyme to be released into the bloodstream, resulting in elevated ALT levels.

4. In Alzheimer's disease, specific pathologic changes occur in the cortex of the _Brain_.

5. Tacrine is particularly damaging to the liver and can result in _Hepatotoxicity_

Activity C   SHORT ANSWERS

A nurse's role in managing patients who are being administered cholinesterase inhibitors involves implementing interventions that aid in their recovery and monitoring the patients for the occurrences of adverse reactions of the drug administration. Answer the following questions which involve the nurse's role in the management of such situations.

1. A patient is administered a cholinesterase inhibitor for treating mild-to-moderate dementia of Alzheimer's disease. What preadministration assessments should the nurse perform in patients who are prescribed cholinesterase inhibitors?

The nurse should assess cognitive abilities, agitation, impulsive behavior, mental status, physical assessments.

2. A patient is administered tacrine for treating mild-to-moderate dementia of Alzheimer's disease.

   a. What interventions should a nurse perform when caring for the patient?

   Monitor for liver damage, check levels of alanine, obtain levels weekly, monitor transaminase g 3 months, monitor adverse reactions.

   b. What adverse reactions of the tacrine administration should the nurse monitor for in the patient?

   Adverse reactions include nausea, vomiting, dizziness, headaches.

Activity D   DOSAGE CALCULATION

1. A physician prescribes 15 mg of donepezil hydrochloride per day for a patient with dementia of Alzheimer's disease. Donepezil is available in the form of 5-mg tablets. How many tablets will the nurse have to administer to the patient in 3 days?

   9 tabs

2. A patient with severe Alzheimer-type dementia is prescribed a total of 200 mg of memantine for a period of 10 days. Memantine hydrochloride is supplied in the form of 10-mg tablets. How many tablets should the nurse administer to the patient in one day?

   2 tabs

3. A physician prescribes a total of 18 mg of rivastigmine tartrate for a patient with moderate Alzheimer-type dementia for a period of 3 days. The drug is to be administered twice a day. Rivastigmine tartrate is supplied in the form of 1.5-mg capsules. How many capsules should the nurse administer to the patient each time?

   2 caps

4. A patient with mild-to-moderate Alzheimer-type dementia is prescribed a total of 120 mg of tacrine HCl for a period of 4 days. Tacrine HCl is supplied in the form of 10-mg capsules. How many capsules should the nurse administer to the patient per day?

   3 caps
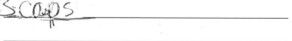

SECTION II: APPLYING YOUR KNOWLEDGE

Activity E CASE STUDY

Ruby Barnes is a 75-year-old Caucasian female. She presents to her physician's office for a follow-up visit. Her husband mentions to the physician that Ruby has been more forgetful lately. One evening after supper, Mr. Barnes noticed Ruby beginning to prepare a roast. When questioned, she said she hadn't yet eaten anything for dinner. She has not wanted to go to church as she has in past and, in converation, asks the same questions multiple times. The physician completes some neurological tests and diagnoses Mrs. Barnes with Alzheimer's disease.

1. Based on her symptoms, in which stage of Alzheimer's disease would Mrs. Barnes be classified?

   Memory difficulty, poor judgement, withdrawl behaviors experienced.

2. The physician writes Mrs. Barnes a prescription for donepezil (Aricept) 5 mg QD. What adverse effects should the nurse review with Mr. and Mrs. Barnes?

   Adverse reactions should be watched for include: headaches, nausea, diarrhea, insomnia and muscle therapy.

SECTION III: PRACTICING FOR NCLEX

Activity F NCLEX-STYLE

Answer the following questions.

1. A patient is prescribed cholinesterase inhibitors for the treatment of dementia. Which of the following adverse reactions should the nurse monitor in the patient?
   a. Diarrhea
   b. High blood pressure
   c. Seizure disorders
   d. Renal dysfunction

2. Patients with Alzheimer's disease are prescribed tacrine so as to slow the progression of dementia. In which of the following cases should tacrine be cautiously used?
   a. Vaginitis
   b. Diabetes mellitus
   c. Cardiovascular problems
   d. Bladder obstruction

3. A patient is prescribed cholinesterase inhibitors for the treatment of dementia. The assigned nurse is required to perform a physical assessment of the patient before administering the cholinesterase inhibitors. Which of the following signs should the nurse monitor during physical assessment? Select all that apply.
   a. Pulse
   b. Respiratory rate
   c. Weight
   d. Brainwaves
   e. Hepatic function

4. A nurse monitoring the ALT levels of a patient administered tacrine reports increased ALT levels to the primary health care provider. The primary health care provider decides to discontinue use of the drug because of the danger of hepatotoxicity. Which of the following could occur in the patient as a result of the abrupt discontinuation of tacrine?
   a. Loss of functional ability
   b. Decline in cognitive functioning
   c. Impulsive behavior
   d. Nervous breakdown

5. A nurse is caring for a patient with dementia of Alzheimer's disease. Which of the following is an effect of the interaction of non-steroidal anti-inflammatory drugs with cholinesterase inhibitors?
   a. Asthma
   b. Sick sinus syndrome
   c. Increased risk of GI bleeding
   d. Increased risk of theophylline toxicity

6. A patient is administered tacrine for treating Alzheimer's disease. Which of the following conditions should the nurse monitor for when caring for the patient?

   a. Cardiovascular disease

   b. Pulmonary disease

   c. Liver damage

   d. Goiter

7. A nurse is caring for a patient receiving cholinesterase inhibitors. The drug is known to cause the adverse reactions of dizziness and syncope that can place the patient at risk for injury. Which of the following interventions should the nurse implement in order to reduce the risk of injury? Select all that apply.

   a. Use side rails

   b. Monitor patient every 12 hours

   c. Keep bed in low position

   d. Use soft bedding

   e. Use night lights

8. A nurse is required to administer the prescribed tacrine to a patient for the treatment of moderate dementia of the Alzheimer type. How should the nurse administer this drug to the patient?

   a. 30 minutes before meals

   b. On an empty stomach

   c. 1 hour after meals

   d. Around the clock intravenously

9. Ginkgo, one of the oldest herbs in the world, is thought to improve memory and brain function and to enhance circulation to the brain, heart, limbs, and eyes. In which of the following patients is the use of ginkgo contraindicated?

   a. Patients receiving monoamine oxidase inhibitors

   b. Patients receiving sedatives and hypnotics

   c. Patients receiving opioid analgesics

   d. Patients receiving anti-cholinergic drugs

10. A nurse is caring for a patient receiving cholinesterase inhibitors for the treatment of Alzheimer's disease. Why is it important for the nurse to provide proper attention to the dosing of medication?

    a. Helps to decrease the adverse GI reactions

    b. Helps the patient to recover faster

    c. Helps the patient to maintain normal temperature

    d. Helps to decrease variations in the pulse rate

11. Cholinesterase inhibitors are utilized for the treatment of which of the following medical conditions?

    a. Myasthenia gravis

    b. Alzheimer's disease

    c. Glaucoma

    d. Urinary retention

12. Which of the following is a cholinesterase inhibitor use to treat dementia which can cause hepatotoxicity?

    a. Tacrine (Cognex)

    b. Rivastigmine (Exelon)

    c. Donepezil (Aricept)

    d. Galantamine (Razadyne)

13. People with memory problems may take which of the following herbal products which has been used to improve mental performance?

    a. Ginseng

    b. Garlic

    c. Kava

    d. Willow bark

14. A nurse observing a patient with Alzheimer's disease will notice difficulty with memory, poor judgment, and withdrawal behaviors in which stage of Alzheimer's disease?

    a. Middle

    b. Pre

    c. Late

    d. Early

15. A nurse caring for an Alzheimer's patient will notice which of the following stages is typically the longest?

    a. Early

    b. Middle

    c. Pre

    d. Late

CHAPTER 29

Antiparkinsonism Drugs

Learning Objectives

- Define the terms *Parkinson's disease* and *Parkinsonism*
- Discuss the uses, general drug action, adverse drug reactions, contraindications, precautions, and interactions of the antiparkinsonism drugs
- Discuss important preadministration and ongoing assessment activities the nurse should perform on the patient taking antiparkinsonism drugs
- List nursing diagnoses particular to a patient taking antiparkinsonism drugs
- Discuss ways to promote an optimal response to therapy, how to manage adverse reactions, and important points to keep in mind when educating patients about the use of the antiparkinsonism drugs

SECTION I: ASSESSING YOUR UNDERSTANDING

Activity A MATCHING

1. **Match the dopaminergic agents in Column A with their adverse reaction in Column B.**

Column A	Column B
1. Amantadine *b*	a. Dysphagia
2. Bromocriptine *d*	b. Orthostatic hypotension
3. Carbidopa/ *a* levodopa	c. Rhinitis
4. Pergolide *c*	d. Epigastria distress

2. **Match the drugs in Column A with their uses in Column B.**

Column A	Column B
1. Bromocriptine *c*	a. Treatment of drug-induced extrapyramidal symptoms
2. Benztropine mesylate *a*	b. Treatment of Parkinson's disease "off" episode
3. Entacapone *d*	c. Treatment of female endocrine imbalances
4. Apomorphine HCl *b*	d. Used as adjunct to levodopa/carbidopa in Parkinson's disease

Activity B FILL IN THE BLANKS

1. ~~parkinson's~~ disease is a degenerative disorder of the central nervous system due to an imbalance of dopamine and acetylcholine within the CNS.

2. Failure of the muscles of the lower esophagus to relax causing difficulty swallowing is known as *achalsia*

3. The *on-off* phenomenon occurs in patients taking levodopa in which the patient may suddenly alternate between improved clinical status and loss of therapeutic effect.

4. *Choreiform* movements are involuntary muscular twitches of the limbs or facial muscles.

5. *pyridoxine* is a milder COMT inhibitor used to help manage fluctuations in the response to levodopa in individuals with Parkinson's disease.

Activity C SHORT ANSWERS

A nurse's role in managing Parkinsonism involves assisting the patients with the administration of antiparkinsonism drugs. The nurse also helps in educating the patients and their family about the treatment regimen. Answer the following questions, which involve the nurse's role in the management of such situations.

1. A nurse is assigned to care for a patient with Parkinson's disease. Under preadministration assessment, the nurse has to evaluate the patient's neuromuscular status. What should the nurse observe to evaluate the neuromuscular status of the patient?

   Nurse should monitor change in gait, tremors, muscular rigidity, speech, face expressions, change in thought process, postural deformities.

2. A nurse has been caring for a patient with Parkinson's disease. What factors should the nurse keep in mind when evaluating the treatment plan for the patient?

   Nurse should keep factors of therapeutic effect, adverse reactions, verbalizing and understanding to, no evidence of injuries.

3. A patient with Parkinson's disease is administered levodopa treatment. The patient's condition is alternating between improved clinical status and loss of therapeutic effect, and the patient is showing an on-off phenomenon. What nursing interventions should the nurse perform when caring for this patient showing an on-off phenomenon?

   The nurse should carefully observe pts muscular rigidity, body temp elevated, mental changes when showing off day phenomenon.

4. A patient with Parkinson's disease is vomiting and experiencing gastrointestinal disturbances. What interventions should the nurse perform when caring for this patient?

   Create a calm environment, serves small frequent meals, monitor pts weight and b/c drug or change if any vomiting or nausea.

5. A nurse has been caring for a patient on Parkinsonism drugs. What information should the nurse include in her family and patient teaching plan when caring for this patient on an outpatient basis?

   Pt takes drug as prescribed, increase/decrease when ordered, if GI occurs to be upset take drug w/ food and avoid driving if dizziness, blurred vision occurs.

Activity D DOSAGE CALCULATION

1. A patient with Parkinson's disease has been recommended amantadine 400 mg/day. The available drug is in the form of a 100-mg capsule. To meet the recommended dose, how many tablets should the nurse administer each day?

   4 tabs

2. A patient is required to take 25 mg of Lodosyn per day with Sinemet. The ratio of carbidopa-levodopa in Sinemet is 1:10. If 25 mg of Lodosyn has to be taken with 100 mg of levodopa in the Sinemet, then how much Lodosyn should the patient consume if the carbidopa ratio in the Sinemet rises to 25 mg?

   62.5 mg of Lodosyn

3. A patient with an "off" episode of Parkinson's disease has been recommended 0.2 mL of benztropine mesylate. The dosage-administering mechanism consists of a pen which can deliver doses in increments of 0.02 mL. To meet the recommended dose, how many increments should the nurse administer the patient each day?

10 increments

4. A physician has prescribed 1000 mg of entacapone to a patient with Parkinson's disease. The available drug is in the form of 200-mg tablets. To meet the recommended dose, how many tablets should the nurse administer the patient each day?

5 tabs

SECTION II: APPLYING YOUR KNOWLEDGE

Activity E CASE STUDY

Marcos Sanchez is an Hispanic male, 54 years of age. He is a newly diagnosed Parkinson's disease patient. He is currently taking carbidopa/levodopa (Sinemet) 300 mg TID. He presents at the clinic for follow-up and has some questions about his disease state and medication.

1. Mr. Sanchez knows that the symptoms of Parkinsonism are caused by a depletion of dopamine in the central nervous system, but he wants to know why he cannot just be given dopamine to supplement the deficiency. What should the nurse answer?

Nurses should say it's hard to supplement dopamine due to blood brain barrier and means it is tightly packed cell walls of the brain capillaries that screen out substances.

2. As this is a follow-up visit for Mr. Sanchez, what should the nurse's ongoing assessment include?

Evaluating pts response to therapy tremors of hands muscular rigidity, gait, facial expression and physical assessments.

SECTION III: PRACTICING FOR NCLEX

Activity F NCLEX-STYLE

Answer the following questions.

1. A nurse is caring for a patient who has been prescribed carbidopa. After administration of the drug, the nurse observes the occurrence of choreiform and dystonic movements in the patient. Which of the following interventions should the nurse perform when caring for this patient?
   a. Monitor vital signs frequently
   b. Withhold the next dose of the drug
   c. Offer frequent sips of water
   d. Observe the patient for nausea and fatigue

2. A nurse is caring for a patient receiving an antiparkinsonism drug. The patient is complaining of constipation. What instructions should the nurse offer the patient to help relieve constipation? Select all that apply.
   a. Decrease the intake of carbohydrates
   b. Use a stool softener
   c. Increase intake of fiber in the diet
   d. Increase intake of fluids in the diet
   e. Increase intake of vitamin C

3. A nurse is assigned to care for a patient with neuroleptic malignant-like syndrome which has occurred due to the abrupt discontinuation of an antiparkinsonism drug. For which of the following symptoms should the nurse monitor the patient? Select all that apply.
   a. Muscular rigidity
   b. Elevated body temperature
   c. Mental changes
   d. Tachycardia
   e. Orthostatic hypotension

4. A nurse is caring for a patient who has been prescribed levodopa for the treatment of Parkinson's disease. The patient informs the nurse that he is taking antacids for the relief of heartburn. What effect of the interaction of the two drugs should the nurse anticipate in the patient?
   a. Increased risk of hypertension
   b. Increased risk of dyskinesia
   c. Increased effect of levodopa
   d. Increased risk of cardiac symptoms

5. A nurse is assigned to care for a patient who has to be administered catechol-O-methyl-transferase (COMT) inhibitors. Which of the following pieces of patient-related information should the nurse obtain to understand that the drug has to be administered cautiously to the patient?
   a. Patient has decreased renal function
   b. Patient has tachycardia
   c. Patient has cardiac arrhythmias
   d. Patient has GI tract problems

6. What should the nurse's plan include when a patient receiving antiparkinsonism drugs is discharged? Select all that apply.
   a. Instruct the patient to avoid taking vitamin B6 with levodopa
   b. Instruct the patient to contact PHCP in case of severe dry mouth
   c. Instruct the patient to avoid consumption of alcohol
   d. Instruct the patient to have small and frequent meals
   e. Encourage the patient to increase intake of vitamin C

7. A nurse is caring for a patient undergoing antiparkinsonism drug therapy. The nurse observes that the patient is vomiting frequently. Which of the following nursing interventions should the nurse perform when caring for this patient?
   a. Change the antiparkinsonism drug
   b. Administer the drug before meals
   c. Administer antacids after meals
   d. Refrain from giving liquids after meals

8. What are the nursing interventions involved when the patient is showing response to therapy with antiparkinsonism drugs?
   a. Change the antiparkinsonism drug to another
   b. Discontinue use of antiparkinsonism drugs
   c. Observe the patient's behavior at frequent intervals
   d. Observe a drug holiday as prescribed

9. A nurse is caring for a patient with Parkinsonism. Which of the following conditions should the nurse observe that may indicate abdominal pain due to constipation in the patient?

   a. Change in facial expression
   b. Change in style of walking
   c. Change in diet intake
   d. Change in sleeping patterns

10. For which category of patient is the use of cholinergic-blocking drugs contraindicated?
    a. Patients with bone marrow depression
    b. Patients with cardiac disorders
    c. Patients with visual impairment
    d. Patients with prostatic hypertrophy

11. Which of the following terms refers to a group of symptoms involving motor movement characterized by tremors, rigidity, and bradykinesia?
    a. Parkinsonism
    b. Myasthenia gravis
    c. Seizure disorder
    d. Anxiety

12. Which of the following drugs is classified as a dopaminergic agent that treats Parkinsonism by supplementing the amount of dopamine in the brain?
    a. Benztropine (Cogentin)
    b. Biperiden (Akineton)
    c. Carbidopa (Lodosyn)
    d. Procyclidine (Kemadrin)

13. Which of the following drugs is classified as a catechol-O-methyltransferase (COMT) inhibitor?
    a. Entacapone (Comtan)
    b. Carbidopa (Lodosyn)
    c. Benztropine (Cogentin)
    d. Biperiden (Akineton)

14. Which of the following drugs is classified as a non-ergot dopamine receptor agonist?
    a. Entacapone (Comtan)
    b. Carbidopa (Lodosyn)
    c. Apomorphine (Apokyn)
    d. Benztropine (Cogentin)

15. Which of the following drugs is classified as a cholinergic-blocking drug used to treat Parkinsonism?
    a. Apomorphine (Apokyn)
    b. Entacapone (Comtan)
    c. Carbidopa (Lodosyn)
    d. Benztropine (Cogentin)

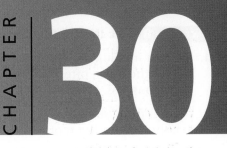

CHAPTER 30

Anticonvulsants

Learning Objectives

- List the different types of drugs used as anticonvulsants
- Discuss the general drug actions, uses, adverse reactions, contraindications, precautions, and interactions of anticonvulsants
- Discuss important preadministration and ongoing assessment activities the nurse should perform with the patient receiving an anticonvulsant
- List nursing diagnoses particular to a patient taking an anticonvulsant
- Discuss ways to promote an optimal response to therapy, how to manage common adverse reactions when administering the anticonvulsants, and important points to keep in mind when educating a patient about the use of anticonvulsants

SECTION I: ASSESSING YOUR UNDERSTANDING

Activity A MATCHING

1. *Match the anticonvulsant drugs in Column A with the uses in Column B.*

Column A	Column B
1. Diamox C	a. Neuropathic pain
2. Lyrica a	b. Preanesthetic
3. Diastat d	c. Altitude sickness
4. Ativan b	d. Anxiety disorders

2. *Match the anticonvulsant drugs in Column A with their adverse reactions in Column B.*

Column A	Column B
1. Epitol C	a. Urinary frequency, pruritus, urticaria
2. Peganone d	b. Ataxia, visual disturbances, rash
3. Klonopin b	c. Unsteady gait, aplastic anemia and other blood cell abnormalities
4. Zarontin a	d. Hypotension, nystagmus, slurred speech

Activity B FILL IN THE BLANKS

1. Sudden involuntary contraction of the muscles of the body, often accompanied by loss of consciousness, is termed as Convulsion.

2. hydantons stabilizes hyperexcitability post-synaptically in the motor cortex of the brain.

3. Oxazolidinediones decreases the repetitive synaptic transmission of nerve impulses.

4. The Succinimide are contraindicated in patients with bone marrow depression or hepatic or renal impairment.

5. The Barbiturates are used with caution in patients with pulmonary disease and in hyperactive children.

Activity C SHORT ANSWERS

A nurse's role in managing a patient who is prescribed an anticonvulsant drug involves assisting the patient with preadministration assessment. The nurse also helps in monitoring patients who are administered with anticonvulsant drugs. Answer the following questions which involve the nurse's role in the management of patients on anticonvulsant therapy.

1. A patient with seizures visits a health care facility and has been prescribed an anticonvulsant drug. What preadministration assessments should the nurse perform before the administration of an anticonvulsant drug?

   Nurse shall check for abnormal behaviors, any seizure disorder, vital signs, run lab tests for seizures if any document type, frequency, description of aura and degree of consciousness.

2. After the preadministration assessment, the patient is administered an anticonvulsant drug for seizure disorders. What is the nurse's role when caring for the patient administered with an anticonvulsant drug?

   Nurse's role includes: Measure regular serum levels of anticonvulsants for toxicity, add a second pill if regimen isn't working, assist primary health provider in evaluation, frequently adjust dosage due to pts response of therapy.

Activity D DOSAGE CALCULATION

1. A patient has been prescribed 400 mg of Zonegran daily. The available drug is in the form of 50-mg capsules. The patient would like to know the total number of capsules he should buy for a 3-day course to meet the prescribed dose. What is the total number of capsules required for this patient?

   24 caps

2. A patient has been prescribed 200 mg of Topamax daily. The availability is 100-mg capsules. The patient has to continue the drug therapy for 2 days. What is the total number of capsules required for this client?

   4 caps

3. A patient is prescribed 500 mg of Depakote to be taken in equal doses 2 times a day orally. On-hand availability is 125-mg tablets. How many tablets should the nurse administer to the patient each time?

   2 tabs

4. A patient has been prescribed 48 mg of Gabitril once a day orally. The drug is available in 12-mg tablets in a pharmacy. How many tablets should the nurse administer to the client?

   4 tabs

5. A patient has been prescribed 400 mg of Mysoline to be taken in 4 divided doses. The drug is available in 50-mg tablets. How many tablets should the nurse administer the patient each time?

   2 tabs

6. A patient has been prescribed 1200 mg of Trileptal to be taken in 2 divided doses. The drug is available in 300-mg tablets. How many tablets should the nurse administer to the patient each time?

   2 tabs

SECTION II: APPLYING YOUR KNOWLEDGE

Activity E CASE STUDY

Frank Miller is an African American male, 44 years of age. Mr. Miller is hospitalized for neurological evaluation after actively seizing while in the ED.

1. What information should the nurse obtain from those who observed the seizure?

   Nurse will obtain, type, description of seizure, average length, aura, degree of impairment and what goes on during seizure.

2. Mr. Miller is started on phynetoin (Dilantin) 100mg TID. His wife brings him back to the ED 1 week later with complaints of slurred speech, ataxia, lethargy, dizziness, and nausea. What might the symptoms Mr. Miller is experiencing indicate?

   Experiencing Phenytoin toxicity

SECTION III: PRACTICING FOR NCLEX

Activity F NCLEX-STYLE

Answer the following questions.

1. A physician has prescribed trimethadione to a patient with epilepsy at a health care facility. Which of the following should the nurse monitor for in the patient while administering trimethadione?
   - **a.** Eye disorders
   - **b.** Bone marrow depression
   - **c.** Hypotension
   - **d.** Myocardial insufficiency

2. A patient with anxiety disorders visits a health care facility. A physician prescribes tranxene to the patient. Which of following adverse drug reactions should the nurse monitor for in the patient?
   - **a.** Dyspepsia
   - **b.** Vomiting
   - **c.** Fatigue
   - **d.** Palpations

3. A nurse at a health care center is assigned to prepare a teaching plan for a patient undergoing hydantoin drug therapy. Which of the following should the nurse include in the teaching plan of the patient? Select all that apply.
   - **a.** Avoid taking the drugs during pregnancy
   - **b.** Brush and floss teeth after each meal
   - **c.** Avoid consumption of discolored capsules
   - **d.** Notify PHCP if blurred vision occurs
   - **e.** Take medication with food

4. A nurse is caring for a patient with tonic-clonic seizures in a health care facility. The physician has prescribed dilantin to the patient. Which of the hematologic changes in the patient should the nurse immediately report to the primary health care provider?
   - **a.** Sinus bradycardia
   - **b.** Sinoatrial block
   - **c.** Thrombocytopenia
   - **d.** Adams-Stokes syndrome

5. A nurse is caring for a patient with disturbed sensory perception. The physician has prescribed Lamictal. What instructions should the nurse provide the patient receiving Lamictal? Select all that apply.
   - **a.** Stay out of sun
   - **b.** Wear sunscreen
   - **c.** Wear protective clothes
   - **d.** Wear light-colored clothes
   - **e.** Place cotton pads soaked in rose water on the eyes

6. A nurse is assigned to care for a patient who has been prescribed phenytoin. In which of the following cases is the use of phenytoin contraindicated?
   - **a.** Patients with history of asthma
   - **b.** Patients with cardiac problems
   - **c.** Patients with hepatic abnormalities
   - **d.** Patients with liver dysfunction

7. A nurse is caring for an elderly patient undergoing diazepam therapy. Which of the following interventions should the nurse perform for the patient?

   a. Examine mouth and gums of the patient

   b. Examine the skin frequently

   c. Observe the patient for throat irritation

   d. Observe the patient for apnea and cardiac arrest

8. A nurse is caring for a patient on analgesic therapy. The patient is also to be administered an anticonvulsant drug. Of which possible effect of the interaction of analgesics with anticonvulsants should the nurse be aware?

   a. Increased carbamazepine levels

   b. Increased seizure activity

   c. Increased blood glucose levels

   d. Increased depressant effect

9. A patient with seizures has been prescribed phenytoin at a health care facility. Which of the following would indicate drug toxicity?

   a. Patient has plasma levels greater than 20 micrograms/mL

   b. Phenytoin plasma levels are greater than 20 micrograms/mL

   c. Patient has plasma levels greater than 30 micrograms/mL

   d. Phenytoin plasma levels are between 10 and 20 micrograms/mL

10. A nurse is caring for a patient on barbiturate therapy for status epilepticus at a health care facility. What ongoing assessment should the nurse perform in the patient? Select all that apply.

    a. Document vital signs of the patient every 4 hours

    b. Document each seizure with regard to the time of occurrence

    c. Measure blood pressure every hour

    d. Measure serum plasma levels of the anticonvulsant

    e. Document each seizure with regard to its duration

11. Simple seizures, motor seizures, and somatosensory seizures are classified as what type of seizure?

    a. Generalized seizures

    b. Tonic-clonic seizures

    c. Partial seizures

    d. Myoclonic seizures

12. Tonic-clonic seizures and myoclonic seizures are classified as what type of seizures?

    a. Generalized seizures

    b. Partial seizures

    c. Somatosensory seizures

    d. Motor seizures

13. Which type of seizure involves a loss of consciousness?

    a. Partial seizures

    b. Somatosensory seizures

    c. Generalized seizures

    d. Motor seizures

14. Which anticonvulsant elicits its effects by stabilizing the hyperexcitability postsynaptically in the motor cortex of the brain?

    a. Valproic acid (Depakote)

    b. Phenytoin (Dilantin)

    c. Ethosuximide (Zarontin)

    d. Zonisamide (Zonegran)

15. Which anticonvulsant elicits its effects by increasing levels of gamma-aminobutyric acid (GABA), which stabilizes cell membranes?

    a. Valproic acid (Depakote)

    b. Pregabalin (Lyrica)

    c. Primidone (Mysoline)

    d. Tiagabine (Gabitril)

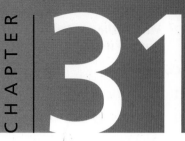

Skeletal Muscle Relaxants and Drugs Used to Treat Bone and Joint Disorders

Learning Objectives

- List the types of drugs used to treat musculoskeletal disorders
- Discuss the uses, general drug actions, adverse reactions, contraindications, precautions, and interactions of the drugs used to treat musculoskeletal disorders
- Discuss important preadministration and ongoing assessment activities the nurse should perform on the patient taking drugs used to treat musculoskeletal disorders
- List nursing diagnoses particular to a patient taking a drug for the treatment of musculoskeletal disorders
- Discuss ways to promote an optimal response to therapy, how to manage adverse reactions, and important points to keep in mind when educating the patient about drugs used to treat musculoskeletal disorders

SECTION I: ASSESSING YOUR UNDERSTANDING

Activity A MATCHING

1. *Match the trade names of drugs used to treat musculoskeletal disorders given in Column A with their uses given in Column B.*

Column A	Column B
1. Rheumatrex *c*	a. Management of symptoms of gout
2. Azulfidine *d*	b. Spasticity due to multiple sclerosis
3. Zyloprim *a*	c. Cancer chemotherapy
4. Lioresal *b*	d. Ulcerative colitis

2. *Match the musculoskeletal disorders in Column A with their description in Column B.*

Column A

1. Synovitis _B_
2. Arthritis _a_
3. Osteoarthritis _d_
4. Paget's disease _c_

Column B

a. Inflammation of a joint involving pain or stiffness

b. Inflammation of the synovial membrane of a joint

c. Chronic bone disorder characterized by abnormal bone remodeling

d. Noninflammatory degenerative joint disease marked by degeneration of the articular cartilage

Activity B FILL IN THE BLANKS

1. The _Bisphosphonates_ are drugs used to treat musculoskeletal disorders such as osteoporosis and Paget's disease.

2. _allopurinol_ reduces the production of uric acid, thereby decreasing serum uric acid levels and the deposit of urate crystals in joints.

3. Antirheumatic drugs have properties to produce _immunosuppression_ which in turn decrease the body's autoimmune response.

4. _Gout_ is a condition in which uric acid accumulates in increased amounts in the blood and is often deposited in the joints.

5. _Colchicine_ reduces the inflammation associated with the deposit of urate crystals in the joints.

Activity C SHORT ANSWERS

A nurse's role in managing a patient who is prescribed a drug for a musculoskeletal disorder involves assisting the patient with a preadministration assessment, and monitoring the patient with the presribed drug. Answer the following questions which involve the nurse's role in the management of patients who are on a drug therapy for a musculoskeletal disorder.

1. A patient with a musculoskeletal disorder is prescribed a drug. What preadministration assessments should the nurse conduct before the administration of a musculoskeletal drug?

Obtain any history of disorders, physical conditions, assess pain, vital signs, weight, perform lab tests and examine affected joints.

2. After the preadministration assessment, the patient is administered a drug for the musculoskeletal disorder. What ongoing assessment should the nurse perform when caring for a patient who is administered a musculoskeletal drug?

Pain relief, adverse reactions, if administered any more toxic drugs, observe any dependence of drugs and evaluate any musculoskeletal disorders seen.

Activity D DOSAGE CALCULATION

1. A physician prescribes 6 mg of the drug tizanidine daily to a patient. On-hand availability of tizanidine is 2-mg tablets. How many tablets should the nurse administer daily to the patient?

3 tabs

2. A physician prescribes 100 mg of orphenadrine daily to a patient. The orphenadrine therapy is to be continued for a period of 4 days. On-hand availability is 100-mg tablets. How many tablets should the nurse administer in total to the patient?

4 tabs

3. A patient has been prescribed 1.5 g of methocarbamol orally. The drug is available as 500-mg tablets. How many tablets should the nurse administer to the patient?

3 tabs

4. A patient recovering from multiple sclerosis has been prescribed 60 mg of cyclobenzaprine. This drug is to be administered orally. On-hand availability of the drug is 30-mg tablets. How many tablets should the nurse administer to the patient each time?

2 tabs

5. A patient recovering from painful musculoskeletal conditions is prescribed 700 mg of carisoprodol per day by a physician. The on-hand availability of the drug is 350-mg tablets. The drugs have to be administered for a period of 3 days. How many tablets should the nurse administer in total to the patient?

6 tabs

SECTION II: APPLYING YOUR KNOWLEDGE

Activity E CASE STUDY

Sophia Morgan is a Caucasian female, 33 years of age. She presents to the ED with complaints of a swollen ankle that is painful to the touch.

1. What assessment should the nurse perform prior to the physician examining the patient?

The appearance of the skins over the joints, any joint enlargement prior to physician examining the pt.

2. The ED physician diagnoses Mrs. Morgan with an acute gout attack. The physician orders colchicine 0.5 mg IV q6h until the attack is aborted. What should the nurse include in the ongoing assessment of Mrs. Morgan?

Inspect the joints every 2 to 3 hrs identify any response or nonresponse to therapy, nurse should questics any relief from pain or any dog adverse reactions.

SECTION III: PRACTICING FOR NCLEX

Activity F NCLEX-STYLE

Answer the following questions.

1. A patient with Paget's disease is administered bisphosphonate drugs. What adverse reactions should the nurse monitor in the patient?
   a. Dyspepsia
   b. Lethargy
   c. Sleepiness
   d. Constipation

2. A patient with Paget's disease is admitted to a local health care facility and is prescribed alendronate. In which of the following types of patients is the use of alendronate contraindicated?
   a. Hypertension patients
   b. Hypocalcemia patients
   c. Insomnia patients
   d. Diabetes patients

3. A patient with rheumatoid arthritis is administered disease-modifying antirheumatic drugs along with sulfa antibiotics. What possible interaction should the nurse monitor in the patient?
   a. Rash
   b. Hepatotoxicity
   c. Methotrexate toxicity
   d. Theophylline toxicity

4. A patient is administered methotrexate for the treatment of rheumatic arthritis. What should the nurse monitor in patients administered methotrexate?
   a. Hematology
   b. Liver function
   c. Renal function
   d. Pancreatic function
   e. Cardiovascular function

5. A patient with rheumatoid arthritis is administered DMARDs. What instructions should the nurse ask the patient to follow while administering DMARDs?
   a. Administer the drugs with food
   b. Drink 10 glasses of water a day
   c. Avoid hazardous tasks in case of drowsiness
   d. Notify PHCP in the case of diarrhea

6. A patient is administered bisphosphonates for a musculoskeletal disorder. What ongoing assessments should a nurse perform for patients receiving bisphosphonates for musculoskeletal disorders?
   a. Obtain the patient's history of disorders
   b. Closely monitor the patient for adverse reactions
   c. Appraise the patient's physical condition and limitations
   d. Assess for pain in upper and lower back or hip

7. A patient is administered hydroxychloro-quine for a musculoskeletal disorder. What nursing interventions are involved when a patient is administered hydroxychloroquine for a musculoskeletal disorder?

   a. Report adverse reactions, especially vision changes

   b. Be alert to reactions such as skin rash, fever, cough, or easy bruising

   c. Encourage liberal fluid intake and measure intake and output

   d. Ask the patient to compensate for missed dosages

   e. Be attentive to patient complaints such as tinnitus, or hearing loss

8. A patient is prescribed sulfinpyrazone for the treatment of rheumatoid arthritis. In which of the following types of patients is the use of sulfinpyrazone contraindicated?

   a. Patients with peptic ulcer disease

   b. Patients with renal disorders

   c. Patients with hepatic disorders

   d. Patients with cardiac disease

9. A patient with rheumatic arthritis is administered the uric acid inhibitor sulfinpyrazone along with oral anticoagulants. What interactions should the nurse monitor for in the patient?

   a. Increased risk of bleeding

   b. Increased risk of hypoglycemia

   c. Increased effect of verapamil

   d. Decreased effectiveness of probenecid

10. A patient with gout is admitted to a local health care facility. What should the nurse examine in a patient with gout?

    a. Appearance of skin over joints

    b. Evidence of hearing loss

    c. Pain in upper and lower back or hip

    d. Mobility of affected joint

11. Which of the following classes of medications are used in the treatment of osteoporosis?

    a. Bisphosphonates

    b. Disease-modifying antirheumatic drugs (DMARDs)

    c. Uric acid inhibitors

    d. Skeletal muscle relaxants

12. Which of the following is an example of a skeletal muscle relaxant?

    a. Allopurinol (Zyloprim)

    b. Alendronate (Fosamax)

    c. Baclofen (Lioresal)

    d. Hydroxychloroquine (Plaquenil)

13. Which of the following is an example of a bisphosphonate?

    a. Zoledronic acid (Zometa)

    b. Cyclobenzaprine (Flexeril)

    c. Allopurinol (Zyloprim)

    d. Etanercept (Enbrel)

14. Which of the following is an example of a bisphosphonate disease-modifying antirheumatic drug (DMARD)?

    a. Allopurinol (Zyloprim)

    b. Carisoprodol (Soma)

    c. Risedronate (Actonel)

    d. Hydroxychloroquine (Plaquenil)

15. Which of the following is the most common adverse reaction to carisoprodol (Soma) that the nurse should discuss with the patient?

    a. Dyspnea

    b. Drowsiness

    c. Hypertension

    d. Tachycardia

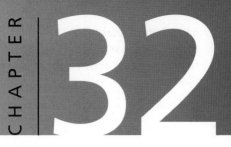
Antitussives, Mucolytics, and Expectorants

Learning Objectives

- Define the terms *antitussive, mucolytic,* and *expectorant*
- Discuss the uses, general drug actions, adverse reactions, contraindications, precautions and interactions of antitussive, mucolytic, and expectorant drugs
- Discuss important preadministration and ongoing assessment activities the nurse should perform on the patient receiving an antitussive, mucolytic, or expectorant drug
- List nursing diagnoses particular to a patient taking an antitussive, mucolytic, or expectorant drug
- Discuss ways to promote an optimal response to therapy, to manage common adverse reactions, and to educate the patient about the use of an antitussive, mucolytic, or expectorant drug

SECTION I: ASSESSING YOUR UNDERSTANDING

Activity A MATCHING

1. *Match the antitussive drugs in Column A with their uses in Column B.*

Column A

1. Codeine sulfate
2. Guaifenesin
3. Diphenhydramine HCl
4. Acetylcysteine

Column B

a. Reduction of pulmonary complication of cystic fibrosis

b. Relief of coughs associated with sinusitis

c. Relief of mild to moderate pain

d. Symptomatic relief of cough caused by bronchial irritation

2. *Match the drugs used to treat the discomfort associated with upper respiratory infection in Column A with their adverse reactions in Column B.*

Column A

1. Codeine sulfate

2. Diphenhydramine

3. Potassium iodide

4. Acetylcysteine

Column B

a. Stomatitis, nausea, vomiting, fever, drowsiness, bronchospasm, irritation of the trachea and bronchi

b. Sedation, nausea, vomiting, dizziness, constipation, CNS depression

c. Iodine sensitivity or iodinism (sore mouth, metallic taste, increased salivation, nausea, vomiting, epigastric pain, parotid swelling, and pain)

d. Sedation, headache, mild dizziness, constipation, nausea, GI upset, skin eruptions, postural hypotension

Activity B FILL IN THE BLANKS

1. _____ is a drug that aids in raising thick, tenacious mucus from the respiratory passages.

2. The _____ antitussives are contraindicated in premature infants or during labor when delivery of a premature infant is anticipated.

3. When _____ is administered with monoamine oxidase inhibitors, patients may experience jerking motions in the leg.

4. The mucolytic acetylcysteine is used to treat _____ due to mucus obstruction.

5. The patient should avoid drinking fluids for 30 minutes after the use of _____ to avoid losing effectiveness of the drug.

6. A mucolytic is a drug that loosens _____ secretions.

Activity C SHORT ANSWERS

A nurse's role in managing a patient receiving an antitussive drug involves monitoring and managing the patient's needs after drug administration. The nurse also educates the patient about use of the drug. Answer the following questions which involve the nurse's role in the management of such situations.

1. A patient with a cough has been prescribed an antitussive drug. What preadministration assessments should the nurse perform for the patient?

_____

_____

2. What should be nurse's role after the patient has been administered antitussives?

_____

_____

Activity D DOSAGE CALCULATION

1. A patient with a cough has been prescribed 120 mg of the codeine sulfate drug daily. The drug is available as 30-mg capsules. How many capsules should a nurse administer the patient daily?

_____

_____

2. A physician has prescribed 600 mg of tessalon every 24 hours. The available drug is in the form of 100-mg tablets. How many tablets should a nurse administer the patient each day?

_____

_____

3. A 15-year-old patient has been prescribed 60 mg of DexAlone for the treatment of a cough. A nurse is required to administer the drug to the patient every 12 hours. The drug is available in 30-mg gelcaps. How many capsules should the nurse administer the patient every 24 hours?

_____

_____

4. A patient has been prescribed 300 mg of organidin, to be taken every 4 hours. The drug is available in 200-mg tablets. How many tablets should a nurse administer the patient every 24 hours?

SECTION II: APPLYING YOUR KNOWLEDGE

Activity E CASE STUDY

Stanley Smith is an African American male, 70 years of age. He has multiple medical conditions including hypertension, type 2 diabetes, and dyslipidemia. His primary care provider is Dr. Jones. Mr. Smith calls Dr. Jones' office today to inquire what he can take for his cough. The triage nurse answers the phone call from Mr. Smith.

1. What information does the triage nurse need to elicit from Mr. Smith?

---

2. Mr. Smith tells the triage nurse he started taking Delsym 1 teaspoonful twice a day about 10 days ago for a dry, hacking cough. His cough is now productive; he has a temperature of 99.8°F, and is having some shortness of breath. What should the triage nurse advise Mr. Smith to do?

SECTION III: PRACTICING FOR NCLEX

Activity F NCLEX-STYLE

Answer the following questions.

1. A patient with a cough visits a health care facility and is prescribed an expectorant. What preadministration assessments should the nurse perform for this patient? Select all that apply.
   a. Ask the patient about throat infection
   b. Assess the respiratory status of the patient
   c. Document the lung sounds of the patient
   d. Examine the pulse rate every 30 minutes
   e. Document the consistency of sputum

2. A nurse at a health care center is assigned to prepare a teaching plan for a patient undergoing antitussive drug therapy. Which of the following instructions should the nurse include in the teaching plan? Select all that apply.
   a. Take the medicine 1 hour before meals
   b. Avoid irritants such as cigarette, dust, or fumes
   c. Avoid drinking fluids for 30 minutes after taking the drug
   d. Take the medicine with milk to enhance absorption
   e. Avoid chewing or breaking open the oral capsules

3. A patient with a cough visits a health care facility and is prescribed an antitussive. Which of the following reactions associated with the antitussive administration should the nurse monitor for in the patient?
   a. Diarrhea
   b. Sedation
   c. Somnolence
   d. Dehydration

4. A nurse is assigned to care for a patient who has been prescribed an antitussive. In which of the following conditions is the use of antitussives contraindicated?
   a. Asthma
   b. Liver dysfunction
   c. Cardiac problems
   d. Hypersensitivity

5. A nurse is caring for a patient who has been prescribed a medication containing potassium. The patient informs the nurse that he is taking a drug containing iodine products. Of whichpossible effect of the interaction of potassium-containing medication with iodine products should the nurse be aware?
   a. Hypokalemia
   b. Hypoglycemia
   c. Hypertension
   d. Hemorrhage

6. A nurse is caring for a patient with ineffective airway clearance at a health care facility. Which of the following is an appropriate nurse's role to promote effective airway clearance?
   a. Suggest avoiding consumption of milk products
   b. Encourage fluid intake of up to 2000 mL per day
   c. Monitor fluid intake of the patient every 8 hours
   d. Encourage taking mucolytics after each coughing episode

7. A nurse is caring for a patient who has been prescribed a eucalyptus product for the treatment of nasal congestion. What instruction should the nurse provide while educating the patient about the use of this herbal medicine?
   a. Take the medicine on an empty stomach
   b. Dilute the medicine before use
   c. Take the drug with warm milk
   d. Warm the medicine before use

8. A patient experiencing a cough takes a non-prescribed cough medicine. Under what conditions should the nurse instruct the patient to consult the PHCP?
   a. Cough lasts more than 10 days
   b. Cough is accompanied by dizziness
   c. Frequency of coughing is 20 minutes
   d. Cough is accompanied by vomiting

9. A nurse is caring for a patient with a severe cough at a health care facility. The physician has prescribed acetylcysteine for the patient. The drug is to be inserted into the tracheostomy. What is the nurse's role in this case?
   a. Ensure that the patient is not receiving any other drug therapy
   b. Ensure that suction equipment is at the patient's bedside
   c. Ensure that the patient gets continuous oxygen supply
   d. Ensure that the patient keeps drinking warm water

10. A nurse is caring for a patient undergoing dextromethorphan therapy. The patient also needs to be administered monoamine oxidase inhibitors for the treatment of depression. What risk associated with the interaction of the two drugs should the nurse observe in the patient?
    a. Hypotension
    b. Dyspepsia
    c. Bronchitis
    d. Opisthotonos

11. A client with cystic fibrosis may use which type of medication to reduce the viscosity of respiratory secretions?
    a. Mucolytic
    b. Centrally acting antitussive
    c. Expectorant
    d. Peripherally acting antitussive
    e. Antihistamine

12. A client is taking levothyroxine 150 mcg daily for hypothyroidism. Which of the following medications should be avoided in this client?
    a. Potassium iodide
    b. Dextromethorphan
    c. Codeine
    d. Benzonatate
    e. Guaifenesin

13. A nurse caring for a client in the hospital is being discharged today with a prescription for benzonatate (Tessalon Perles) 200 mg 1 capsule 3 times daily. What would you tell the patient about this prescription during discharge counseling? Select all that apply.

    a. Benzonatate can cause GI upset and sedation.
    b. Benzonatate capsules should be sucked on like a lozenge.
    c. The patient should drink plenty of fluids.
    d. Consumption of alcohol is permitted while taking benzonatate.
    e. Benzonatate can be taken more frequently than prescribed if needed.

14. What information should be obtained from the client by the nurse and documented prior to the administration of antitussive? Select all that apply.

    a. Type of cough
    b. Presence of sputum
    c. Color and amount of sputum
    d. Home remedies used to treat the cough
    e. Vital signs

15. Expectorants elicit their effect by which of the following mechanisms?

    a. Thinning respiratory secretions
    b. Breaking down thick mucus in the lower lungs
    c. Depressing the cough center in the brain
    d. Anesthetizing stretch receptors in the respiratory passages

CHAPTER 33

Antihistamines and Decongestants

Learning Objectives

- Discuss the uses, general drug action, general adverse reactions, contraindications, precautions, and interactions of the antihistamines and decongestants
- Discuss important preadministration and ongoing assessment activities the nurse should perform on the patient taking an antihistamine or a decongestant
- List nursing diagnoses particular to a patient taking an antihistamine or a decongestant
- Discuss ways to promote an optimal response to therapy, how to manage common patient needs (e.g., adverse reactions), and important points to keep in mind when educating a patient about the use of an antihistamine or a decongestant

SECTION I: ASSESSING YOUR UNDERSTANDING

Activity A MATCHING

1. *Match the medications that interact with antihistaminic drugs in Column A with the effect of the interaction in Column B.*

Column A	Column B
1. Rifampin	a. Causes additive central nervous system (CNS) depressant effect
2. Monoamine oxidase inhibitors	b. Increases the risk of cardiovascular effects
3. Beta-blockers	c. Reduces the absorption of certain antihistamines
4. Opioid analgesics	d. Decreases the concentration of the antihistamine in the blood
5. Aluminum-based antacids	e. Increases the anticholinergic and sedative effects of antihistamines

2. *Match the trade names of the medications in Column A with their generic names in Column B.*

Column A	Column B
1. Clarinex	**a.** Clemastine fumarate
2. Aller-Chlor	**b.** Diphenhydramine hydrochloride
3. Tavist	**c.** Promethazine hydrochloride
4. Benadryl	**d.** Desloratidine
5. Phenergan	**e.** Chlorpheniramine maleate

Activity B FILL IN THE BLANKS

1. In allergic or hypersensitivity reactions, histamine is released from the _____ cells.

2. A _____ is a drug that reduces the swelling of the nasal passages, which, in turn, opens clogged nasal passages and enhances drainage of the sinuses.

3. Nasal decongestants produce localized _____ of the small blood vessels of the nasal membranes.

4. _____ is produced from the amino acid histidine.

5. Antihistamines that penetrate the blood-brain barrier minimally exhibit fewer _____ effects.

Activity C SHORT ANSWERS

A nurse's role in managing patients who are being administered antihistamines and decongestants involves monitoring and implementing interventions that aid in their recovery. Answer the following questions which involve the nurse's role in the management of such situations.

1. A patient with mild angioneurotic edema is prescribed an antihistamine to relieve his symptoms. What teaching should the nurse provide to the patient and his family?

_____

_____

2. A patient with sinusitis is on a decongestant medication. He wants to know about the possible side effects of the medication. What should the nurse inform him regarding the possible side effects of this medication?

_____

_____

Activity D DOSAGE CALCULATION

1. A child, aged 10 years, is prescribed 30 mg of pseudoephedrine to relieve nasal congestion. The syrup contains 15 mg/5 mL (1 teaspoon) of pseudoephedrine. How many teaspoonsful of the syrup should the nurse administer?

_____

_____

2. A 30-year-old patient has been prescribed 12 mg of brompheniramine for a runny nose due to hay fever. Each tablet contains 4 mg of brompheniramine. How many such tablets per dose does the nurse need to give him?

_____

_____

3. A 17-year-old patient has been prescribed 4 mg of chlorpheniramine maleate every 6 hours. Chlorpheniramine maleate is available as 4-mg tablets. How many such tablets does the nurse need to give the patient in a single day?

_____

_____

4. An 8-year-old girl is prescribed 1.25 mg of clemastine fumarate twice daily for allergic rhinitis. The syrup contains 0.5 mg/5 mL of the medication. Each teaspoonful is 5 mL. How many teaspoonsful of the medication should the nurse give her as a single dose?

_____

_____

5. A patient has been prescribed 100 mg of hydroxyzine as a sedative. How many 25-mg tablets should the nurse give her?

_____

_____

6. A patient is prescribed 25 mg of promethazine hydrochloride to relieve the symptoms of nausea. Each tablet contains 12.5 mg of promethazine hydrochloride. How many such tablets does the nurse need to give the patient?

_____

_____

SECTION II: APPLYING YOUR KNOWLEDGE

Activity E CASE STUDY

Kimberly Jones is a Caucasian female, 47 years of age. Her current medical conditions include hypertension and dyslipidemiaHer current medications include metoprolol succinate (Toprol XL) 50 mg QD, hydrochlorathiazide 25 mg QAM, simvastatin (Zocor) 2 mg QD. Dr. Langdon is her primary care provider. Mrs. Jones calls Dr. Langdon's office today to inquire what she can take for her nasal congestion. The triage nurse takes her call and tells Mrs. Jones she will talk with Dr. Langdon and call her back. Mrs. Jones tells the triage nurse she has not taken anything to treat her nasal congestion. She checked her blood pressure at home today and it was 125/80 mm Hg and her pulse was 70 bpm. She reported no other symptoms.

1. Was Mrs. Jones' call warranted?

_____

_____

2. What information does the triage nurse need to elicit from Mrs. Jones?

_____

_____

SECTION III: PRACTICING FOR NCLEX

Activity F NCLEX-STYLE

Answer the following questions.

1. A patient has been prescribed an antihistamine for urticaria. He wants to know about the possible side effects of the drug. Which of the following are the possible side effects with this medication? Select all that apply.

   a. Thickening of bronchial secretions

   b. Disturbed coordination

   c. Increased frequency of micturition

   d. Anaphylactic shock or urticaria

   e. Excessive sweating and salivation

2. A nurse is required to care for a patient who is prescribed an antihistamine for the treatment of Parkinsonism. Antihistamines need to be used cautiously in certain conditions. In which of the following conditions should the nurse administer the drug with caution?

   a. Acute conjunctivitis

   b. Allergic rhinitis

   c. Angle-closure glaucoma

   d. Hypotension

3. A 70-year-old patient with acute sinusitis has been prescribed decongestant medication. At this age, he is at a greater risk of developing side effects due to overdosage. Which of the following symptoms of overdosage should the nurse monitor for when caring for the patient? Select all that apply.

   a. Hallucination

   b. Dyspnea

   c. Convulsion

   d. Depression

   e. Fatigue

4. A patient has been prescribed a nasal decongestant to relieve symptoms of nasal congestion. The nurse needs to educate the patient about how to administer the drug. Which of the following procedures should be followed?

a. Administer the nasal spray by reclining on the bed with the head hanging

b. Administer the nasal drop by sitting upright and sniffing hard

c. Administer the nasal spray by touching the tip to the nasal mucosa

d. Administer the inhaler by warming it in hand before use

5. Promethazine is prescribed to a patient who is also receiving an opioid analgesic. Which of the following factors should the nurse assess in the patient before administering promethazine?

a. Bone density

b. Urine output

c. Blood pressure

d. Skin turgidity

6. A patient has been prescribed an antihistamine drug to be given parenterally. Which of the following parenteral routes of drug administration should the nurse prefer?

a. Intravenous

b. Intramuscular

c. Subcutaneous

d. Intradermal

7. Given below, in a random order, are the steps of inflammatory response to injury. Arrange the inflammatory response in the order they most likely occur in most situations.

a. Dilatation of arterioles

b. Increased capillary permeability

c. Release of histamine

d. Escape fluid from blood vessels

e. Localized redness

f. Localized swelling

8. A 40-year-old patient is prescribed an antihistamine medication. The nurse needs to educate the patient about certain other drugs that he takes concomitantly that can interact with the antihistamine to either enhance or reduce its effects. Which of the following drugs reduces the effect of antihistamines?

a. Beta-blocking agents

b. Opioid analgesics

c. Magnesium-based antacids

d. Monoamine oxidase inhibitors

9. A patient is prescribed a decongestant for allergic rhinitis. In which of the following conditions should the nurse administer the drug cautiously? Select all that apply.

a. Hypertension

b. Hyperthyroidism

c. Conjunctivitis

d. Nephropathy

e. Glaucoma

10. Which of the following instructions should the nurse provide a patient who is prescribed an antihistamine for hay fever? Select all that apply.

a. Take an antacid 1 hour before the drug

b. Avoid the use of alcohol and other sedatives

c. Crush the sustained release tablet before use

d. Take the drug with food to avoid gastric upset

e. Take frequent sips of water or suck on hard candy

11. Which of the following elicits its antihistamine effects by nonselectively binding to central and peripheral H_1 receptors?

a. Cetirizine

b. Fexofenadine

c. Diphenhydramine

d. Loratadine

12. Which of the following elicits its antihistamine effects by selectively binding to peripheral H_1 receptors?

a. Diphendydramine

b. Desloratadine

c. Brompheniramine

d. Clemastine

13. Why are antihistamines administered intramuscularly instead of subcutaneously?

   a. Antihistamines irritate subcutaneous tissue

   b. Antihistamines are not absorbed from subcutaneous tissue

   c. Antihistamines result in more side effects when administered subcutaneously

   d. Antihistamines cause hypertension when administered subcutaneously

14. Antihistamines can be used to treat which of the following conditions? Select all that apply.

   a. Allergic rhinitis

   b. Treatment of Parkinsonism

   c. Relief of nausea

   d. Relief of dry mouth

   e. Reversal of sedation

15. Decongestants elicit their effect by which of the following mechanisms?

   a. Selectively binding to peripheral H_1 receptors

   b. Nonselectively binding to central and peripheral H_1 receptors

   c. Anesthetizing stretch receptors in the respiratory passages

   d. Vasoconstriction of small blood vessels of the nasal membranes

Bronchodilators and Antiasthma Drugs

Learning Objectives

- Describe the uses, general drug action, general adverse reactions, contraindications, precautions, and interactions of the bronchodilators and antiasthma drugs
- Discuss important preadministration and ongoing assessment activities the nurse should perform on the patient taking bronchodilators or antiasthma drugs
- List nursing diagnoses particular to a patient taking a bronchodilator or an antiasthma drug
- Discuss ways to promote an optimal response to therapy, how to manage common adverse reactions, and important points to keep in mind when educating a patient about the use of a bronchodilator or an antiasthma drug

SECTION I: ASSESSING YOUR UNDERSTANDING

Activity A MATCHING

1. *Match the bronchodilator and antiasthmatic drugs given in Column A with their class given in Column B.*

Column A	Column B
1. Albuterol	a. Leukotriene receptor antagonist
2. Theophylline	b. Leukotriene formation inhibitor
3. Flunisolide	c. Xanthine derivative
4. Zafirlukast	d. Sympathomimetic bronchodilator
5. Zileuton	e. Corticosteroid

2. *Match the interactant drugs in Column A with their interactions with sympathomimetic agents in Column B.*

Column A	Column B
1. Adrenergic drugs	**a.** Increased pressor response
2. Monoamine oxidase inhibitor	**b.** Possible additive effects
3. Methyldopa	**c.** Possible severe hypotension
4. Uterine stimulants	**d.** Increased risk of cardiotoxicity
5. Theophylline	**e.** Risk of severe headache and hypertensive crisis

Activity B FILL IN THE BLANKS

1. Methylxanthines stimulate the central nervous system to promote _____ of the bronchi.

2. In asthma, the airways become narrow and extra _____ clogs the smaller airways.

3. The three most common symptoms of asthma are cough, dyspnea, and _____.

4. Cromolyn sodium acts by preventing _____ ions from entering mast cells, thus preventing the release of inflammatory mediators.

5. Terbutaline is a bronchodilator with β_2 receptor _____ activity.

Activity C SHORT ANSWERS

A nurse's role in managing patients who are being administered bronchodilators and antiasthma drugs involves monitoring and implementing interventions that aid in recovery. Answer the following questions which involve the nurse's role in the management of such situations.

1. A patient has been prescribed theophylline for the symptomatic relief of bronchial asthma.

_____

_____

a. What possible adverse effects of the drug should the nurse inform the patient about?

b. What points should the nurse include in the patient teaching plan in such a case?

2. A patient with chronic bronchitis has been prescribed a bronchodilator agent. What preadministration assessments should the nurse implement when caring for the patient?

_____

_____

Activity D DOSAGE CALCULATION

1. A patient has been advised to take 4 mg of albuterol 3 times a day for the prevention of bronchospasm. The oral syrup available contains 2 mg/5 mL of albuterol. How many teaspoonfuls of the syrup should the nurse administer in a single dose?

_____

_____

2. Child weighing 25 kg has been prescribed 0.5 mg/kg of ephedrine sulfate as a subcutaneous injection for bronchial asthma. The strength of the injection is 50 mg/mL. What volume of the injection should the nurse administer?

_____

_____

3. A 35-year-old patient has bronchospasm during anesthesia. He is prescribed 0.01 mg of isoproterenol as a bolus IV injection. The 1 mL ampoule contains 0.2 mg of the drug. The nurse dilutes the contents of the ampoule with 10 mL of Sodium Chloride Injection USP. How much of the diluted solution should be injected?

_____

_____

4. A 13-year-old patient is prescribed 0.25 mg of Terbutaline SC for the reversal of bronchospasm. Each ampoule contains 1 mg of the drug in 1 mL of solution. What volume of the solution should the nurse administer?

_____

_____

5. A patient weighing 30 kg is prescribed dyphylline 10 mg/kg for the symptomatic relief of bronchial asthma. How much of the drug should the nurse administer in a single dose?

_____

_____

6. A patient is prescribed 0.5 mg of epinephrine solution SC for respiratory distress. The solution contains 5 mg/mL of epinephrine. How much of the solution should the nurse administer?

_____

_____

SECTION II: APPLYING YOUR KNOWLEDGE

Activity E CASE STUDY

Joshua Jackson is a Caucasian male, 27 years of age. He was diagnosed with asthma at 8 years of age. He presents to the physician's office complaining of increased shortness of breath and coughing, especially at night, despite using his albuterol (Proventil) inhaler 1 or 2 inhalations every 4 to 6 hours as needed. The physician classifies Mr. Jackson's asthma as step 3 persistent.

1. What medications are recommended to treat Mr. Jackson's asthma?

_____

_____

2. What environmental controls can Mr. Jackson use to help control his asthma?

_____

_____

SECTION III: PRACTICING FOR NCLEX

Activity F NCLEX-STYLE

Answer the following questions.

1. A pregnant client is admitted to a health care facility with acute respiratory distress. Which of the following drugs should the nurse consider as relatively safe for such a patient?

   a. Albuterol
   b. Epinephrine
   c. Terbutaline
   d. Salmeterol

2. A patient is prescribed aminophylline for the symptomatic relief of bronchial asthma. The nurse is required to inform the patient about other drugs that may interact with aminophylline. Which of the following drugs increases the effects of aminophylline?
   a. Ketoconazole
   b. Rifampin
   c. Loop diuretics
   d. Beta-blockers

3. A patient is prescribed aminophylline for emphysema. Which of the following factors should the nurse assess to check for the occurrence of any adverse effects?

a. Electrocardiographic changes

b. Fluid intake and output

c. Consistency of the stool

d. Changes in blood hemoglobin

4. A patient is admitted to a health care facility with complaints of cough, difficulty breathing, and a wheezing sound during respiration. The patient is diagnosed as having asthma. Which of the following additional symptoms will the nurse observe in the patient?

a. Decreased blood pressure

b. Increased sweating

c. Decreased pulse rate

d. Increased urination

5. A patient is prescribed the antiasthmatic drug zafirlukast. The patient's medical history indicates that the patient is on aspirin for the pain relief of arthritis. Which of the following possible drug interactions should the nurse monitor for?

a. Increased thrombolytic effect of aspirin

b. Increased plasma levels of zafirlukast

c. Decreased absorption of zafirlukast

d. Decreased plasma levels of aspirin

6. Given below, in random order, are the steps involved in the progress of chronic inflammation seen in asthma. Arrange the steps in the correct order.

a. Decreased airflow to the lungs

b. Bronchospasm and inflammation

c. Release of histamine from the mast cells

d. Increased mucus production and edema of the airway

e. Narrowing and clogging of the airways

7. A patient has been prescribed a multi-drug regimen for the treatment of asthma. Which of the following drugs may be given as adjuncts to bronchodilator therapy in such a case? Select all that apply.

a. Corticosteroids

b. Leukotriene formation inhibitors

c. Uricosuric agents

d. Mast cell stabilizers

e. Leukotriene receptor antagonists

8. A patient with asthma has been prescribed a corticosteroid agent by inhalation for the reduction of inflammation in the airways. Which of the following drugs are corticosteroid agents? Select all that apply.

a. Cromolyn

b. Flunisolide

c. Beclomethasone

d. Ipratropium

e. Triamcinolone

9. A patient complains of nausea after receiving antiasthmatic medication. Which of the following instructions should the nurse provide to alleviate the patient's condition? Select all that apply.

a. Keep head end of bed elevated

b. Eat frequent small meals

c. Suck on sugarless candy

d. Limit fluids with meals

e. Rinse mouth properly after food

10. A patient with asthma has been prescribed the use of montelukast orally. When should the nurse instruct the patient to take the drug?

a. Once a day

b. Twice a day

c. Three times a day

d. Four times a day

11. Which of the following is an example of a short-acting beta 2 agonist (SABA)?

a. Formoterol

b. Salmeterol

c. Albuterol

d. Arformoterol

12. Which of the following may increase the risk of asthma-related death?

a. Long-acting β_2 agonists

b. Inhaled corticosteroids

c. Short-acting β agonists

d. Mast cell stabilizers

13. Asthma exacerbations are usually preceded by an increase in which of the following symptoms? Select all that apply.

a. Cough

b. Chest tightness

c. Nasal congestion

d. Bradypnea

e. Dyspnea

14. A client was using a nicotine patch to stop smoking when he was started on theophylline for emphysema. He has successfully stop smoking and has stopped using his nicotine patch. Which of following would be warranted?

a. Theophylline dose should be decreased

b. Theophylline should be discontinued

c. Theophylline dose should be increased

d. Theophylline dose should remain the same

15. Xanthine derivatives elicit their effect by which of the following mechanisms?

a. Stimulation of beta-adrenergic receptors

b. Stimulation of the central nervous system

c. Reduction of airway hyper-responsiveness

d. Stabilization of mast cell membranes

Antihyperlipidemic Drugs

- Define cholesterol, HDL, LDL, and triglyceride levels and how they contribute to the development of heart disease
- Define therapeutic life changes and how they affect cholesterol levels
- Discuss the uses, general drug actions, general adverse reactions, contraindications, precautions, and interactions of antihyperlipidemic drugs
- Discuss important preadministration and ongoing assessment activities the nurse should perform on the patient taking an antihyperlipidemic drug
- List nursing diagnoses particular to a patient taking an antihyperlipidemic drug
- Discuss ways to promote an optimal response to therapy, how to manage common adverse reactions, and important points to keep in mind when educating patients about the use of an antihyperlipidemic drug

SECTION I: ASSESSING YOUR UNDERSTANDING

Activity A MATCHING

1. *Match the antihyperlipidemic drugs in Column A with their adverse reactions in Column B.*

Column A	Column B
1. Rosuvastatin	a. Coughing
2. Ezetimibe	b. Tingling
3. Niacin	c. Vertigo
4. Gemfibrozil	d. Pharyngitis

2. *Match the antihyperlipidemic drugs in Column A with their uses in Column B.*

Column A	Column B
1. Cholestyramine	a. Reduction of elevated serum triglycerides levels
2. Atorvastatin	b. Secondary prevention of cardiovascular events
3. Fluvastatin	c. Relief from partial biliary obstruction
4. Lovastatin	d. Slowed progression of coronary artery disease

Activity B FILL IN THE BLANKS

1. _____ is an increase in the lipids, which are a group of fats or fatlike substances in the blood.

2. Atherosclerosis is a disorder in which _____ deposits accumulate on the lining of the blood vessels.

3. High-density lipoproteins take cholesterol from the peripheral cells and transport it to the _____.

4. A substance that accelerates a chemical reaction without itself undergoing a change is called a _____.

5. _____ is a condition in which muscle damage results in the release of muscle cell contents into the bloodstream.

Activity C SHORT ANSWERS

A nurse's role in managing a patient who has been prescribed an antihyperlipidemic drug involves performing preadministration and ongoing assessments during the course of the drug therapy. The nurse also monitors the patients for any occurrence of adverse reactions. Answer the following questions which involve the nurse's role in the management of patients on antihyperlipidemic drug therapy.

1. A nurse is caring for a patient with hyperlipidemia. What preadministration assessments should the nurse perform before the administration of a prescribed antihyperlipidemic drug?

   _____

   _____

2. What is the nurse's role after an antihyperlipidemic drug is administered to a patient?

   _____

   _____

Activity D DOSAGE CALCULATION

1. A patient with partial biliary obstruction has been prescribed 16 g of cholestyramine to be taken 4 times a day in equal doses. The drug is available in 4-g packets. How many packets would be required for 1 day?

   _____

   _____

2. A patient with hyperlipidemia has been prescribed 5 g of colestipol to be taken every day. Colestipol is available as 1-g tablets. How many tablets should be administered to the patient in a day?

   _____

   _____

3. A patient with hyperlipidemia has been prescribed 80 g of atorvastatin per day. The drug is available in 40-mg tablets. How many tablets should the nurse administer to the patient every day?

   _____

   _____

4. A patient with mixed dyslipidemia has been prescribed 60 mg of fluvastatin to be consumed per day. The drug is available as 20-mg capsules. How many capsules should the nurse administer to the patient in a day?

   _____

   _____

5. An adolescent patient with hypercholesterolemia has been prescribed 40 mg of lovastatin per day. The drug is available in the form of 10-mg tablets. How many tablets should the nurse administer to the patient daily?

   _____

   _____

SECTION II: APPLYING YOUR KNOWLEDGE

Activity E **CASE STUDY**

Susan Smith is a 40-year old African American female admitted to the hospital after having a myocardial infarction. She has a history significant for diabetes, hypertension, and smoking (1 ppd). She is being discharged today. The only new prescription she will be leaving with is pravastatin (Pravachol) 40 mg, with directions to take 1 tablet daily at bedtime. The physician has asked the nurse to go over discharge instructions with Mrs. Smith. During the discharge counseling Mrs. Smith inquires about her new medication.

1. What class of antihyperlipidemic medication is pravastatin and what should Mrs. Smith be told about the medication?

   _____

   _____

2. What lifestyle modification should Mrs. Smith be encouraged to follow?

   _____

   _____

SECTION III: PRACTICING FOR NCLEX

Activity F **NCLEX-STYLE**

Answer the following questions.

1. A nurse is caring for a patient undergoing ezetimibe drug therapy at a health care facility. What instruction should the nurse provide to the patient if the drug is to be taken with cholestyramine, a bile acid sequestrant?
   a. Take the drug 2 hours before a bile acid sequestrant
   b. Ensure a time gap of 1 hour between the intake of these two drugs
   c. Take both drugs 30 minutes before meals
   d. Take the bile acid sequestrant with warm water

2. The nurse is required to initiate an atorvastatin drug therapy for a patient. For which of the following conditions of the patient is atorvastatin contraindicated?
   a. Visual disturbances
   b. Biliary obstruction
   c. Serious liver disorders
   d. Renal dysfunction

3. A nurse is caring for a patient with primary hypercholesterolemia who is undergoing ezetimibe drug therapy. What adverse reaction to the drug should the nurse monitor for in the patient?
   a. Vertigo
   b. Headache
   c. Cholelithiasis
   d. Arthralgia

4. A patient is undergoing gemfibrozil drug therapy for high serum triglyceride levels. The patient is also receiving an anticoagulant as a blood thinner. What effect of the interaction of these two drugs should the nurse observe for in the patient?
   a. Increased hypoglycemic effects
   b. Increased risk of severe myopathy
   c. Enhanced effect of the anticoagulant
   d. Increased risk of hypertension

5. A nurse at a health care facility is caring for a patient who has been prescribed HMG-CoA reductase inhibitors. For which of the following patient conditions should the nurse use the prescribed drug cautiously? Select all that apply.
   a. Peptic ulcer
   b. Acute infection
   c. Visual disturbances
   d. Unstable angina
   e. Endocrine disorders

6. A nurse is caring for a patient receiving garlic therapy for lowering serum cholesterol and triglyceride levels. The patient is also taking warfarin as an anticoagulant. What should the nurse monitor for in this patient?
   a. Bleeding
   b. Peptic ulcers
   c. Irritation
   d. Skin rashes

7. A nurse is caring for an elderly patient undergoing bile acid sequestrants therapy. What should the nurse monitor for in the patient? Select all that apply.

   a. Difficulty in passing stools

   b. Hard dry stools

   c. Complains of constipation

   d. Complains of mouth dryness

   e. Complains of urinary hesitancy

8. A nurse is caring for a patient receiving an antihyperlipidemic drug. The nurse observes a paradoxical elevation of blood lipid levels in the patient. What should be the nurse's intervention in such a situation?

   a. Notify the PHCP for a different antihyperlipidemic drug

   b. Collect blood samples for further examination

   c. Administer next dose of the drug with milk

   d. Record the fluid intake and output every hour

9. A patient informs the nurse that he has been taking flax powder for improving the blood lipid profile. Which toxic reaction associated with the consumption of flax should the nurse relay to the patient?

   a. Abdominal pain

   b. Dyspnea

   c. Cramps

   d. Dyspepsia

10. A nurse is caring for a patient who has been prescribed colestipol for the treatment of hyperlipidemia. This drug is known to cause constipation. What instructions should the nurse provide to the patient to help prevent constipation? Select all that apply.

    a. Exercise daily

    b. Consume foods high in dietary fiber

    c. Take the drug one hour after meals

    d. Increase fluid intake

    e. Take oral vitamin K supplements

11. Which of the following are examples of modifiable risk factors for hyperlipidemia? Select all that apply.

    a. Weight

    b. Diet

    c. Post-menopause

    d. Age older than 55 years (women)

    e. Age older than 45 years (men)

12. Increased levels of low-density lipoprotein (LDL) combined with certain risk factors can lead to the development of which medical condition?

    a. Diabetes

    b. Glaucoma

    c. Hypertension

    d. Heart disease

13. Which of the following herbal products has shown in studies to lower serum cholesterol and triglycerides?

    a. Ginseng

    b. Hawthorne berry

    c. Garlic

    d. Feverfew

    e. Black cohosh

14. Which of the following classes of medications are used to treat hyperlipidemia? Select all that apply.

    a. HMG-CoA reductase inhibitors

    b. Fibric acid derivatives

    c. Bile acid resins

    d. Calcium channel blockers

    e. Angiotensin II receptor blockers

15. Bile acid resins can decrease serum levels of several medications, primarily via which mechanism?

    a. Inhibition of hepatic enzymes

    b. Decreased gastrointestinal absorption

    c. Induction of hepatic enzymes

    d. Increased renal excretion

Antihypertensive Drugs

Learning Objectives

- Discuss the various types of hypertension and risk factors involved
- Identify normal and abnormal blood pressure levels for adults
- List the various types of drugs used to treat hypertension
- Discuss the general drug actions, uses, adverse reactions, contraindications, precautions, and interactions of the antihypertensive drugs
- Discuss important preadministration and ongoing assessment activities the nurse should perform for the patient taking an antihypertensive drug
- Explain why blood pressure determinations are important during therapy with an antihypertensive drug
- List nursing diagnoses particular to a patient taking an antihypertensive drug
- Discuss ways to promote an optimal response to therapy, how to manage adverse reactions, and important points to keep in mind when educating patients about the use of an antihypertensive drug

SECTION I: ASSESSING YOUR UNDERSTANDING

Activity A MATCHING

1. *Match the terms associated with hypertension given in Column A with their correct description given in Column B.*

Column A

1. Hypertension
2. Essential hypertension
3. Hypertensive emergency
4. Secondary hypertension
5. Prehypertension

Column B

a. Blood pressure rise with no known, discernable cause. It has been associated with certain risk factors such as diet and lifestyle.

b. Rise in blood pressure in which the cause is discernable.

c. Blood pressure that remains elevated over a period of time.

d. Rise in blood pressure wherein the systolic pressure is between 120 and 139 mm Hg or the diastolic pressure is between 80 and 89 mm Hg.

e. Rise in blood pressure to extremely high levels, which can lead to damage of target organs such as kidney, eye, and heart, if not lowered.

2. *Match the antihypertensive drugs in Column A with their mode of action in Column B.*

Column A

1. Propranolol
2. Prazosin
3. Amlodipine
4. Captopril
5. Losartan

Column B

a. An angiotensin-converting enzyme inhibitor (ACEI)

b. A beta-adrenergic blocking drug

c. An angiotensin II receptor antagonist

d. An alpha-adrenergic blocking drug

e. A calcium channel blocker

Activity B FILL IN THE BLANKS

1. Angiotensin I is converted to angiotensin II, which is a powerful _____.

2. Furosemide and hydrochlorothiazide are examples of _____ agents used in the treatment of hypertension.

3. Diazoxide and nitroprusside are drugs used in the management of _____ emergencies.

4. Aldosterone promotes the retention of _____ and water, which contributes to the rise in blood pressure.

5. Electrolyte imbalance such as _____, which is a low blood sodium level, occurs with diuretic usage.

Activity C SHORT ANSWERS

A nurse's role in managing patients who are being administered antihypertensive drugs involves monitoring and implementing interventions that aid in the recovery of the patients. Answer the following questions, which involve the nurse's role in the management of such situations.

1. A patient has been prescribed antihypertensive therapy with captopril for hypertension. During the course of the therapy, what assessments should the nurse carry out?

_____

_____

2. A patient is prescribed amlodipine for hypertension. What points should the nurse include in the patient teaching plan?

_____

_____

Activity D DOSAGE CALCULATION

1. A patient is advised to take 200 mg of captopril daily, in two divided doses, for hypertension. It is available as 25-mg tablets. How many tablets should the patient take in a day?

_____

_____

2. A patient is prescribed 40 mg of hydralazine IV to be given for hypertensive emergency management. Each ampule contains 20 mg of hydralazine. How many ampules should the nurse break to give the required dosage?

_____

_____

3. A patient is prescribed 100 mg of losartan daily for hypertension. The tablets are available in 50-mg strength. How many tablets should the patient take daily?

_____

_____

4. A nurse should give 150 mg of atenolol to a patient with hypertension. The tablets are available in 50-mg strength. How many tablets should the nurse administer?

_____

_____

5. A patient requires 1.2 mg of clonidine for hypertension management. The strength available is 0.3 mg per tablet. How many tablets should the nurse administer daily?

_____

_____

6. A doctor prescribes 2 mg of doxazosin daily for hypertension. The drug is available in 4-mg tablets. What fraction of the tablet should the patient consume?

_____

_____

SECTION II: APPLYING YOUR KNOWLEDGE

Activity E CASE STUDY

James Dunn is a 40-year-old African American male who presents to the physician's office complaining of headache. His vital signs during triage are as follows: BP 165/90 mm Hg, HR 80 bpm, temperature 98.5°F, WT 125 kg (275 lb) and HT 5 ft 11 in. He currently has no other diagnosed medical conditions. The physician gives Mr. Dunn a prescription for lisinopril/hctz (Prinzide) 10/12.5 mg, 1 tablet by mouth daily in the morning.

1. In which stage of hypertension would you place Mr. Dunn?

   _____

   _____

2. What lifestyle modification should Mr. Dunn be encouraged to follow?

   _____

   _____

SECTION III: PRACTICING FOR NCLEX

Activity F NCLEX-STYLE

Answer the following questions.

1. When assessing a 40-year-old patient, the nurse observes an increase in the patient's blood pressure. Which of the following changes in blood pressure is indicative of prehypertension?
   a. Systolic pressure between 120 and 139 mm Hg
   b. Systolic pressure between 100 and 119 mm Hg
   c. Systolic pressure between 80 and 99 mm Hg
   d. Systolic pressure between 60 and 79 mm Hg

2. A patient is diagnosed with renal impairment and hypertension. Which of the following drugs is contraindicated in renal impairment?
   a. Doxazosin
   b. Captopril
   c. Hydralazine
   d. Minoxidil

3. A nurse is monitoring a patient admitted to the emergency department with hypertensive emergency. Which of the following drugs should be administered in such situations?
   a. Amlodipine
   b. Acebutolol
   c. Diltiazem
   d. Nitroprusside

4. A patient with diabetes mellitus and hypertension is on insulin and enalapril for hypertension. Which of the following risks would occur with the simultaneous administration of both drugs?
   a. Increased risk of hypersensitivity reaction
   b. Increased risk of electrolyte imbalance
   c. Increased risk of hypoglycemia
   d. Increased risk of hypotensive effect

5. A patient has developed a headache following the use of prazosin for hypertension. Which of the following instructions should the nurse provide the patient receiving prazosin? Select all that apply.
   a. Lie down and elevate legs above head level
   b. Withhold consumption of prazosin
   c. Apply a cool cloth over the forehead
   d. Engage in progressive body relaxation
   e. Take an analgesic drug for the pain

6. A nurse is monitoring a patient on minoxidil for hypertension. Which of the following changes should the nurse report to the practitioner in patients on minoxidil? Select all that apply.
   a. Swelling of the face
   b. Pulse rate more than 10 beats per minute
   c. Rapid weight gain of 1 pound
   d. Difficulty breathing
   e. Angina and severe indigestion

7. A nurse is caring for a patient receiving captopril for hypertension. Which of the following precautions should the nurse take when administering captopril?

   a. Administer captopril 1 hour before or 2 hours after food

   b. Rub the patient's back before administering captopril

   c. Ensure that the patient exercises before administering captopril

   d. Take captopril along with antacids

8. A patient receiving terazosin for orthostatic hypertension complains of dizziness. Which of the following instructions should the nurse give the patient? Select all that apply.

   a. Rise slowly from a sitting or lying position

   b. Increase fluid intake

   c. Apply a cool cloth over the forehead

   d. Rest on the bed for 1 or 2 minutes before rising

   e. Stand still for a few minutes after rising

9. A nurse is required to educate patients on the consequences of hypertension. Which of the following will develop as a consequence of hypertension? Select all that apply.

   a. Adrenal tumor

   b. Blindness

   c. Stroke

   d. Heart diseases

   e. Obesity

10. A nurse is educating a patient with hypertension about the adverse effects associated with hawthorn use. Which of the following should the nurse include as the adverse effects of hawthorn? Select all that apply.

    a. Hypotension

    b. Arrhythmia

    c. Pruritus

    d. Neutropenia

    e. Sedation

11. A nurse checks a client's blood pressure and finds it to be 130/82 mm Hg. This client should be classified as having which stage of hypertension?

    a. Prehypertension

    b. Stage 1 hypertension

    c. Stage 2 hypertension

    d. Normotensive

    e. Hypotensive

12. Which of the following lowers blood pressure primarily via suppression of the rennin-angiotensin-aldosterone system?

    a. Verapamil (Calan)

    b. Diltiazem (Cardizem)

    c. Lisinopril (Prinivil)

    d. Furosemide (Lasix)

13. Hypertension increases a person's risk for which of the following? Select all that apply.

    a. Heart failure

    b. Stroke

    c. Blindness

    d. Kidney disease

    e. Liver disease

14. Once a client develops primary hypertension, therapy should last for how long?

    a. Until blood pressure is 120/80 mm Hg

    b. 1 year

    c. For life

    d. 5 years

15. Bile acid resins can decrease serum levels of several medications, primarily via which mechanism?

    a. Decreased gastrointestinal absorption

    b. Inhibition of hepatic enzymes

    c. Induction of hepatic enzymes

    d. Increased renal excretion

CHAPTER 37

Antianginal Drugs

Learning Objectives

- List the two types of antianginal drugs
- Discuss the general actions, uses, adverse reactions, contraindications, precautions, and interactions of antianginal drugs
- Discuss important preadministration and ongoing assessment activities the nurse should perform on the patient taking an antianginal drug
- List nursing diagnoses particular to a patient taking an antianginal drug
- Discuss ways to promote an optimal response to therapy, how to manage common adverse reactions, and important points to keep in mind when educating patients about the use of antianginal drugs

SECTION I: ASSESSING YOUR UNDERSTANDING

Activity A MATCHING

1. *Match the antianginal and vasodilator drugs in Column A with their appropriate uses in Column B.*

Column A	Column B
1. Verapamil	a. Used to provide symptomatic relief in intermittent claudication
2. Amyl nitrite	b. Used in the treatment of cardiac arrhythmias
3. Cilostazol	c. Used to control blood pressure in perioperative hypertension associated with surgical procedures
4. Nitroglycerin, intravenous	d. Used for the relief of angina pectoris
5. Nifedipine	e. Used in the treatment of myocardial ischemia complicated with arrhythmias
6. Isoxsuprine hydrochloride	f. Used in the treatment of Prinzmetal's variant angina
7. Papaverine hydrochloride	g. Used in the treatment of peripheral vascular disease

2. *Match the terms associated with angina in Column A with their correct descriptions in Column B.*

Column A	Column B
1. Atherosclerosis	a. Condition in which there is reduced blood supply to an area
2. Angina	b. Characterized by the presence of fatty plaque deposits on the inner wall of the arteries
3. Ischemia	c. Characterized by chest pain occurring as a result of decreased oxygen supply to the heart muscles

Activity B FILL IN THE BLANKS

1. Antianginal drugs relieve chest pain by dilating _____ arteries and thereby increasing the blood supply to the cardiac musculature.

2. The contractions of cardiac and vascular smooth muscles depend on the movement of extracellular _____ ions through specific ion channels.

3. Nitrates act by relaxing the _____ muscle layer of the blood vessels.

4. Contact _____ may occur with the use of transdermal nitrate.

5. Intermittent _____ is a group of symptoms characterized by pain in the calf muscle brought on by walking and relieved by rest.

Activity C SHORT ANSWERS

A nurse's role in managing patients who are being administered antianginal drugs involves monitoring and implementing interventions that aid in the patient's recovery. Answer the following questions, which involve the nurse's role in the management of such situations.

1. A patient has been admitted to a health care facility with severe anginal attacks. What instructions should the nurse provide the patient on discharge?

_____

_____

2. A nurse is monitoring a patient admitted to the primary health care facility for treatment of Raynaud's disease. What assessments should the nurse undertake during the therapy with peripheral vasodilators?

_____

_____

Activity D DOSAGE CALCULATION

1. A patient is prescribed 20 mg of isoxsuprine hydrochloride daily for Raynaud's disease. The tablet is available in 10-mg strength. How many tablets should the nurse administer to give the correct dosage?

_____

_____

2. A nurse has to administer 40 mg of isosorbide dinitrate orally to a patient for the treatment of angina. The tablet is available in 20-mg strength. How many tablets should the nurse administer to the patient?

_____

_____

3. A patient is prescribed 10 mg of amlodipine for Prinzmetal's angina. The tablet is available in 5-mg strength. How many tablets should the patient take to relieve his angina?

_____

_____

4. A patient has been prescribed 12.5 mg of IV diltiazem for atrial fibrillation. Each ampoule contains 5 mL of solution in the strength of 5 mg/ mL. What amount of the solution should the nurse draw from the ampoule to give the correct dosage?

_____

_____

5. A patient requires 50 mg of nifedipine daily for the treatment of chronic stable angina. The drug is available in the strength of 25 mg per tablet. How many tablets should the patient consume daily?

_____

_____

6. The physician has prescribed 100 mg of cilostazol daily to a patient with peripheral vascular disease. The drug is available in 100-mg strength. How many tablets should the patient buy for a week?

_____

_____

SECTION II: APPLYING YOUR KNOWLEDGE

Activity E CASE STUDY

Harold Rollins is a 75-year-old Caucasian male who has a history significant for hypertension, hyperlipidemia, and diabetes. He is being discharged from the hospital today, and was given a prescription for nitroglycerin (Nitrostat) tablets.

1. Mr. Rollins asks the nurse, "What is this new tablet for?"

_____

_____

2. How should Mr. Rollins be instructed to use the nitroglycerin sublingual tablets?

_____

_____

SECTION III: PRACTICING FOR NCLEX

Activity F NCLEX-STYLE

Answer the following questions.

1. A patient has been admitted to a health care facility for the treatment of severe acute angina. A nurse is administering sublingual nitroglycerin to the patient every 5 minutes. After administrating how many doses of nitroglycerin should the nurse report to the practitioner if there has been no improvement?

   a. 3 doses in a 15-minute period

   b. 5 doses in a 30-minute period

   c. 7 doses in a 30-minute period

   d. 9 doses in a 60-minute period

2. A nurse is caring for a patient who has been prescribed cilostazol for intermittent claudication. Which of the following interventions should the nurse implement when administering cilostazol?

   a. Powder and mix cilostazol with food

   b. Administer cilostazol with grape juice

   c. Administer cilostazol in supine position

   d. Administer cilostazol 30 minutes before food

3. A nurse is required to care for a patient receiving L-arginine for peripheral vascular disease. Which of the following functions should the nurse identify as the mode of action of L-arginine?

   a. Promotes sodium retention

   b. Increases nitric oxide levels

   c. Blocks calcium ion channels

   d. Blocks alpha adrenergic receptors

4. A nurse is caring for a patient with peripheral vascular disease who has delivered a baby 2 hours before. The patient complains of severe cramping in her calf muscles. Which of the following drugs should not be given in the immediate postpartum period?

   a. Isosorbide dinitrate

   b. Nitroglycerin

   c. Isoxsuprine

   d. Nifedipine

5. A patient has been admitted for the management of peripheral vascular disease (PVD). Which of the following drugs can be given in PVD?

   a. Papaverine

   b. Nitroglycerin

   c. Isosorbide mononitrate

   d. Amyl nitrite

6. A nurse is educating a group of nursing students on the various effects of calcium channel-blockers on the heart. Which of the following are the effects of calcium channel-blockers on the heart? Select all that apply.

   a. Increase the heart rate

   b. Retard the conduction velocity

   c. Depress myocardial contractility

   d. Cause rapid atrial muscle contraction

   e. Dilate the coronary arteries

7. A patient is admitted to a health care center for angina management and is started on IV diltiazem. Which of the following adverse effects should the nurse monitor for in the patient? Select all that apply.

   a. Hypertension

   b. Tachycardia

   c. Arrhythmia

   d. Asthenia

   e. Flushing

8. A nurse is caring for a patient with Raynaud's disease who is receiving cilostazol. Which of the following indicates improvement following treatment with cilostazol? Select all that apply.

   a. Increase in the coldness of the affected limb

   b. Increase in painless walking distance

   c. Decreased pain and cramping in the legs

   d. Decreased amplitude of the peripheral pulse

   e. Decreased scaling of the affected area

9. A patient has been admitted for the treatment of arteriosclerosis obliterans and is started on isoxsuprine. Which of the following adverse effects should the nurse monitor for in patients on isoxsuprine? Select all that apply.

   a. Hypertension

   b. Sedation

   c. Flushing

   d. Bradycardia

   e. Headache

10. A patient is prescribed translingual nitrates for the management of angina. What instructions should the nurse give for a patient taking translingual nitrates? Arrange them in the correct sequence.

    a. If pain is not relieved after taking 3 metered doses in a 15-minute period, report to the health care provider immediately.

    b. Read the instructions for the use of translingual nitrates supplied with the product.

    c. At the occurrence of chest pain, spray 1 or 2 metered doses onto or under the tongue.

    d. Use the drug prophylactically 5–10 minutes before engaging in strenuous activities.

11. Which of the following statements are true in regards to nitrates? Select all that apply.

    a. Nitrates relax the smooth muscle layer of blood vessels

    b. Nitrates increase the lumen of the artery or arteriole

    c. Nitrates slow the conduction velocity of the cardiac impulse

    d. Nitrates depress myocardial contractility

    e. Nitrates increase the amount of blood flowing through the vessel

12. Nitrates are available in which of the following dosage forms? Select all that apply.

    a. Sublingual

    b. Transdermal

    c. Parenteral

    d. Rectal

    e. Via inhalation

13. Which of the following is true of calcium channel-blockers? Select all that apply.

    a. Calcium channel-blockers slow the conduction velocity of the cardiac impulse

    b. Calcium channel-blockers depress myocardial contractility

    c. Calcium channel-blockers increase the amount of blood flowing through the vessel

    d. Calcium channel-blockers relax the smooth muscle layer of blood vessels

    e. Calcium channel-blockers dilate coronary arteries and arterioles

14. Nitrates can result in which of the following adverse reactions? Select all that apply.

    a. Headache

    b. Flushing

    c. Diarrhea

    d. Hypotension

    e. Blurred vision

15. Nitrates should not be used in clients with which of the following?

    a. Closed-angle glaucoma

    b. Asthma

    c. Diabetes

    d. Hypertension

Anticoagulant and Thrombolytic Drugs

- Describe hemostasis and thrombosis
- Discuss the uses, general drug actions, adverse reactions, contraindications, precautions, and interactions of anticoagulant, antiplatelet, and thrombolytic drugs
- Discuss important preadministration and ongoing assessment activities the nurse should perform on the patient taking an anticoagulant, antiplatelet, or thrombolytic drug
- List nursing diagnoses particular to a patient taking an anticoagulant, antiplatelet, or thrombolytic drug
- Discuss ways to promote an optimal response to therapy, how to manage common adverse reactions, and important points to keep in mind when educating patients about the use of an anticoagulant, antiplatelet, or thrombolytic drug

SECTION I: ASSESSING YOUR UNDERSTANDING

Activity A MATCHING

1. *Match the drugs in Column A with their adverse reactions in Column B.*

Column A	Column B
1. Heparin	**a.** Dyspepsia
2. Cilostazol	**b.** Pallor
3. Ticlopedine	**c.** Heart alpitations
4. Treprostinil	**d.** Chills

2. *Match the antiplatelet drugs in Column A with their uses in Column B.*

Column A	Column B
1. Clopidogrel	**a.** Intermittent claudication
2. Ticlopidine	**b.** Recent myocardial infarction
3. Cilostazol	**c.** Pulmonary arterial hypertension
4. Treprostinil	**d.** Thrombotic stroke

Activity B FILL IN THE BLANKS

1. _____ is essential for the clotting of blood.

2. Venous _____ can develop as the result of venous stasis, injury to the vessel wall, or altered blood coagulation.

3. _____ thrombosis can occur because of atherosclerosis or arrhythmias.

4. Drugs that help to eliminate clots are known as _____.

5. Glycoprotein receptor blockers work to prevent _____ production.

6. The use of an adapter and tubing to stay in the vein for intermittent IV administration is called a _____ lock.

Activity C SHORT ANSWERS

A nurse's role in managing patients who are being administered anticoagulant and thrombolytic drugs involves monitoring the patients and implementing interventions that aid in their recovery. Answer the following questions, which involve the nurse's role in the management of such situations.

1. A nurse has been caring for a client with deep venous thrombosis (DVT). Post-treatment, the nurse has to evaluate the effectiveness of the treatment plan. What factors should the nurse consider to determine the success of the treatment plan?

   _____

   _____

2. A nurse is caring for a patient who has been prescribed enoxaparin sodium for the treatment of pulmonary emboli (PE). What instructions should the nurse provide to help the patient cooperate with the prescribed therapy?

   _____

   _____

Activity D DOSAGE CALCULATION

1. A patient undergoing treatment for venous thrombosis has been prescribed 250 mg of anifsindione per day orally. The drug is available in 50-mg compressed tablets. How may tablets should the nurse administer to the patient in a day?

   _____

2. A patient has been prescribed 7.5 mg of warfarin per day for the prophylaxis of venous thrombosis. On-hand availability of the drug is 2.5-mg tablets. How many tablets should the nurse administer to the patient every day?

   _____

3. A patient with intermittent claudication has been prescribed 100 mg of cilostazol to be administered orally twice a day. The drug is available in the form of 50-mg tablets. How many tablets should be administered to the patient in a day?

   _____

4. A patient has been prescribed a single loading dose containing 300 mg of clopidogrel per day for treatment of acute coronary syndrome. The drug is available in 75-mg tablets. How many tablets should the nurse administer to the patient in the course of 1 day?

   _____

5. A patient undergoing treatment for thrombotic stroke is prescribed ticlopidine drug therapy. The physician has instructed the nurse to administer 250 mg of ticlopidine twice a day to the patient. The drug is available in 250-mg tablets. How many tablets should the nurse get for the course of 3 days?

   _____

SECTION II: APPLYING YOUR KNOWLEDGE

Activity E CASE STUDY

Rita Simms is a 28-year-old Caucasian female being discharged from the hospital today after a recent DVT. She is being discharged with a prescription for warfarin (Coumadin) 5 mg with directions to take 1 tablet daily at 5 PM. The physician has asked the nurse to complete discharge counseling with Ms. Simms.

1. How often will Ms. Simms need her PT/INR drawn?

   _____

   _____

2. What are the signs of warfarin overdosage?

   _____

   _____

SECTION III: PRACTICING FOR NCLEX

Activity F NCLEX-STYLE

Answer the following questions.

1. Alteplase has been prescribed to a patient with acute ischemic stroke. Which of the following adverse reactions associated with the drug administration should the nurse monitor for in the patient? Select all that apply.
   a. Gingival bleeding
   b. Erythema
   c. Epistaxis
   d. Ecchymosis
   e. Anemia

2. A nurse is caring for a patient who has been prescribed abciximab for coronary angioplasty. The patient is also taking aspirin for pain relief. What effects of the interaction between these two drugs should the nurse observe for in the patient?
   a. Decreased effectiveness of aspirin
   b. Increased effectiveness of abciximab
   c. Increased risk of bleeding
   d. Decreased absorption of abciximab

3. A nurse is required to start anticoagulant drug therapy for a patient. In which of the following conditions of the patient is an anticoagulant contraindicated? Select all that apply.
   a. Diabetic retinopathy
   b. Tuberculosis
   c. GI bleeding
   d. Leukemia
   e. Hemorrhagic disease

4. A nurse is caring for a patient who is undergoing anifsindione drug therapy for the treatment of venous thrombosis. What assessment should the nurse perform during the course of the therapy?
   a. Draw blood for a complete blood count
   b. Determine the international normalized ratio
   c. Draw blood for a baseline PT/INR test
   d. Continually assess for any signs of bleeding

5. A nurse is caring for a patient taking antiplatelet drugs. What instruction should the nurse include in the teaching plan for this patient?
   a. Use a soft toothbrush
   b. Take foods high in vitamin K
   c. Take medication with food
   d. Take drug at a different time each day

6. A patient is undergoing warfarin drug therapy. After taking the drug, the patient develops signs of GI bleeding. Which of the following interventions should the nurse perform for this patient?
   a. Inspect urine for red-orange color
   b. Monitor vital signs every 4 hours
   c. Inspect for bright red to black stools
   d. Monitor patient's fluid intake and output

7. A nurse is caring for a patient who has been administered heparin after the administration of a thrombolytic drug to prevent another thrombus from forming. What should the nurse monitor for in the patient after the administration of heparin?
   a. Internal bleeding
   b. Difficulty in breathing
   c. Excessive perspiration
   d. Skin rash

8. A nurse is required to administer heparin to a patient. What should the nurse do to avoid the possibility of the development of local irritation, pain, or hematoma?

a. Avoid application of firm pressure after the injection

b. Avoid administration sites such as buttocks and lateral thighs

c. Use an area within 2 inches of the umbilicus for drug administration

d. Avoid intramuscular (IM) administration of the drug

9. A nurse is caring for a patient receiving parenteral anticoagulant drug therapy. The nurse notices overdosage of the drug. What intervention should the nurse perform if administration of this drug is necessary?

a. Measure the patient's body temperature every hour

b. Monitor the patient's pulse rate every 2 hours

c. Observe the patient for new evidence of bleeding

d. Administer the drug to the patient via the IV route

10. A patient is administered a thrombolytic drug. The drug is known to cause bleeding. Which of the following symptoms of internal bleeding should the nurse monitor for in the patient? Select all that apply.

a. Black tarry stools

b. Hematuria

c. Chest pain

d. Petechiae

e. Coffee-ground emesis

11. Which of the following is used to treat a warfarin (Coumadin) overdose?

a. Protamine

b. Urokinase

c. Phytonadione

d. Alteplase

12. Use of St. John's wort during warfarin therapy can result in which of the following?

a. Increased risk of bleeding

b. Increased risk of thrombus formation

c. Increase blood pressure

d. Increased platelet count

13. When should the nurse administer a 300-mg dose of clopidogrel (Plavix) to a patient, instead of the 75-mg dose?

a. As a maintenance dose

b. In treatment of myocardial infarction

c. In treatment of stroke

d. As a loading dose

14. Thrombolytic drugs are contraindicated in which of the following? Select all that apply.

a. Active bleeding

b. History of stroke

c. Active infection

d. History of aneurysm

e. Recent abdominal surgery

15. Enoxaparin (Lovenox) should be administered via which route?

a. Subcutaneous injection

b. Intramuscular injection

c. Intravenous infusion

d. Orally

CHAPTER 30

Cardiotonics and Miscellaneous Inotropic Drugs

- Discuss heart failure in relationship to left ventricular failure, right ventricular failure, neurohormonal activity, and treatment options
- Discuss the uses, general drug action, general adverse reactions, contraindications, precautions, and interactions of the cardiotonic and inotropic drugs
- Discuss the use of other drugs with positive inotropic action
- Discuss important preadministration and ongoing assessment activities the nurse should perform on the patient taking a cardiotonic or inotropic drug
- List nursing diagnoses particular to a patient taking a cardiotonic or inotropic drug
- Identify the symptoms of digitalis toxicity
- Discuss ways to promote an optimal response to therapy, how to manage common adverse reactions, and important points to keep in mind when administering a cardiotonic

SECTION I: ASSESSING YOUR UNDERSTANDING

Activity A MATCHING

1. *Match the drugs which interact with cardiotonics in Column A with the effect of their interaction with digitalis in Column B.*

Column A	Column B
1. Amiodarone	a. Decreases plasma digitalis levels
2. Antacids	b. Results in electrolyte imbalance
3. Thyroid hormones	c. Increases plasma digitalis levels
4. Loop diuretics	d. Decreases effectiveness of digoxin

2. *Match the terms associated with congestive heart failure in Column A with their descriptions in Column B.*

Column A

1. Ejection fraction
2. Nocturia
3. Congestive heart failure
4. Cardiotonics
5. Cardiac hypertrophy
6. Orthopnea

Column B

a. Inability of the heart to pump sufficient quantities of blood to meet tissue demands

b. Enlargement of cardiac musculature

c. Agents that bring about an increase in heart contraction

d. Amount of blood ejected by the ventricles per beat in relation to amount of blood available to eject

e. Difficulty in breathing when lying flat

f. A need to urinate frequently at night

Activity B FILL IN THE BLANKS

1. When cardiotonics are given by the _____ method, the site should be inspected for redness and infiltration.

2. _____ ventricular dysfunction results in pulmonary symptoms, which include dyspnea and moist cough.

3. Fetal toxicity and _____ death have been reported from the maternal overdosage of digoxin.

4. During digoxin therapy if severe _____ develops, atropine may be given.

5. Patients started on cardiotonic drug therapy are said to be _____.

Activity C SHORT ANSWERS

A nurse's role in managing patients who are being treated with digoxin involves careful monitoring and implementing interventions that aid in recovery. Answer the following questions, which involve the nurse's role in the management of such situations.

1. A patient is diagnosed with heart failure and requires digoxin therapy. What physical assessment should a nurse carry out in a patient before starting digoxin?

_____

_____

2. A patient had rapid digitalization for heart failure. He is required to continue taking digitalis for a prolonged period. What teaching plan should the nurse implement for patients taking digitalis?

_____

_____

Activity D DOSAGE CALCULATIONS

1. A doctor prescribes 0.25 mg of digoxin to a patient with heart failure. The available digoxin tablet is 0.125 mg. How many tablets should a nurse administer to the patient?

_____

_____

2. A doctor has prescribed 1.25 mg of digoxin as the loading dose for a patient with atrial fibrillation. Each ampoule contains 1 mL of digoxin in the strength of 0.25 mg/mL. How many ampoules of digoxin should the nurse administer?

_____

_____

3. A patient with heart failure has been prescribed 600 mg of digoxin immune fab for digoxin toxicity to be given IV. The patient's parents have brought 25 vials. Each vial contains 40 mg of the drug. How many of the vials need to be returned after the correct dose has been given?

_____

_____

4. A patient with severe heart failure has been prescribed 50 mg of milrinone lactate to be given IV. Each vial contains 100 mg of milrinone lactate/10 mL. What volume of the injection should the nurse administer?

_____

_____

5. A doctor has prescribed 40 mg of inamrinone lactate to be given as IV bolus for a patient with heart failure. Each vial contains 5 mg of inamrinone/mL. How many vials of inamrinone should the nurse administer?

_____

_____

6. A doctor has prescribed 0.75 mg of digoxin to be given IV for a patient with atrial flutter. Each ampoule contains 1 mL of digoxin in the strength of 0.25 mg/ampoule. How many ampoules of digoxin should a nurse administer?

_____

_____

SECTION II: APPLYING YOUR KNOWLEDGE

Activity E CASE STUDY

Mr. Jackson was hospitalized today for heart failure. The physician orders a loading dose of digoxin 0.75 mg to be given intravenously. The digoxin is available in a solution of 0.5 mg/mL.

1. How many milliliters should the nurse prepare?

_____

_____

2. What should the nurse do before administering the IV dose?

_____

_____

SECTION III: PRACTICING FOR NCLEX

Activity F NCLEX-STYLE

Answer the following questions.

1. A patient arrives at a community health care center complaining of dyspnea and a hacking cough. The nurse assessing the patient notes that there are distended jugular veins, edema of the extremities, and reduced ejection fraction. Which of the following conditions do these symptoms indicate?
   a. Heart failure
   b. Glomerulonephritis
   c. Pulmonary disease
   d. Hypothyroidism

2. A patient is diagnosed with heart failure and is started on digoxin. The patient informs the nurse that he is taking benzodiazepine for seizures. Which of the following interventions should the nurse implement?
   a. Increase the dosage of digoxin
   b. Monitor for signs of digoxin toxicity
   c. Increase the dosage of benzodiazepine
   d. Monitor for signs of reduced effectiveness of digoxin

3. A nurse is educating a group of nursing students on the uses of digitalis. For which of the following conditions may digitalis be used?
   a. Ventricular tachycardia
   b. Atrioventricular block
   c. Atrial fibrillation
   d. Ventricular failure

4. When caring for a patient on digoxin, the nurse observes that the patient's pulse rate is 56 bpm. The patient is also complaining of nausea and vomiting. Which of the following is the most appropriate intervention in this situation?
   a. Administer milrinone lactate
   b. Increase the rate of digoxin infusion
   c. Give a gastrointestinal suction
   d. Withhold the drug and notify the practitioner

5. A nurse is caring for a patient who requires rapid digitalization for his heart failure. What amount of the total dose should the nurse administer as the first dose?

a. Quarter of the total dose

b. Half of the total dose

c. Three-quarters of the total dose

d. The complete dose

6. A patient has been admitted for heart failure and is on digoxin. The nurse monitoring the patient notes that the serum digoxin level is 2.5 mg/mL. Which of the following signs should a nurse assess for in the case of digoxin toxicity? Select all that apply.

a. Anorexia

b. Headache

c. Weakness

d. Blurred vision

e. Vomiting

7. A patient is being digitalized for congestive heart failure. The practitioner assessing the patient orders an analysis of serum electrolytes to be done. Which of the following electrolyte changes indicates toxicity and needs to be reported? Select all that apply.

a. Hyponatremia

b. Hypokalemia

c. Hypomagnesemia

d. Hypocalcemia

e. Hypophosphatemia

8. A nurse is caring for a patient on digitalis. The patient complains of nausea and vomiting after 2 days of digitalis administration. Which of the following is the appropriate nursing intervention in this situation? Select all that apply.

a. Ensure that the patient takes double the drug dosage

b. Ensure the patient consumes small frequent meals

c. Ensure the patient intakes fluid 1 hour before meals

d. Ensure that the patient rinses his or her mouth after the consumption of meals

e. Restrict fluid consumption at meal times

9. A patient is admitted to a health care center with atrial flutter. The patient complains of headache after the first dose of digitalis is administered. Which of the following adverse effects of digitalis should a nurse assess for in such a situation? Select all that apply.

a. Hepatotoxicity

b. Angina

c. Drowsiness

d. Vomiting

e. Arrhythmia

10. A patient with heart failure has been advised to maintain digoxin therapy. Prior to discharge, the nurse teaches the steps of calculating the pulse. Arrange the steps involved in calculating the pulse in correct order.

a. Record the number of times the pulse beats in a minute

b. Place the non-dominant arm on a table or armchair

c. Place index and third fingers of the other hand on wrist bone

d. Feel for the beating or pulsing sensation, which is the pulse

e. If pulse rate more than 100 beats per minute, notify the practitioner

11. Cardiotonic drugs are used to treat which medical condition? Select all that apply.

a. Heart failure

b. Hypothyroidism

c. Hyperlipidemia

d. Atrial fibrillation

e. Hypertension

12. Milrinone (Primacor) is a miscellaneous inotropic drug used in the shortterm management of heart failure. What is the only way this drug is approved to be administered?

a. Intravenously

b. Intramuscularly

c. Subcutaneously

d. Orally

13. Which of the following symptoms would most likely be present in a client with right ventricular dysfunction? Select all that apply.

    a. Peripheral edema

    b. Neck vein distention

    c. Orthopnea

    d. Weight loss

    e. Nocturia

14. Which of the following classes of medications are currently used as first-line treatments of heart failure? Select all that apply.

    a. Angiotensin-converting enzyme inhibitors (ACEIs)

    b. Loop diuretics

    c. Cardiotonics

    d. Beta-blockers

    e. Angiotensin II receptor blockers (ARBs)

15. Which of the following is the result of positive inotropic activity?

    a. Increased cardiac output

    b. Decreased heart rate

    c. Increased preload

    d. Increased conduction velocity

40

Antiarrhythmic Drugs

Learning Objectives

- Describe various types of cardiac arrhythmias
- Discuss the uses, general drug actions, general adverse reactions, contraindications, precautions, and interactions of the antiarrhythmic drugs
- Discuss important preadministration and ongoing assessments the nurse should perform on a patient taking an antiarrhythmic drug
- List nursing diagnoses particular to a patient taking an antiarrhythmic drug
- Discuss ways to promote an optimal response to therapy, how to manage common adverse reactions, and important points to keep in mind when educating patients about the use of antiarrhythmic drugs

SECTION I: ASSESSING YOUR UNDERSTANDING

Activity A MATCHING

1. *Match the terms associated with cardiac arrhythmias in Column A with their brief description in Column B.*

Column A	Column B
1. Arrhythmia	a. Hearing loss and ringing sensation in the ears due to quinidine toxicity
2. Cinchonism	b. Movement of positive ions into nerve cell and negative ions to outside of cell
3. Polarization	c. Movement of positive ions to outside and negative ions to inside of nerve cell
4. Depolarization	d. Disturbance or irregularity in heart rate, rhythm, or both
5. Repolarization	e. Positive ions on outside and negative ions on inside of cell membrane when they are at rest

2. *Match the interactant drugs in Column A with effects of their interaction with antiarrhythmic agents in Column B.*

Column A

1. Fluoroquinolones

2. Anticholinergics

3. Local anesthetics

4. Warfarin

5. Rifampin

Column B

a. Additive antivagal effects on atrioventricular (AV) conduction

b. Decreased levels of antiarrhythmic agent

c. Risk of life-threatening arrhythmias

d. Possible increased risk of CNS side effects

e. Increased prothrombin time

Activity B FILL IN THE BLANKS

1. _____ is a term applied to any stimulus of the lowest intensity that will give rise to a response in a nerve fiber.

2. Beta-adrenergic blocking agents reduce the influence of the _____ nervous system in the heart and kidney.

3. All antiarrhythmic drugs may cause new arrhythmias or worsen existing arrhythmias, even though they are administered to resolve an existing arrhythmia. This phenomenon is called the _____ effect.

4. Flecainide depresses fast _____ channels, decreases the height and rate of rise of action potentials, and slows conduction of all areas of the heart.

5. A transient increase in arrhythmias and _____ may occur within 1 hour after initial therapy with bretylium is begun.

Activity C SHORT ANSWERS

A nurse's role in managing patients who are being administered antiarrhythmic drugs involves monitoring and implementing interventions that aid in recovery. Answer the following questions, which involve the nurse's role in the management of such situations.

1. A patient with paroxysmal atrial tachycardia is admitted to a health care facility. The patient is prescribed disopyramide.

_____

_____

a. What side effects of the drug should the nurse inform the patient about?

b. What conditions, if present, necessitate a cautious use of the drug?

2. A nurse is caring for a patient who has been prescribed an antiarrhythmic agent for atrial tachycardia. What assessments should the nurse perform before administering the drug to the patient?

_____

_____

Activity D DOSAGE CALCULATIONS

1. A patient with paroxysmal atrial tachycardia is prescribed disopyramide 150 mg orally every 6 hours. The Norpace (disopyramide) tablets from the pharmacy are each 100 mg disopyramide base. How many tablets should the nurse instruct the patient to take per dose?

_____

_____

2. A patient was prescribed mexiletine for the treatment of life-threatening ventricular tachycardia. By observing the patient's response, the health care provider has transferred to the 12-hour dosage schedule to improve compliance and convenience and has prescribed 300 mg of mexiletine every 12 hours. How many 150-mg tablets of mexiletine should the nurse administer in a single dose?

_____

_____

3. A patient weighing 55 kg has been prescribed 0.1 mL/kg of ibutilide fumarate for atrial fibrillation. How much of the drug should the nurse administer to the patient?

_____

_____

4. A patient with angina pectoris is prescribed propranolol hydrochloride 240 mg/d orally in 3 divided doses. How much of the drug should the nurse instruct the patient to take in each dose?

_____

_____

5. A patient weighing 70 kg has supraventricular arrhythmia. He receives a loading dose of IV esmolol hydrochloride. This is to be followed by an infusion of 50 mg/kg/min IV for 4 minutes. How much of the drug should the nurse infuse during these 4 minutes?

_____

_____

6. A patient with hypertension has been prescribed the drug acebutolol hydrochloride 390 mg/d in two divided doses orally. How much of the drug should the nurse instruct him to take in each dose?

_____

_____

SECTION II: APPLYING YOUR KNOWLEDGE

Activity E CASE STUDY

Mrs. Simpson was hospitalized today for a ventricular arrhythmia. The physician orders procainamide (Procanbid) to be given orally at a dose of 50mg/kg/day in divided doses every 3 hours. Mrs. Simpson weighs 176 lb.

1. How many milligrams should the nurse give Mrs. Simpson in one dose?

_____

_____

2. Procainamide is available in a 250-mg capsule. How many capsules would Mrs. Simpson need per dose?

_____

_____

SECTION III: PRACTICING FOR NCLEX

Activity F NCLEX-STYLE

Answer the following questions.

1. When educating a group of nursing students on the class IA antiarrhythmic drugs, the nurse cites which of the following drugs as an example of a class IA antiarrhythmic drug?
   a. Lidocaine
   b. Disopyramide
   c. Propafenone
   d. Amiodarone

2. A patient is prescribed flecainide for the treatment of cardiac arrhythmia. Which of the following channels in the heart does the drug depress?
   a. Calcium
   b. Chloride
   c. Oxygen
   d. Sodium

3. A patient has been prescribed an antiarrhythmic drug for cardiac arrhythmia. Which of the following possible adverse effects of the drug should the nurse inform the patient about?
   a. Hypertension
   b. Insomnia
   c. Lightheadedness
   d. Urinary frequency

4. A patient on amiodarone reports that she is pregnant. The primary health care provider informs her to stop use of the drug as it might cause fetal harm. Which of the following FDA Pregnancy Categories does amiodarone belong to?
   a. Category B
   b. Category C
   c. Category D
   d. Category X

5. A nurse is required to assess the vital signs of a patient with paroxysmal atrial tachycardia who is on an antiarrhythmic agent. Which of the following pulse rates alerts the nurse to inform the primary health care provider immediately?

   a. 82 bpm
   b. 92 bpm
   c. 102 bpm
   d. 122 bpm

6. A patient who is on antiarrhythmic drug therapy complains of nausea after taking the drug. Which of the following instructions should the nurse provide the patient to help alleviate nausea?

   a. Take the drug 2 hours before taking food
   b. Lie down flat for at least 1 hour after taking the drug
   c. Eat small frequent meals rather than large meals
   d. Drink lots of water after taking the medicine

7. A nurse caring for a patient who has been prescribed disopyramide for the treatment of arrhythmia is required to obtain the patient's drug history. Which of the following drugs, if taken concurrently, can decrease the serum levels of disopyramide?

   a. Erythromycin
   b. Quinidine
   c. Thioridazine
   d. Rifampicin

8. A nurse is required to closely monitor a patient with arrhythmia receiving IV lidocaine. Which of the following blood levels of lidocaine should the nurse report to the health care provider?

   a. 1.5 mcg/mL
   b. 3.0 mcg/mL
   c. 4.5 mcg/mL
   d. 6.0 mcg/mL

9. A patient has been admitted to a health care facility with the symptoms of cardiac arrhythmia. The patient is prescribed an antiarrhythmic agent. Which of the following adverse effects are possible with the use of an antiarrhythmic agent? Select all that apply.

   a. Weakness
   b. Hypertension
   c. Insomnia
   d. Arrhythmias
   e. Lightheadedness

10. A nurse is caring for an 86-year-old patient on antiarrhythmic drugs. Which of the following signs, if present, indicates the development of heart failure in the patient?

    a. Decrease in weight
    b. Shortness of breath
    c. Increased volume of urine
    d. Chills and fever

11. Which of the following types of arrhythmias is described as rapid contraction of the atria (up to 300 bpm) at a rate too rapid for the ventricles to pump efficiently?

    a. Atrial fibrillation
    b. Premature ventricular contraction
    c. Atrial flutter
    d. Ventricular fibrillation

12. Urinary retention during administration of disopyramide (Norpace) is caused by which of the following?

    a. Anticholinergic effects
    b. Bladder obstruction
    c. Decreased input
    d. Renal failure

13. All antiarrhythmic medications can cause which of the following? Select all that apply.

    a. New arrhythmias
    b. Increased blood pressure
    c. Increased blood glucose
    d. Worsen existing arrhythmias
    e. Increased body temperature

14. Which of the following medications are class II antiarrhythmics? Select all that apply.
    a. Acebutolol (Sectral)
    b. Amiodarone (Cordarone)
    c. Ibutilide (Corvert)
    d. Verapamil (Calan)
    e. Propranolol (Inderal)

15. Flecainide (Tambocor) is classified as which type of antiarrhythmic?
    a. Class IA
    b. Class IB
    c. Class IC
    d. Class II

CHAPTER 41

Drugs That Affect the Upper Gastrointestinal System

Learning Objectives

- Discuss the general drug actions, uses, adverse reactions, contraindications, precautions, and interactions of drugs used to treat conditions of the upper gastrointestinal system
- Discuss important preadministration and ongoing assessment activities the nurse should perform with the patient receiving a drug used to treat conditions of the upper gastrointestinal system
- List nursing diagnoses particular to a patient receiving a drug used to treat conditions of the upper gastrointestinal system
- Use the nursing process when administering drugs used to treat conditions of the upper gastrointestinal system

SECTION I: ASSESSING YOUR UNDERSTANDING

Activity A MATCHING

1. *Match the drugs in Column A with the disorders for which they are used in Column B.*

Column A	Column B
1. Aluminum carbonate gel C	a. Cystic fibrosis
2. Calcium carbonate e	b. Hypersecretory conditions
3. Lansoprazol a	c. Hyperphosphatemia
4. Pantoprazole b	d. Gastric ulcers
5. Misoprostol d	e. Osteoporosis

2. *Match the drugs in Column A with the effect of their interaction with the antacids listed in Column B.*

Column A

1. Chlorpromazine *B*
2. Tetracycline *C*
3. Corticosteroids *a*
4. Salicylates *e*
5. Amphetamines *d*

Column B

a. Decreased effectiveness of antiinflammatory properties

b. Decreased absorption of the interactant drug

c. Decreased effectiveness of antiinfective

d. Interactant drug is excreted slowly from the urine

e. Pain reliever is excreted rapidly from the urine

Activity B FILL IN THE BLANKS

1. The Gastrointestinal system is a long tube within the body where ingested food and fluids are prepared for absorption and ultimate replenishment of nutrients to the cells.

2. The esophagus connects the mouth to the stomach where food is mixed with acids and enzymes to become a solution for absorption.

3. Forceful expulsion of gastric contents through the mouth is known as vomiting.

4. Dronabinol is the only medically available cannabinoid prescribed for antiemetic use.

5. Proton pump inhibitors are particularly important in the treatment of *Helicobacter pylori* in patients with active Duodenal ulcers.

Activity C SHORT ANSWERS

A nurse's role in managing patients receiving a drug for an upper GI disorder involves assisting the patient for preadministration assessment. The nurse also monitors the patient for the occurrence of any adverse reactions. Answer the following questions, which involve the nurse's role in the management of such situations.

1. A patient with severe nausea and vomiting has been prescribed an antiemetic drug. What preadministration assessments should the nurse perform for the patient?

Ask pt type of pain and symptoms felt, record vitals, assess Electrolyte balance fluid, document fluid and vomiting.

2. After the preadministration assessment, the patient is administered an antiemetic drug. What is the nurse's role after administration of the drug?

Monitor vitals, I & O, signs & symptoms of complaints pain) Electrolyte imbalance a nausea. Document and notify provider of any problems.

Activity D DOSAGE CALCULATIONS

1. A physician has prescribed 2.5 mg of dronabinol to a patient as an HIV appetite stimulant, to be taken twice a day. The drug is available in the form of 2.5-mg capsules at the facility's pharmacy. How many capsules should the nurse administer to the patient during the treatment course of 3 days?

6 capsules

2. A physician has prescribed 40 mg esomeprazole magnesium to a patient daily for the treatment of erosive esophagitis. The drug is available as 20-mg capsules at a pharmacy store. How many capsules should the nurse administer to the patient per day?

2 capsules

3. A patient has been prescribed 1600 mg of cimetidine for the treatment of gastric ulcers, to be consumed orally per day. The drug is available as 400-mg tablets. How many tablets should the nurse administer to the patient per day?

4 tablets

4. A patient has been prescribed 600 mg of ranitidine per day for the treatment of erosive esophagitis. The drug is available as 150-mg tablets. How many tablets should the nurse administer to the patient daily?

4 tablets

5. A patient has been prescribed 30 mg of the lansoprazole drug daily for the treatment of cystic fibrosis. The drug is available as 15-mg capsules. How many capsules should the nurse administer to the patient for the treatment course of 3 days?

6 tablets

SECTION II: APPLYING YOUR KNOWLEDGE

Activity E CASE STUDY

Lauren Myers is a 19-year-old college student. She presents to the physician's office for her yearly physical. While in the office she mentions she is going on a cruise for spring break next week. Last time she was on a boat she suffered a bout of motion sickness and asks the nurse what she can do to prevent it.

1. What product can be used prophylactically to prevent motion sickness?

Medications such as promethizane, cyclizine, meclizine and buclizine.

2. The physician writes Ms. Myers a prescription for scopolamine (Transderm-Scop). How should the nurse advise Ms. Myers to use the patch?

Patch applied behind the ear approx 4 hrs before continuous effect as needed, discard any disk that becomes displaced re apply behind opposite ear, you need to wash hands thoroughly after applying patch also be sure you avoid drug contact of eyes and know the disk lasts about 3 days and can be removed if needed but only use one disk at a time. Can be dangerous when driving or any hazardous tasks when on medicine.

SECTION III: PRACTICING FOR NCLEX

Activity F NCLEX-STYLE

Answer the following questions.

1. A patient has been administered dronabinol for the prevention of chemotherapy-induced nausea. Which of the following adverse reactions should the nurse monitor for in the patient?
   a. Sedation
   b. Hypoxia
   c. Euphoria
   d. Asthenia

2. A nurse is caring for a patient who has been administered antacids for the treatment of gastric ulcer. The patient informs the nurse that he is also taking opioid analgesics for pain relief. What effect of interaction between the two drugs should the nurse assess for in the patient?
   a. Increased risk of respiratory depression
   b. Decreased white blood cell count
   c. Increased risk of bleeding
   d. Increased risk of dehydration

3. A physician has asked a nurse to start promethazine therapy for a patient with nausea. For which of the following conditions in the patient should the nurse administer the drug with caution? Select all that apply.
   a. Hypertension
   b. Sleep apnea
   c. Glaucoma
   d. Epilepsy
   e. Viral illness

4. A nurse has administered aluminum hydroxide gel to a patient for the relief of stomach hyperacidity. What should the nurse monitor for in the patient after administration of the drug?
   a. Complaints of headache
   b. Coffee-ground–colored emesis
   c. Signs of electrolyte imbalance
   d. Amount of fluid lost

5. A patient undergoing antacid drug therapy is to be discharged from a health care facility. What should the nurse include in the teaching plan for the patient?

  a. Increase frequency of dose if symptoms worsen

  b. Avoid direct exposure to sunlight

  c. Take other drugs 1 hour before taking the antacid

  d. Avoid driving when taking the drug

6. A nurse is caring for a patient who has intentionally ingested a poison. The nurse is required to administer an emetic drug to the patient. What information should the nurse obtain from a family member or friend of the patient before administration of the drug? Select all that apply.

  a. Substances that have been ingested

  b. Cause for ingesting the poison

  c. Approximately when the substances were ingested

  d. Patient's mental status before taking poison

  e. Symptoms noted before seeking medical treatment

7. A nurse is caring for a patient experiencing nausea and vomiting. The physician has prescribed an antiemetic drug therapy for the patient. What symptoms of dehydration, which is a serious concern associated with nausea and vomiting, should the nurse monitor in the patient? Select all that apply.

  a. White streaks in stool

  b. Decreased urinary output

  c. Concentrated urine

  d. Decreased respiratory rate

  e. Dry mucous membranes

8. A patient who has undergone surgery is prescribed acid-reducing drugs through IV. What should the nurse monitor during administration of the drug to the patient?

  a. Rate of infusion at frequent intervals

  b. Body temperature every hour

  c. Irritation due to drug administration

  d. Blood pressure every 2 hours

9. A nurse is caring for a patient undergoing antacid drug therapy. The patient complains of diarrhea after taking the drug. What interventions should the nurse perform in this case?

  a. Remove items with strong odor

  b. Change to a different antacid

  c. Record the patient's temperature every hour

  d. Record the patient's fluid intake and output

10. A nurse is caring for a patient undergoing antiemetic drug therapy to prevent nausea. The patient reports loss of appetite due to nausea. What should the nurse do to enhance the patient's appetite?

  a. Suggest consumption of milk products

  b. Suggest physical exercises

  c. Remove items with strong smell and odor

  d. Avoid giving frequent oral rinses to the patient

11. Which of the following drugs treat heartburn by neutralizing the acidity of the stomach, combining with hydrochloric acid (HCl) and increasing the pH of the stomach acid?

  a. Omeprazole (Prilosec)

  b. Famotidine (Pepcid)

  c. Magaldrate (Riopan)

  d. Metoclopramide (Reglan)

12. The nurse should warn a patient taking magnesium- and sodium-containing antacids about which of the following adverse effects?

  a. Diarrhea

  b. Constipation

  c. Dehydration

  d. Flatulence

13. The nurse should warn a patient taking aluminum- and calcium-containing antacids about which of the following adverse effects?

  a. Diarrhea

  b. Dehydration

  c. Flatulence

  d. Constipation

14. Which of the following antacids is contraindicated in patients with congestive heart failure?

a. Sodium bicarbonate (Bellans)
b. Calcium carbonate (Tums)
c. Magnesium hydroxide (Milk of Magnesia)
d. Aluminum hydroxide (ALternaGEL)

15. Administering an antacid to a patient taking which of the following medications will decrease the absorption of the medication and results in a decreased drug effect? (Choose one)

a. Quinidine
b. Digoxin
c. Dextroamphetamine
d. Simvastatin

CHAPTER 42

Drugs That Affect the Lower Gastrointestinal System

Learning Objectives

- Describe how inflammatory bowel disease alters function of the lower gastrointestinal system
- List the types of drugs prescribed or recommended for lower gastrointestinal disorders
- Discuss the uses, general drug actions, general adverse reactions, contraindications, precautions, and interactions associated with lower gastrointestinal drugs
- Discuss important preadministration and ongoing assessment activities the nurse should perform on the patient taking a lower gastrointestinal drug
- List nursing diagnoses particular to a patient taking a lower gastrointestinal drug
- Discuss ways to promote an optimal response to therapy, how to manage common adverse reactions, and important points to keep in mind when educating patients about the use of lower gastrointestinal drugs

SECTION I: ASSESSING YOUR UNDERSTANDING

Activity A MATCHING

1. *Match the drugs in Column A with their uses in Column B.*

Column A	Column B
1. Loperamide C	a. Prevents the formation of gas pockets in the intestine
2. Simethicone a	b. Irritable bowel syndrome
3. Lactulose d	c. Treatment of chronic diarrhea associated with IBD
4. Psyllium b	d. Reduction of blood ammonia levels in hepatic encephalopathy

2. *Match the drugs used in managing lower GI disorders in Column A with their adverse reactions in Column B.*

Column B

1. Infliximab *d*
2. Difenoxin *b*
3. Olsalazine *a*
4. Sulfasalazine *c*

Column B

a. Abdominal crampin
b. Constipation
c. Anorexia
d. Sore throat

Activity B FILL IN THE BLANKS

1. Transit of contents rapidly through the bowel is called Diarrhea

2. Chamomile herb protects against the development of stomach ulcers.

3. For short-term relief or prevention of constipation, a laxative is prescribed.

4. Charcoal may be used in the prevention of nonspecific pruritus associated with kidney dialysis treatment.

5. Amino salicylate used to treat Crohn's disease and ulcerative colitis.

Activity C SHORT ANSWERS

A nurse's role in managing patients who have been prescribed drugs for lower GI disorder involves performing preadministrative and ongoing assessments during the course of drug therapy. The nurse also monitors the patients for the occurrence of any adverse reactions after administration of the drug. Answer the following questions, which involve the nurse's role in the management of such situations.

1. A patient with dyspepsia has been prescribed simethicone. What preadministration assessments should the nurse perform before administration of the simethicone drug?

Ask pt type of pain intensity, symptoms, where located, listen to bowel sounds, palpate abdomen, you should monitor pt for any discomfort or pain noticed + felt.

2. What is the nurse's role after administering the drug to the patient?

Asses pt for relief of pain + symptoms felt, notify physician if meds don't work, monitor vital signs frequent, observe pt for any adverse drug reactions, you also need to evaluate pts response to therapy used for treatment did it work.

Activity D DOSAGE CALCULATIONS

1. A patient with active ulcerative colitis is prescribed balsalazide by the physician. The nurse needs to administer 2250 g of balsalazide on a daily basis. The drug is available in the form of 750-mg capsules. How many capsules should the nurse administer to the patient to complete a course of 8 weeks?

168 capsules

2. A patient with proctitis has been prescribed mesalamine. The physician has prescribed the patient 200 mg of mesalamine to be taken 4 times a day. The drug is available in 400-mg tablets. How many tablets should the nurse administer the patient every day?

2 tablets

3. A patient has been prescribed 1 g of olsalazine daily in 2 doses for the maintenance of remission of ulcerative colitis. The drug is available as 250-mg capsules. How capsules should the nurse administer in each dose?

2 capsules

4. A nurse is caring for a patient with rheumatoid arthritis. The physician has prescribed the patient 4 g of sulfasalazine daily in divided doses. The drug is available in the form of 500-mg tablets. How many tablets will the nurse require to complete the course of 3 days?

24 tablets

5. A physician has prescribed 10 mg of bisacodyl on a daily basis to a patient for the relief of constipation. The drug is available as 5-mg tablets. How may tablets should the nurse administer the patient every day?

2 tablets

SECTION II: APPLYING YOUR KNOWLEDGE

Activity E CASE STUDY

Wilbert Jackson is an African American male, 67 years of age. He presents to the physician's office for a follow-up appointment. His chief complaint today is hard stools and straining to have a bowel movement. His current medications include: amitriptyline (Elavil) 25 mg QHS for sleep, ferrous sulfate (Feosol) 325 mg TID for anemia, and lisinopril/HCTZ (Prinizide) 20/25 mg QD for high blood pressure.

1. Which of Mr. Jackson's medication may be contributing to his constipation?

   Opiods, phenothiazines, antihistamine, non opiods, antidepressants and antacids.

2. What nonpharmacological steps can Mr. Jackson take to relieve his constipation?

   Non pharmacological therapys to relieve constipation would be to increase daily fluid one after so its consistent and exersise would help increase GI motility.

SECTION III: PRACTICING FOR NCLEX

Activity F NCLEX-STYLE

Answer the following questions.

1. A nurse is caring for a patient with proctosigmoiditis. The physician has prescribed mesalamine to the patient. The patient informs the nurse that he is also taking hypoglycemic drugs for the management of diabetes mellitus. What condition should the nurse monitor in this patient as a result of the interaction of the two drugs?
   a. Decreased absorption of hypoglycemic drugs
   b. Increased risk of bleeding
   c. Increased blood glucose level
   d. Reduced effect of mesalamine

2. A nurse is caring for a patient with acute diarrhea who has been prescribed loperamide. Which of the following adverse reactions to the drug should the nurse monitor in the patient?
   a. Cramping
   b. Constipation
   c. Anorexia
   d. Sore throat

3. A physician has prescribed bismuth subsalicylate to a patient with abdominal cramps. For which of the following conditions in the patient should the nurse administer the drug with caution?
   a. Hepatic impairment
   b. Intestinal obstruction
   c. Acute appendicitis
   d. Rectal bleeding

4. A patient undergoing simethicone drug therapy for a peptic ulcer is to be discharged from the health care facility. What instruction should the nurse offer the patient regarding self-administration of the drug at home?
   a. Take the drug early in the morning
   b. Chew the tablets thoroughly
   c. Drink a glass of water after taking the drug
   d. Take the drug with a glass of juice

5. A nurse is caring for a patient with chronic diarrhea. The physician has prescribed diphenoxylate to the patient. What intervention should the nurse perform when caring for this patient?
   a. Encourage the patient to drink extra fluids
   b. Avoid the use of commercial electrolytes
   c. Encourage the patient to take food high in fiber
   d. Encourage the patient to exercise

6. A nurse is caring for an outpatient undergoing antidiarrheal therapy for diarrhea. Which of the following instructions should the nurse include in the teaching plan for this patient? Select all that apply.
   a. Get sufficient exercise
   b. Observe caution when driving
   c. Avoid the use of alcohol
   d. Eat foods high in roughage
   e. Avoid the use of nonprescription drugs

7. A nurse is to instruct an outpatient in the right method of administering mineral oil for constipation. Which of the following should the nurse instruct the patient for optimal response to therapy?
   a. Take it half an hour after a meal
   b. Take it before breakfast
   c. Take it at bedtime after dinner
   d. Take it on an empty stomach in the evening

8. A nurse is caring for a patient undergoing methylcellulose therapy for the treatment of irritable bowel syndrome. The overuse of the drug results in constipation in the patient. What instruction should the nurse offer the patient to avoid constipation?
   a. Take commercial electrolytes
   b. Take the drug with food
   c. Eat foods high in roughage
   d. Avoid milk products

9. A nurse is caring for an outpatient undergoing laxative therapy. Which of the following is an effect of the prolonged use of a laxative that the nurse should inform the client about?
   a. Obstruction of small intestine
   b. Serious electrolyte imbalances
   c. Fecal impaction
   d. Renal impairment

10. A nurse needs to start antidiarrheal drug therapy for a patient. For which of the following categories of patients is an antidiarrheal contraindicated?
   a. Patient with constipation
   b. Patient with nausea
   c. Patient with obstructive jaundice
   d. Patient with abdominal distention

11. Patients with a sulfonamide allergy should avoid the use of which of the following to treat an ulcerative colitis flare?
   a. Infliximab (Remicade)
   b. Famotidine (Pepcid)
   c. Mesalamine (Asacol)
   d. Metoclopramide (Reglan)

12. Which of the following herbal products has been used to treat digestive upset and stomach ulcers?
   a. Chamomile
   b. Kava
   c. Ginger
   d. Valerian

13. Which of the following is an antidiarrheal that decreases intestinal peristalsis?
   a. Loperamide (Imodium)
   b. Sodium bicarbonate (Bellans)
   c. Diphenoxylate (Lomotil)
   d. Omeprazole (Prilosec)

14. The nurse should counsel a patient to discontinue use of over-the-counter antidiarrheals and seek treatment from a physician if diarrhea persists for how long?
   a. 1 day
   b. 12 hours
   c. 2 days
   d. 7 days

15. Which of the following medicationS could the nurse recommend a patient purchase overthecounter to treat flatulence?
   a. Loperamide (Imodium)
   b. Simethicone (Mylicon)
   c. Olsalazine (Dipentum)
   d. Psyllium (Metamucil)

CHAPTER 43

Antidiabetic Drugs

Learning Objectives

- Describe the two types of diabetes mellitus
- Discuss the types, uses, general drug actions, adverse reactions, contraindications, precautions, and interactions of the antidiabetic drugs
- Discuss important preadministration and ongoing assessment activities the nurse should perform with the patient taking an antidiabetic drug
- List nursing diagnoses particular to a patient taking an antidiabetic drug
- Discuss ways to promote an optimal response to therapy, how to manage common adverse reactions, and important points to keep in mind when educating patients about the use of the antidiabetic drugs

SECTION I: ASSESSING YOUR UNDERSTANDING

Activity A MATCHING

1. **Match the antidiabetic drugs in Column A with their uses in Column B.**

Column A		Column B
1. Rosiglitazone	*b*	a. Hypoglycemia
2. Diazoxide	*c*	b. Type 2 diabetes
3. Glucagon	*a*	c. Hypoglycemia due to hyperinsulinism

2. **Match the antidiabetic drugs in Column A with their adverse reactions in Column B.**

Column A		Column B
1. Acetohexamide	*c*	a. Aggravated diabetes
2. Metformin	*d*	b. Fluid retention
3. Pioglitazone HCl	*a*	c. Heartburn
4. Diazoxide	*b*	d. Asthenia

Activity B FILL IN THE BLANKS

1. Diabetes mellitus is a chronic disorder characterized by insufficient __Insulin__ production by the beta cells of the pancreas.
2. Increased urination is termed __polyuria__.
3. Insulin stimulates the synthesis of __glycogen__ by the liver.
4. Insulin is used to treat __hypokalemia__ in combination with glucose.
5. Elevated blood glucose or sugar level is termed __hyperglycemia__
6. When blood glucose levels are high, glucose molecules attach to __hemoglobin__ in the red blood cells.
7. Diabetic __ketoacidosis__ is a potentially life-threatening deficiency of insulin.

Activity C SHORT ANSWERS

A nurse's role in managing patients who are being administered oral antidiabetic drugs involves monitoring the patients and implementing interventions that aid in their recovery. Answer the following questions, which involve the nurse's role in the management of such situations.

1. A nurse is caring for a patient with type 2 diabetes. The nurse evaluates the effectiveness of the treatment plan. What factors should the nurse consider to determine its success?

   Pt verbalizes willingness to agree w/ plan, Pt shows understanding, anxiety is decreased and normal fluid level (glucose) are maintained

2. A nurse has been caring for a patient with type 2 diabetes. The nurse has to ensure that the patient complies with the drug regimen. What instructions should the nurse offer to the patient and patient's family to decrease the chance of noncompliance by the patient?

   You take drug correct time, Any diet follow, avoid alcohol, maintain health, hygiene, healthy food and test blood glucose for any ketones.

Activity D DOSAGE CALCULATION

1. A patient with type 2 diabetes has been prescribed 30 mg of pioglitazone HCl (Actos) by a physician at a health care facility. The physician has instructed the nurse to continue the drug therapy for 2 days. The drug is available in 15-mg tablets at a pharmacy. How many tablets should the nurse administer the patient during the entire therapy?

   4 tablets

2. A patient diagnosed with type 2 diabetes has been prescribed 10 mg of repaglinide to be taken once daily. The drug is available in 2-mg tablets. How many tablets should the nurse administer the patient daily?

   5 tablets

3. A patient at a health care facility has been prescribed nateglinide 120 mg (Starlix) to be given 3 times a day. The drug is available in 60-mg tablets. How many tablets should the nurse administer the patient through the entire day?

   6 tablets

4. A patient has been prescribed 2650 mg of metformin to be taken orally. The tablets on hand are 850 mg. How many tablets should the nurse administer the patient daily?

   3 tablets

5. A patient with type 2 diabetes has been prescribed miglitol drug therapy. The physician has instructed the nurse to administer 100 mg of the drug 3 times a day. The drug is available in 50-mg tablets. How many tablets should the nurse administer the patient daily?

   6 tablets

SECTION II: APPLYING YOUR KNOWLEDGE

Activity E CASE STUDY

Emma Arthur is a Caucasian female, 56 years of age. She has type 2 diabetes, hypertension, and dyslipidemia. Her current medications include glyburide/metformin (Glucovance) 5/500 mg 2 tabs BID, pioglitazone (Actos) 45 mg QD, simvastatin 20 mg QHS, and losartan/hctz (Hyzaar) 100/25 mg QD. She presents to the physician's office for a follow-up appointment. Her home blood glucose readings are 250–350 mg/dL 2 hours after meals and 130–160 mg/dL fasting.

1. After examining Mrs. Arthur and looking at her home blood glucose readings, the physician starts Mrs. Arthur on insulin glargine (Lantus) 10 mg QHS subcutaneously. The physician asks the nurse to teach Mrs. Arthur to properly inject the insulin. What should the nurse tell Mrs. Arthur about injecting insulin and injection site rotation?

   Injections can be given in upper arm, abdomen 2 inches from ablicous, below the waist, upper thighs. Clean site w/ alcohol pad, and top of vial of insulin, draw up right dose and inject insulin into the skin at 45°. If any infections you need to rotate sites used no scars or a bruise mg

2. The nurse should also discuss hypoglycemia with Mrs. Arthur, as she is more likely to experience a hypoglycemic episode while on insulin. What information should the nurse provide Mrs. Arthur about hypoglycemia?

hypoglycemia is low blood sugar under 60 mg/dl. signs/symptoms are confusion, dizziness, fatigue and sweaty skin, rapid 3 shallow breathing as well.

SECTION III: PRACTICING FOR NCLEX

Activity F NCLEX-STYLE

Answer the following questions.

1. A patient at a health care facility has been prescribed pioglitazone HCl for the treatment of type 2 diabetes. What adverse reaction to the drug should the nurse monitor for in the patient?
   a. Congestive heart failure
   b. Myalgia
   c. Sodium retention
   d. Glycosuria

2. A nurse refers to the medical history of a patient who is to be administered chlorpropamide sulfonylureas. In which of the following preexisting conditions is the use of chlorpropamide sulfonylureas contraindicated?
   a. Coronary artery disease
   b. Chronic intestinal diseases
   c. Colonic ulceration
   d. Inflammatory bowel disease

3. A nurse is caring for a female patient with gestational diabetes. The patient asks the nurse during which stage of pregnancy the need for insulin is greatest. Which of the following should the nurse reply?
   a. Immediately after conception
   b. First trimester of pregnancy
   c. Third trimester of pregnancy
   d. Immediately after delivery

4. A nurse is assigned to administer a regular insulin dosage to a patient with type 1 diabetes mellitus. What care should be taken by the nurse before administering insulin?
   a. Administer 15 minutes before a meal
   b. Administer 30 to 60 minutes before a meal
   c. Administer once at bedtime via SC route
   d. Administer within 5 to 10 minutes of a meal

5. A patient has been prescribed miglitol. The administration of miglitol causes hypoglycemia in the patient. What should be the nurse's intervention in such a situation?
   a. Discuss the disease and methods of control with the patient
   b. Administer acetohexamide with insulin to the patient
   c. Administer the patient dextrose rather than sugar
   d. Obtain capillary blood specimens from the patient

6. A nurse is to administer an insulin mixture of insulin lispro and long-acting insulin. What care should the nurse take with regard to preparing the solution?
   a. Confirm with the PHCP whether the solution is to be mixed in the same syringe
   b. Draw up insulin lispro first in the syringe while preparing the solution
   c. Confirm if the ratio of insulin to be administered is 70/30 or 50/50
   d. Keep the mixture for 1 hour if the patient has difficulty controlling diabetes

7. A nurse is preparing a teaching plan for a patient who has been prescribed α-glucosidase inhibitors. What instruction should the nurse include in the teaching plan for this patient?
   a. Avoid drug administration in case of a skipped meal
   b. Report respiratory distress or muscular aches to the PHCP
   c. Keep a source of glucose ready for signs of low blood glucose
   d. Take the drug at different times each day

8. A nurse is required to administer insulin to a patient who has undergone a renal transplantation. Which method of insulin delivery should the nurse adopt for the patient?

    a. Needle and syringe method

    b. Jet injection system method

    c. Syringe with prefilled cartridge

    d. Insulin pump method

9. A nurse at a health care facility is preparing an insulin solution to be administered to a diabetic patient. What precaution should the nurse take before withdrawing the syringe from the insulin vial?

    a. Eliminate air bubbles from the syringe barrel

    b. Shake the vial vigorously just before withdrawal

    c. Ensure the vial has been undisturbed for an hour

    d. Use a syringe labeled with a higher concentration

10. A pregnant diabetic patient with early long-term complications is administered insulin with an insulin pump. Which of the following should the nurse instruct the patient?

    a. Monitor blood glucose levels twice per day

    b. Ensure that the needle is changed every 1 to 3 days

    c. Inject the same amount of insulin each time

    d. Use a mixture of isophane and regular insulin

11. Glycosylated hemoglobin measures average blood glucose over what time period?

    a. Past 12 to 24 hours

    b. Past 7 to 10 days

    c. Past 1 or 2 months

    d. Past 3 or 4 months

12. Insulin is produced by which organ in the human body?

    a. Pancreas

    b. Spleen

    c. Liver

    d. Kidney

13. Which of the following is an example of rapid-acting insulin?

    a. Insulin lispro (Humalog)

    b. Insulin Glargine (Lantus)

    c. Insulin detemir (Levemir)

    d. Isophane insulin suspension (Humulin N)

14. Which of the following is an example of long-acting insulin?

    a. Insulin lispro (Humalog)

    b. Insulin glargine (Lantus)

    c. Insulin aspart (Apidra)

    d. Isophane insulin suspension (Humulin N)

15. During insulin teaching, when should the nurse advise the patient to administer insulin aspart (Apidra)?

    a. Immediately before a meal

    b. At bedtime

    c. 30 to 60 minutes before a meal

    d. Immediately after a meal

Pituitary and Adrenocortical Hormones

Learning Objectives

- List the hormones produced by the pituitary gland and the adrenal cortex
- Discuss general actions, uses, adverse reactions, contraindications, precautions, and interactions of the pituitary and adrenocortical hormones
- Discuss important preadministration and ongoing assessment activities the nurse should perform with a patient taking the pituitary and adrenocortical hormones
- List nursing diagnoses particular to a patient taking a pituitary or adrenocortical hormone
- Discuss ways to promote an optimal response to therapy, how to manage common adverse reactions, and important points to keep in mind when educating patients about the use of pituitary or adrenocortical hormones

SECTION I: ASSESSING YOUR UNDERSTANDING

Activity A MATCHING

1. *Match the drugs in Column A with their uses in Column B.*

Column A		Column B
1. Desmopressin acetate	*b*	a. Treatment of Parkinson's disease
2. Bromocriptine mesylate	*a*	b. Treatment of von Willebrand's disease
3. Budesonide	*d*	c. Partial replacement therapy for Addison's disease
4. Fludrocortisone acetate	*c*	d. Treatment of Crohn's disease

2. *Match the drugs in Column A with their adverse reactions in Column B.*

Column A		Column B
1. Octreotide acetate	*c*	a. Ovarian enlargement
2. Vasopressin	*d*	b. Arthralgia
3. Somatropin	*b*	c. Sinus bradycardia
4. Clomiphene citrate	*a*	d. Tremor

Activity B FILL IN THE BLANKS

1. ACTH stimulates the adrenal cortex to secrete the _Corticosteroids_

2. Anterior pituitary hormone _Prolactin_ is the only hormone that is not used medically.

3. Follicle-stimulating hormone and luteinizing hormone are called _Gonadotropins_ because they influence the organs of reproduction.

4. The nasal tube delivery system comes with a flexible calibrated plastic tube called a _Rhibyle_.

5. _Menotropins_ is used in an assisted reproductive technology (ART) program to stimulate multiple follicles for in vitro fertilization.

Activity C SHORT ANSWERS

A nurse's role in managing patients receiving growth hormones involves assisting them in order to promote an optimal response to growth hormone therapy. The nurse also helps patients in educating them and their families about the successful implementation of therapy. Answer the following questions, which involve the nurse's role in the management of such situations.

1. A 10-year-old patient has enrolled in a growth hormone program. What is the nurse's role in promoting an optimal response to the growth hormone therapy?

2. What is the nurse's role in educating the patient and his family about the growth hormone therapy?

Activity D DOSAGE CALCULATION

1. A physician has prescribed 2 g of aminoglutethimide on a daily basis to a patient for suppressing adrenal function. The drug is available as 250-mg tablets. How may tablets should the nurse administer the patient every day?

   8 tablets

2. A patient has been recommended 1 mg of cabergoline twice weekly for the treatment of acromegaly. The drug is available as 0.5-mg tablets. How many tablets should the nurse administer to the patient to complete the 3 week course?

   12 tablets

3. A nurse is caring for a patient with salt-losing adrenogenital syndrome. The physician has prescribed 0.2 mg of fludrocortisone acetate daily for 5 days. The drug is available as 0.1-mg tablets. How many tablets will the nurse require to complete the course of drug administration?

   10 tablets

4. A physician has prescribed 50 mg of cortisone on a daily basis as a treatment for systemic dermatomyositis. The drug is available as 25-mg tablets. How many tablets will the nurse need to complete a 3-day treatment course?

   6 tablets

5. A nurse is caring for a patient with psoriatic arthritis. The physician has prescribed 20 mg of prednisone on a daily basis. The drug is available as 10-mg tablets. How many tablets should the nurse administer to the patient in 2 days?

   4 tablets

1. nurse should administer the hormone sc, do not shake vial containing the hormone, nurse should swirl the hormone contained, give the drug at bedtime, divide dosage up 3 to doses a wk and not to administer solution if these 3, cloudy.

2. Nurses role of educating is to show and explain proper therapeutic regimen increasing hormone growth, Explain proper injection technique if administered at home not at the clinic, and encourage pt to watch for any unnormal symptoms, lack of growth and report it.

SECTION II: APPLYING YOUR KNOWLEDGE

Activity E CASE STUDY

Jerry Smallwood is an African American male, 45 years of age. He presents to the physician's office today with complaints of frequent urination and increased thirst. After a thorough exam, the physician diagnoses Mr. Smallwood with diabetes insipidus.

1. The physician prescribes intranasal desmopressin (DDAVP) to Mr. Smallwood. How should the nurse instruct Mr. Smallwood to use the intranasal spray?

   The nurses should advise Mr Smallwood to tip bottle upward, insert nares of the nose and squeeze one spray into his nose.

2. What adverse effects should the nurse discuss with Mr. Smallwood?

   Adverse effects would be signs of a headache, nausea, abdominal cramps, water intoxication and nasal congestion.

SECTION III: PRACTICING FOR NCLEX

Activity F NCLEX-STYLE

Answer the following questions.

1. A nurse is caring for a patient who has been prescribed corticotropin for acute exacerbations of multiple sclerosis. In which of the following types of patients should the nurse administer the drug cautiously? Select all that apply.
   a. Patients with diverticulosis
   b. Patients with sinus bradycardia
   c. Patients with febrile infections
   d. Patients with arthralgia
   e. Patients with myasthenia gravis

2. A nurse is caring for a patient with abnormal urination and thirst. The physician has prescribed vasopressin to the patient. The patient informs the nurse that he is also taking oral anticoagulants for blood thinning. What effect of interaction between these two drugs should the nurse inform the patient about?
   a. Increased risk of hypokalemia
   b. Increased need for antidiabetic medication

   c. Decreased muscle function
   d. Decreased antidiuretic effect

3. A patient with mycosis fungoides is prescribed dexamethasone. Which of the following adverse reactions to the drug should the nurse monitor in the patient? Select all that apply.
   a. Nasal congestion
   b. Acneiform eruptions
   c. Increased sweating
   d. Perineal itch
   e. Abdominal cramps

4. A physician has prescribed adrenocorticotropic hormone (ACTH) to the patient with non-suppurative thyroiditis. What intervention should the nurse perform as a part of ongoing assessment during the course of treatment?
   a. Record the patient's abdominal girth
   b. Monitor for a rise in blood glucose level
   c. Measure the specific gravity of the urine
   d. Monitor bone age periodically

5. A physician prescribes hydrocortisone to a patient with regional enteritis. The patient informs the nurse of gastric irritation after taking the drug. Which of the following interventions should the nurse perform while managing the needs of the patient?
   a. Give drug with a full glass of water
   b. Administer enema before first dose of drug
   c. Supply with large amounts of drinking water
   d. Auscultate the abdomen

6. A patient undergoing a replacement therapy for primary adrenocortical deficiency is prescribed fludrocortisone acetate by a physician. Which of the following adverse reactions should the nurse monitor in the patient?
   a. Joint pain
   b. Hypothyroidism
   c. Hypertension
   d. Insulin resistance

7. A physician has prescribed ganirelix acetate to an infertile patient. During the course of the treatment, the patient complains of visual disturbances. Which of the following precautionary measures should the nurse take?

   a. Discontinue the drug therapy
   b. Administer the drug with food
   c. Perform a CBC test as ordered by the PHCP
   d. Assess skin integrity

8. A patient in a health care facility is prescribed glucocorticoids for systemic lupus erythematosus. What should the nursing diagnoses checklist include for this patient?

   a. Pain related to abdominal distention
   b. Deficient fluid volume related to inability to replenish fluid intake
   c. Disturbed body image related to adverse reactions
   d. Risk for infection related to masking of signs of infection

9. A patient is prescribed vasopressin for diabetes insipidus, and the physician also instructs the patient to undergo abdominal roentgenography. Which of the following interventions should the nurse perform for implementing the process?

   a. Give enema before first dose
   b. Check stools for evidence of bleeding
   c. Monitor patient for rash, urticaria, and hypotension
   d. Provide daily oral drug doses before 9AM

10. A nurse is caring for a patient with congenital adrenal hyperplasia. The physician has prescribed prednisone to the patient. During the course of the treatment, the patient undergoes an overdose of prednisone. Which of the following conditions is the nurse most likely to observe in the patient as a result of the overdose of prednisone? Select all that apply.

    a. Swelling
    b. Buffalo hump
    c. Muscle pain
    d. Moon face
    e. Weight gain

11. Which of the following hormones is secreted by the posterior pituitary gland?

    a. Vasopressin
    b. Gonadotropin
    c. Somatropin
    d. Adrenocorticotropic hormone (ACTH)

12. Diabetes insipidus is treated with replacement of which of the following hormones?

    a. Gonadotropin
    b. Somatropin
    c. Vasopressin
    d. Adrenocorticotropic hormone (ACTH)

13. Which of the following hormones is responsible for the regulation of reabsorption of water by the kidneys?

    a. Vasopressin
    b. Gonadotropin
    c. Somatotropin
    d. Adrenocorticotropic hormone (ACTH)

14. Which of the hormones is responsible for the growth of the body during childhood, especially the growth of muscles and bones?

    a. Vasopressin
    b. Somatotropin
    c. Gonadotropin
    d. Adrenocorticotropic hormone (ACTH)

15. Which of the following medications binds to estrogen receptors, decreasing the amount of available estrogen receptors and causing the anterior pituitary to increase secretion of FSH and LH?

    a. Clomiphene (Clomid)
    b. Medroxyprogesterone (Provera)
    c. Estradiol (Estrace)
    d. Estropipate (Ogen)

CHAPTER 45

Thyroid and Antithyroid Drugs

Learning Objectives

- Identify the hormones produced by the thyroid gland
- Discuss the uses, general drug actions, adverse reactions, contraindications, precautions, and interactions of thyroid and antithyroid drugs
- Discuss important preadministration and ongoing assessment activities the nurse should perform with the patient taking thyroid and antithyroid drugs
- List the signs and symptoms of iodism (too much iodine) and iodine allergy
- Discuss ways to promote an optimal response to therapy, how to manage adverse reactions, and important points to keep in mind when educating patients about the use of thyroid and antithyroid drug.

SECTION I: ASSESSING YOUR UNDERSTANDING

Activity A MATCHING

1. **Match the drugs in Column A with their adverse reactions in Column B.**

Column A

1. Levothyroxine sodium (T_4) *b*
2. Methimazole *C*
3. Sodium iodine (^{131}I) *a*

Column B

a. Hives
b. Palpitations
c. Agranulocytosis

2. **Match the interactant drugs in Column A with the effect of their interaction with the thyroid hormones in Column B.**

Column A

1. Digoxin *C*
2. Insulin *a*
3. Oral anticoagulants *d*
4. Antidepressant *b*

Column B

a. Increased risk of hypoglycemia
b. Decreased effectiveness of thyroid drug
c. Decreased effectiveness of cardiac drug
d. Prolonged bleeding

Activity B FILL IN THE BLANKS

1. _hyperthyroidism_ is an increase in the amount of thyroid hormones manufactured and secreted.

2. Thyroid hormones are used as replacement therapy when the patient is _hypothyroid_.

3. _Iodine_ is an essential element for the manufacture of the thyroxine (T_4) and tri-iodothyronine (T_3) hormones.

4. Enlargement of a normal thyroid gland is called the _euthyroid_ goiter.

5. _Antithyroid_ drugs inhibit the manufacture of thyroid hormones.

Activity C **SHORT ANSWERS**

A nurse's role in managing patients who are being administered thyroid hormones involves monitoring the patients and implementing interventions that aid in their recovery. Answer the following questions, which involve the nurse's role in the management of such situations.

1. A patient undergoing thyroid hormone replacement therapy is discharged. What information should the nurse provide to the patient and family emphasizing the importance of taking the replacement therapy?

   Replacement therapy is for rest of your life, do not skip, increase, decrease, contact provider if any side affects occur and watch your weight.

2. A nurse is caring for a patient undergoing thyroid hormone therapy. Post-therapy, the nurse needs to evaluate the effectiveness of the therapy. What factors should the nurse consider to determine the success of the therapy?

   Therapeutic effect is successful, pt verbalizes importance, understanding of regimen, adverse reactions are advised, family and pt understand drug regimen.

Activity D **DOSAGE CALCULATION**

1. A primary health care provider has prescribed 75 micrograms per day of levothyroxine sodium to be administered orally in 3 doses. The drug is available as 25-microgram tablets. How many tablets should the nurse administer to the patient per day?

   3 tablets

2. A patient is prescribed methimazole for the treatment of hyperthyroidism. The primary health care provider instructs the nurse to administer 10 mg of the drug in 8-hour intervals daily. The available tablets are 5 mg. How many tablets should the nurse administer to the patient in a day?

   6 tablets

3. A patient is prescribed 900 mg of propylthiouracil daily for the treatment of hyperthyroidism. The drug is available in the form of 100-mg tablets. The nurse needs to administer the divided doses at 8-hour intervals. How many tablets should the nurse administer to the patient in each dose?

   3 tablets

4. A patient with hypothyroidism is prescribed thyroid USP. The primary health care provider has prescibed 30 mg of the drug initially each day to the patient. the drug is available in 15-mg tablets. How many tablets should the nurse administer to the patient per day?

   2 tablets

5. A primary health care provider prescribes 1 tablet of Thyrolar-1 daily to the patient for treatment of hypothyroidism. How much of the drug liotrix (T_3) does the patient receive per day?

   2 1/2 mcg

SECTION II: APPLYING YOUR KNOWLEDGE

Activity E **CASE STUDY**

Miranda Higgs is a Caucasian female, 25 year of age, who presents to the physician's office today with complaints of weight gain, cold intolerance, sleepiness, and dry skin. The physician checks her TSH and diagnoses Ms. Higgs with hypothyroidism. She is given a prescription for levothyroxine (Synthroid) 50 mcg QD.

1. How should the nurse instruct Ms. Higgs to take the levothyroxine (Synthroid)?

   The nurse advises Ms. Higgs to take medication in the am, empty stomach, for full effect of absorption.

2. How long can it take for Ms. Higgs to see the effects of the levothyroxine (Synthroid)?

   She may not feel effects for several wks but could as soon as w/in 48 hrs.

SECTION III: PRACTICING FOR NCLEX

Activity F NCLEX-STYLE

Answer the following questions.

1. A patient is administered methimazole for the treatment of hyperthyroidism. Of which of the following adverse reactions to the drug should the nurse notify the primary health care provider?
   a. Tachycardia
   b. Agranulocytosis
   c. Weight loss
   d. Fatigue

2. A nurse is caring for a patient receiving thyroid hormones. The patient informs the nurse that he is also taking digoxin for a cardiac problem. What effect of drug interaction should the nurse observe in the patient?
   a. Decreased effectiveness of the cardiac drug
   b. Increased risk of prolonged bleeding
   c. Decreased effectiveness of the thyroid drug
   d. Increased potential for bleeding

3. A nurse is caring for a patient undergoing thyroid hormone therapy. What signs of therapeutic response should the nurse monitor after the thyroid hormone is administered to the patient?
   a. Agranulocytosis
   b. Headache
   c. Mild diuresis
   d. Loss of hair

4. A nurse is assessing a patient with hypothyroidism. Which of the following symptoms should the nurse document during the preadministration assessment? Select all that apply.
   a. Weight loss
   b. Cold intolerance
   c. Confusion
   d. Sweating
   e. Unsteady gait

5. A patient undergoing propylthiouracil drug therapy is discharged from the health care facility. What instruction should the nurse include in the teaching plan?
   a. Take the drug at regular intervals
   b. Take the drug before breakfast
   c. Record weight twice a week
   d. Notify the PHCP if palpitations occur
   e. Avoid taking the drug in larger doses

6. A patient with cardiovascular disease is administered thyroid hormones. Of which symptoms should the nurse notify the primary health care provider to reduce the patient's dosage of thyroid hormones?
   a. High fever
   b. Chest pain
   c. Sweating
   d. Headache

7. A patient is administered an antithyroid drug by the primary health care provider. What signs of thyroid storm should the nurse monitor for in the patient during the ongoing assessment?
   a. Nervousness
   b. Increased pulse rate
   c. Anxiety
   d. Altered mental status

8. A patient is prescribed an iodine procedure for the treatment of hyperthyroidism. What interventions should the nurse perform before administering the iodine procedure to the patient?
   a. Record history of allergies to seafood
   b. Monitor signs of agranulocytosis
   c. Assess patient for mouth infection
   d. Monitor patient's stool color

9. A patient is prescribed thyroid hormone therapy. In which of the following conditions of the patient is the drug contraindicated?
   a. Agranulocytosis
   b. Adrenal cortical insufficiency
   c. Granulocytopenia
   d. Hypoprothrombinemia

10. A health care provider administers thyroid hormone therapy to a patient. Which of the following signs of hyperthyroidism should the nurse report to the primary health care provider before the next dose is due? Select all that apply.

    a. Moist skin
    b. Easy bruising
    c. Moderate hypertension
    d. Increased appetite
    e. Sore throat

11. Which of the following is an essential element for the manufacturing of thyroxine and triiodothyronine?

    a. Iodine
    b. Sodium
    c. Hydrogen
    d. Potassium

12. Which of the following is the drug of choice for hypothyroidism because it is relatively inexpensive, requires once-a-day dosing, and has a more uniform potency than do other thyroid hormone replacement drugs?

    a. Propylthiouracil (PTU)
    b. Methimazole (Tapazole)
    c. Levothyroxine (Synthroid)
    d. Liotrix (Thyrolar)

13. When should the nurse advise a patient to take levothyroxine (Synthroid)?

    a. In the morning on an empty stomach
    b. In the morning on a full stomach
    c. In the evening on an empty stomach
    d. In the evening on a full stomach

14. A nurse should be cautious not to administer levothyroxine (Synthroid) to a patient who has recently had which of the following?

    a. Myocardial infarction
    b. Cataract surgery
    c. Seizure
    d. Hypoglycemic episode

15. Levothyroxine (Synthroid) is classified in which pregnancy category?

    a. Category A
    b. Category B
    c. Category C
    d. Category X

CHAPTER 46

Male and Female Hormones

Learning Objectives

- Discuss the medical uses, actions, adverse reactions, contraindications, precautions, and interactions of the male and female hormones
- Discuss important preadministration and ongoing assessment activities the nurse should perform with the patient taking male or female hormones
- List nursing diagnoses particular to a patient taking male or female hormones
- Discuss ways to promote an optimal response to therapy, how to manage adverse reactions, and important points to keep in mind when educating the patient about the use of male or female hormones

SECTION I: ASSESSING YOUR UNDERSTANDING

Activity A MATCHING

1. *Match the hormones and their related drugs in Column A with the conditions they are used for in Column B.*

Column A		Column B
1. Androgens	C	a. Anemia of renal insufficiency
2. Anabolic steroids	a	
3. Androgen hormone inhibitors	e	b. Endometriosis
		c. Male hypogonadism
4. Progestins	b	d. Atrophic vaginitis
5. Estrogens	d	e. Benign hypertrophy of the prostate

2. *Match the drugs used in hormonal therapy for cancer in Column A with their common adverse effects in Column B*

Column A		Column B
1. Mitotane	e	a. ECG changes
2. Testolactone	c	b. Hematuria
3. Goserelin acetate	d	c. Maculopapular erythema
4. Leuprolide acetate	a	d. Breast atrophy
5. Bicalutamide	b	e. Leukocytosis

Activity B FILL IN THE BLANKS

1. The age of onset of first menstruation is called **menarche**

2. Hormones produced by the body are called **endogenous** hormones.

3. **Catabolism** is called reverse tissue-depleting processes of the body.

4. The development of the **prostate** gland is dependent on the potent androgen 5(α)-dihydrotestosterone (DHT).

5. Testosterone and its derivatives are collectively called **androgens**.

Activity C SHORT ANSWERS

A nurse's role in managing patients who are receiving hormone therapy involves monitoring and implementing interventions that aid in recovery. Answer the following questions, which involve the nurse's role in the management of such situations.

1. A nurse is caring for a patient who is on androgen therapy. What assessments should the nurse implement when monitoring for excess fluid volume in the patient?

   Nurse should observe other signs of edema, from too much sodium, weight is important & should be noted before therapy, do weight daily basis important.

2. A nurse is educating a patient who plans to take oral contraceptives as a method of birth control. What points should the nurse include in the teaching plan when educating the patient regarding oral contraceptives?

   When to take it, carefully insert it, if pill missed take pills on those missed days 1 day take 1 pill 2 pills 2 pills etc, no smoking any headaches or problems contact provider.

Activity D DOSAGE CALCULATION

1. A female patient has been prescribed 20 mg of Halotestin (fluoxymesterone) per day as a palliative therapy for advanced inoperable breast cancer. How many of the 5-mg tablets does she need to take in a single dose?

   4 tablets

2. A patient with anemia weighing 30 kg has been prescribed 5 mg/kg of Anadrol-50 (oxymetholone) orally per day. Anadrol-50 is available as 50-mg tablets. How many of such tablets should the patient take each day?

   3 tablets

3. A patient with primary ovarian failure has been prescribed 1.5 mg of estropipate as a daily dose. How many of the Ortho-Est tablets (0.75 mg estropipate) should the nurse instruct the patient to take daily?

   2 tablets

4. A patient with endometriosis has been prescribed Aygestin (norethindrone acetate) to be taken at a dose of 5 mg/day for the first 2 weeks and 7.5 mg/day for the next 2 weeks. How many of the 5-mg tablets should the nurse instruct the patient to take during the third and the fourth week?

   1 1/2 tablets

5. A patient has been prescribed 200 mg of oral progesterone daily for the prevention of endometrial hyperplasia. How many of the 100-mg progesterone capsules should the patient take daily?

   2 capsules

6. A patient with prostate cancer weighing 75 kg has been prescribed 14 mg/kg/day of estramustine phosphate sodium in divided doses. How many of the 140-mg tablets does the patient need to take daily?

   7 1/2 tablets in a day

SECTION II: APPLYING YOUR KNOWLEDGE

Activity E CASE STUDY

Melissa Murphy is a Caucasian female, 21 years of age. She presents to the health clinic at the university she attends to obtain emergency contraception after contraceptive failure. She has no medical conditions and takes no medications.

1. It is important for the nurse to question a patient seeking emergency contraception about when the unprotected intercourse or contraceptive failure occurred, as emergency contraception needs to be taken soon after the event. How long after unprotected intercourse or contraceptive failure occurs should high-dose levonorgestrel (Plan B) be administered?

   High dose should be given w/in 72 hrs after unprotected intercourse or if birth control fails.

2. How should levonorgestrel (Plan B) be taken?

   First dose w/in 72 hrs, 2nd dose 12 hrs after if nausee and vomiting occurs w/in an hr later taken after dose provider should be contacted immediately.

SECTION III: PRACTICING FOR NCLEX

Activity F NCLEX-STYLE

Answer the following questions.

1. A patient has been prescribed androgen therapy. Which of the following conditions should the nurse consider to be an indication for such a prescription?
   a. Adrenal cortical cancer
   b. Testosterone deficiency
   c. Benign prostatic hypertrophy
   d. Male pattern baldness

2. Following a major road accident and disability 2 years ago, a patient had profound weight loss. The patient tells the nurse that he had been prescribed a certain drug to promote weight gain during that time. To which of the following groups should the nurse consider that the drug might have belonged?
   a. Androgen hormones
   b. Progestins
   c. Conjugate estrogens
   d. Anabolic steroids

3. A patient with obesity is receiving anticoagulant therapy as a prophylaxis for thromboembolism following an appendectomy. Which of the following interactions may be seen when androgens or androgen hormone inhibitors are used concomitantly in this patient?
   a. Increased antidiuretic effect
   b. Decreased anticoagulant effect
   c. Increased risk of hypoglycemia
   d. Increased risk of paranoia

4. A nurse caring for a male patient with hypogonadism who has been prescribed androgen therapy is required to educate the patient about the use of the drug and its possible adverse effects. Which of the following is an adverse effect of androgen therapy?
   a. Enlargement of testes
   b. Gynecomastia
   c. Virilization
   d. Frequent urination

5. A 44-year-old female patient complains of severe vasomotor symptoms of menopause such as hot flushes and excessive sweating. The patient is prescribed estrogen to treat menopausal symptoms along with a concurrent use of progestins. Which of the following is the reason for the concurrent use of progestins?
   a. Reduce GI irritation caused by estrogen
   b. Treat associated atrophic vaginitis
   c. Reduce risk of endometrial carcinoma
   d. Decrease risk of postmenopausal osteoporosis

6. A 46-year-old woman is experiencing symptoms of menopause and is taking black cohosh, a herb, to alleviate these symptoms. Concerning which of the following possible adverse effects of the herb should the nurse caution the patient?
   a. Low blood pressure
   b. Ringing in the ears
   c. Impaired vision
   d. Weight loss

7. A 30-year-old female patient arrives at the health care center complaining of abnormal uterine bleeding. Diagnosis indicates endometrial hyperplasia and the patient is prescribed Depo-Provera (medroxyprogesterone acetate). Which of the following should the nurse keep in mind when administering this drug?
   a. The drug is implanted in the subdermal tissue
   b. Drug is to be shaken vigorously before use
   c. First dose is given on the 10th day of a menstrual cycle
   d. The drug provides contraception for 5 years

8. A woman taking oral contraceptives has heard about health benefits associated with oral contraceptive use, apart from contraception, and is eager to know more about it. Which of the following risks are reduced with oral contraceptive use? Select all that apply.
   a. Iron-deficiency anemia
   b. Ovarian cancer
   c. Cervical erosion
   d. Osteoporosis
   e. Vaginal candidiasis

9. A 20-year-old woman taking oral contraceptives is anxious that she has missed 1 day's dose. Which of the following instructions should the nurse offer the patient?
   a. Discontinue the drug and use another form of birth control untilthe next cycle
   b. Take 2 tablets for the next 2 days and continue with the normal schedule
   c. Remember to take 1 tablet the next day and forget about the missed dose
   d. Take the missed dose as soon as remembered or take 2 tablets the next day

10. When educating a group of nursing students regarding the various female hormones, the nurse identifies which of the following hormones as a synthetic estrogen which is available only as a drug?
    a. Estradiol
    b. Estrone
    c. Estriol
    d. Estropipate

11. Which of the following is an example of an androgen hormone inhibitor that is used to treat patients with benign prostatic hypertrophy?
    a. Dutasteride (Avodart)
    b. Oxymetholone (Anadrol-50)
    c. Oxandrolone (Oxandrin)
    d. Methyltestosterone (Testred)

12. Which of the following is an example of an androgen that can be used to treat hypogonadism?
    a. Fluoxymesterone
    b. Nandrolone
    c. Dutasteride
    d. Oxymetholone

13. Which of the following medications can be used to treat anemia?
    a. Fluoxymesterone
    b. Oxymetholone
    c. Finasteride
    d. Dutasteride

14. Which of the following is an example of an anabolic steroid?
    a. Nandrolone
    b. Fluoxymesterone
    c. Testosterone
    d. Dutasteride

15. The androgen testosterone is available in several dosage forms. In which of the following routes is testosterone not able to be given?
    a. Intravenously
    b. Topically
    c. Orally
    d. Subcutaneously

Drugs Acting on the Uterus

- Discuss the actions, uses, adverse reactions, contraindications, precautions, and interactions of drugs acting on the uterus
- Discuss important preadministration and ongoing assessment activities the nurse should perform with the patient taking an oxytocic or tocolytic drug
- List some nursing diagnoses particular to a patient taking an oxytocic or tocolytic drug
- Discuss ways to promote an optimal response to therapy, how to manage adverse reactions, and important points to keep in mind when educating patients about the use of an oxytocic or tocolytic drug

SECTION I: ASSESSING YOUR UNDERSTANDING

Activity A MATCHING

1. **Match the drugs acting on the uterus in Column A with their adverse reactions in Column B.**

Column A	Column B
1. Indomethacin	a. Diplopia
2. Oxytocin	b. Anaphylactic reactions
3. Magnesium sulfate	c. Vertigo
4. Ritodrine hydrochloride	d. Hypokalemia
5. Terbutaline	e. Fluid in the lungs

2. *Match the drugs acting on the uterus in Column A with their contraindications in Column B.*

Column A

1. Tocolytics
2. Oxytocin
3. Ergonovine and methylergonovine
4. Magnesium sulfate
5. Indomethacin

Column B

a. Before delivery of placenta
b. Eclampsia
c. Cephalopelvic disproportion
d. With nonsteroidal anti-inflammatory drugs (NSAIDs)
e. Myocardial damage

Activity B FILL IN THE BLANKS

1. Oxytocic drugs are used antepartum to induce uterine _____.

2.

3. Oxytocin is an endogenous hormone produced by the _____ pituitary gland.

4.

5. A complication of pregnancy characterized by convulsive seizures and coma is known as _____.

6. Overdosage of ergonovine is known as _____.

7. Oxytocin leads to water intoxication due to its _____ effect.

Activity C SHORT ANSWERS

A nurse's role in managing patients who are being administered drugs acting on the uterus involves monitoring and implementing interventions that aid in recovery. Answer the following questions, which involve the nurse's role in the management of such situations.

1. A nurse is required to monitor the uterine contractions in a patient who is receiving oxytocin infusion. What conditions would alert the nurse to discontinue the oxytocin infusion?

   _____

   _____

2. What ongoing assessment should the nurse engage in when caring for a patient receiving tocolytic drugs?

   _____

   _____

Activity D DOSAGE CALCULATION

1. A doctor prescribes a patient 40 units of oxytocin in 1000 mL IV solution to induce labor. The available 1-mL ampoule contains 10 units of oxytocin. How many ampoules will the nurse need to administer to the patient in 1000 mL of IV solution?

   _____

   _____

2. A patient in preterm labor has been prescribed 2 g of magnesium sulfate intramuscularly. Each mL of the 50% solution for injection contains 0.5 g of magnesium sulfate. What volume of the solution should be administered to the patient?

   _____

   _____

3. A patient with postpartum bleeding has been prescribed 0.4 mg of methylergonovine maleate. The available methylergonovine maleate tablet is 0.2 mg. How many such tablets should the nurse administer to the patient?

   _____

   _____

4. A doctor prescribes 50 mg of indomethacin oral suspension to a patient in preterm labor. The available solution contains 25 mg of indomethacin per 5 ml. What volume of the solution should the nurse administer to the patient?

   _____

   _____

5. A doctor prescribes 0.25 mg of Brethine (terbutaline) to a patient in preterm labor. Each ampoule contains 1 mg of Brethine per 1 mL of solution. What volume of the available solution should the nurse administer to the patient?

   _____

   _____

6. A patient with postpartum bleeding has been prescribed 5 units of oxytocin. The available 1 mL ampoule contains 10 units of oxytocin. What volume of the solution should the nurse administer to the patient?

_____

_____

SECTION II: APPLYING YOUR KNOWLEDGE

Activity E CASE STUDY

Stella Stevens is an African American female, 25 years of age. She is admitted to the labor and delivery floor of the hospital to give birth to her first child. She is preeclamptic and the physician has ordered her to receive oxytocin (Pitocin) IV to induce labor.

1. Before the nurse starts the IV oxytocin (Pitocin), what information should be obtained from Mrs. Stevens?

_____

_____

2. Once the oxytocin (Pitocin) is started IV, for which adverse effects should the nurse monitor Mrs. Stevens?

_____

_____

SECTION III: PRACTICING FOR NCLEX

Activity F NCLEX-STYLE

Answer the following questions.

1. A 32-year-old woman has been prescribed oxytocin intranasally to stimulate the milk ejection reflex. In which of the following positions should the nurse place the patient when administering oxytocin intranasally?
   a. Upright position
   b. Supine position
   c. Lateral position
   d. Standing position

2. A patient is receiving oxytocin to induce labor and is concerned about the use of the drug. Which of the following interventions should the nurse implement to help alleviate the patient's anxiety? Select all that apply.
   a. Explain the purpose of the IV infusion
   b. Do not inform the patient of the expected outcome
   c. Administer an antianxiety drug to the patient
   d. Offer encouragement and reassurance
   e. Spend time with the patient

3. A patient has been administered ergonovine after expulsion of the placenta following childbirth. The nurse observes that the patient's uterus is not responding well to the drug. Which of the following interventions is most appropriate in this situation?
   a. Increase the dosage of the drug
   b. Administer magnesium sulfate by IV injection
   c. Administer calcium by IV injection
   d. Administer terbutaline by SC route

4. A pregnant woman in her 28th week of gestation is admitted to a health care center with preterm labor. In which of the following conditions is magnesium sulfate contraindicated?
   a. Cephalopelvic disproportion
   b. Hypertension
   c. Total placenta previa
   d. Eclampsia

5. A 31-year-old patient in her 28th week of gestation is experiencing preterm labor. The patient has been administered IV magnesium sulfate to prolong the pregnancy. Which of the following factors has to be monitored by the nurse when administering tocolytics?
   a. Urine output
   b. Pedal edema
   c. Cardiac function
   d. Vaginal bleeding

6. A 32-year-old pregnant woman is admitted to a hospital with labor pains. The patient is prescribed ergonovine during the third stage of labor after the placenta has been delivered. In which of the following conditions is this drug strictly contraindicated?

   a. Renal disease
   b. During lactation
   c. Heart disease
   d. Hypertension

7. A nurse is advised to administer methylergonovine to a patient with postpartum hemorrhaging. Which of the following nursing interventions should the nurse implement when administering the drug? Select all that apply.

   a. Monitor vital signs every 4 hours
   b. Discontinue the drug if the patient develops severe cramping
   c. Notify the health care provider if abdominal cramping is severe
   d. Note character and amount of vaginal bleeding
   e. Place the patient in a lateral position

8. When caring for a pregnant patient, the nurse observes signs of excess fluid volume in the patient. Which of the following drugs leads to the danger of an excessive fluid volume (water intoxication)?

   a. Oxytocin
   b. Ergonovine
   c. Magnesium sulfate
   d. Methylergonovine

9. When caring for a pregnant woman receiving ergonovine to increase uterine contractions during labor, the nurse is required to monitor for signs and symptoms of ergotism. Which of the following symptoms are manifestations of ergotism? Select all that apply.

   a. Dyspnea
   b. Diplopia
   c. Hallucinations
   d. Water intoxication
   e. Tachycardia

10. A patient in her 28th week of gestation is experiencing preterm labor and is prescribed magnesium sulfate. Which of the following is the property of magnesium sulfate?

   a. It is a calcium antagonist
   b. It blocks the production of prostaglandins
   c. It has an antidiuretic action
   d. It acts as a uterine stimulant

11. Which of the following is used antepartum to induce uterine contractions?

   a. Oxytocin (Pitocin)
   b. Ritodrine (Yutopar)
   c. Indomethacin (Indocin)
   d. Terbutaline (Brethine)

12. Oxytocin is an endogenous hormone produced by which of the following?

   a. Adrenal gland
   b. Posterior pituitary gland
   c. Uterus
   d. Corpus luteum

13. How would the nurse administer oxytocin (Pitocin) to a patient to stimulate the milk ejection reflex?

   a. Intranasally
   b. Topically
   c. Intramuscularly
   d. Orally

14. A nurse should monitor a patient receiving oxytocin (Pitocin) for which of the following adverse effects?

   a. Cardiac arrhythmias
   b. Hypotension
   c. Headache
   d. Dizziness

15. Which of the following is an adverse effect caused by all uterine stimulants because of their antidiuretic effect?

   a. Dehydration
   b. Hypotension
   c. Water intoxication
   d. Polydipsia

Diuretics

- List the 5 general types of diuretics
- Discuss the uses, general drug actions, adverse reactions, contraindications, precautions, and interactions of the diuretics
- Describe important preadministration and ongoing assessment activities the nurse should perform with the patient taking a diuretic
- List nursing diagnoses particular to a patient taking a diuretic
- Discuss ways to promote an optimal response to therapy, how to manage common adverse reactions, and important points to keep in mind when educating patients about the use of diuretics

SECTION I: ASSESSING YOUR UNDERSTANDING

Activity A MATCHING

1. *Match the diuretics in Column A with their uses in Column B.*

Column A

1. Ethacrynic acid
2. Mannitol
3. Urea
4. Amiloride
5. Metolazone

Column B

a. Treatment of cerebral edema

b. Reduction of intracranial pressure

c. Prevention of polyuria with lithium use

d. Hypertension, edema due to CHF, cirrhosis, corticosteroid and estrogen therapy

e. Short-term management of ascites caused by lymphedema

2. *Match the interactant loop diuretic with their interactant drugs in Column A with the results given in Column B.*

Column A	Column B
1. Loop diuretics + thrombolytics	**a.** Increased risk of lithium toxicity
2. Loop diuretics + lithium	**b.** Increased risk of arrhythmias
3. Loop diuretics + aminoglycosides	**c.** Increased risk of bleeding
4. Loop diuretics + digitalis	**d.** Increased risk of ototoxicity

Activity B FILL IN THE BLANKS

1. Retention of excess fluid in the tissue or body is known as _____.

2. _____ anhydrase inhibition, which is the action of a diuretic drug, results in the excretion of sodium, potassium, bicarbonate, and water.

3. Increase in the _____ in the blood is known as hyperkalemia.

4. Extremity _____, meaning numbness, tingling or flaccid muscles, may indicate hypokalemia, which is an adverse reaction to diuretics.

5. _____ reactions to diuretics involve rash and photosensitivity.

Activity C SHORT ANSWERS

A nurse's role in managing patients who are prescribed a diuretic involves performing preadministrative and ongoing assessments during the course of the drug therapy. The nurse also monitors the patients administered with diuretic drugs for the occurrence of any adverse reactions. Answer the following questions which involve the nurse's role in the management of patients on diuretic drug therapy.

1. A patient with edema is prescribed a diuretic drug. What preadministration assessments should the nurse perform before administration of this diuretic drug?

_____

_____

2. What is the nurse's role after the administration of a diuretic drug to a patient?

_____

_____

Activity D DOSAGE CALCULATION

1. A patient with edema has been prescribed acetazolamide. The physician instructs the nurse to administer 250 mg of the drug every 4 hours. The drug is available in 500-mg tablets. How many tablets should the nurse administer to the patient daily?

_____

_____

2. A patient with glaucoma is undergoing methazolamide drug therapy. The physician has prescribed the patient 100 mg of the drug to be taken twice in a day. How many tablets should the nurse administer if the drug is available in 50-mg tablets?

_____

_____

3. A patient with edema due to cirrhosis of the liver has been prescribed 6 mg bumetanide (Bumex) on a daily basis. The drug is available in 2-mg tablets. How many tablets should the nurse administer the client every day?

_____

_____

4. A physician has prescribed 500 mg of chlorothiazide (Diuril) for a patient to be taken twice a day. The physician has instructed the nurse to administer the drug through the IV route. The drug is available in the form of 250 mg of chlorothiazide per 5 mL. How much solution should the nurse prepare for this patient per day?

_____

_____

5. A patient has been prescribed 200 mg of furosemide (Lasix) per day by the physician. On-hand availability of the drug is 80-mg tablets. How many tablets should the nurse administer the patient every day?

_____

_____

SECTION II: APPLYING YOUR KNOWLEDGE

Activity E CASE STUDY

Richard Morton is an African American male, 70 years of age. He is admitted to the hospital for treatment of significant edema associated with heart failure. The physician has ordered furosemide (Lasix) IV 1 mg/kg Q6 hours.

1. If Mr. Morton weighs 150 lb, how many mL should the nurse administer every 6 hours if furosemide (Lasix) is available in a 20 mg/mL vial?

   _____

   _____

2. During the administration of furosemide (Lasix), for what adverse reactions should the nurse observe Mr. Morton?

   _____

   _____

SECTION III: PRACTICING FOR NCLEX

Activity F NCLEX-STYLE

Answer the following questions.

1. A nurse is caring for a patient with edema. What assessments should the nurse perform on this patient to promote optimal response to therapy? Select all that apply.
   a. Measure and record patient's weight daily
   b. Check the pupils every 2 hours for dilation
   c. Measure fluid intake and output every 8 hours
   d. Assess respiratory rate every 4 hours
   e. Check the patient's response to light

2. A nurse is caring for a patient receiving diuretics. During assessment, the nurse observes that the patient is experiencing a GI upset after taking the prescribed drug. Which of the following interventions should the nurse perform when caring for this patient?
   a. Ensure that the drug is taken on an empty stomach
   b. Ensure that the drug is taken with food or milk

   c. Instruct the patient to reduce fluid intake
   d. Avoid any consumption of fibrous food by the patient

3. A nurse is caring for a patient with edema due to congestive heart failure (CHF). The physician has prescribed a spironolactone drug to the patient. Which of the following adverse reactions to the drug should the nurse monitor for in the patient?
   a. Vertigo
   b. Paresthesias
   c. Hyperkalemia
   d. Anorexia

4. A physician has prescribed a chlorothiazide drug to a patient with hypertension. The patient informs the nurse that he is also taking an antidiabetic drug for controlling diabetes. What effect of the interaction between these two drugs should the nurse monitor for in the patient?
   a. Increased risk of ototoxicity
   b. Increased risk of hyperglycemia
   c. Increased hypersensitivity to antidiabetic
   d. Increased chlorothiazide effect

5. A primary health care provider has prescribed treatment with an antihypertensive drug along with a diuretic to a patient as a treatment for hypertension. The patient informs the nurse about his preference for herbal extracts over medical drugs. What information regarding herbal extracts should the nurse provide to the patient? Select all that apply.
   a. No herbal diuretic should be taken unless approved by the PHCP
   b. Some herbal extracts have been associated with renal damage
   c. Herbal extracts are more effective than caffeine
   d. Most plant and herbal extracts available as diuretics are nontoxic
   e. After consulting the PHCP, consume diuretic teas like juniper berries

6. A nurse is caring for a patient showing signs of excess fluid retention. The nurse knows that which of the following has caused this condition in the patient?
   a. Endocrine disturbances
   b. Hyperkalemia
   c. Hematological changes
   d. Gastric distress

7. A nurse is caring for a patient with renal dysfunction. The physician has prescribed a metolazone drug for the patient. What should the nurse monitor in the patient before administering the drug? Select all that apply.
   a. Serum potassium levels
   b. Levels of serum electrolytes
   c. Fluid loss every hour
   d. Creatinine clearance levels
   e. Blood urea nitrogen level

8. A nurse is caring for a patient who complains of cramps and muscle pains. Assessment reveals that the patient is also experiencing oliguria, hypotension, and GI disturbances. Which of the following conditions is the patient experiencing?
   a. Hyperkalemia
   b. Electrolyte imbalance
   c. Hypercalcemia
   d. Hyponatremia

9. A patient is prescribed amiloride (Midamor), a potassium-sparing diuretic, by the physician. In which of the following conditions should the nurse discontinue the drug?
   a. If the patient experiences gout attacks
   b. If the patient's urine tests positive for glucose
   c. If patient's serum potassium levels exceed 5.3 mEq/mL
   d. If excess fluid has been removed from the patient's body

10. Which of the following is an example of a loop diuretic?
    a. Furosemide (Lasix)
    b. Hydrochlorothiazide (Microzide)
    c. Acetazolamide (Diamox)
    d. Spironolactone (Aldactone)

11. Which of the following diuretics exerts its effect by inhibiting the enzyme carbonic anhydrase?
    a. Furosemide (Lasix)
    b. Acetazolamide (Diamox)
    c. Hydrochlorothiazide (Microzide)
    d. Spironolactone (Aldactone)

12. Which of the following exerts its diuretic effects by increasing the density of the filtrate in the glomerulus?
    a. Mannitol (Osmitrol)
    b. Furosemide (Lasix)
    c. Hydrochlorothiazide (Microzide)
    d. Spironolactone (Aldactone)

13. Which of the following exerts its diuretic effect by antagonizing the action of aldosterone?
    a. Spironolactone (Aldactone)
    b. Furosemide (Lasix)
    c. Hydrochlorothiazide (Microzide)
    d. Acetazolamide (Diamox)

14. Which of the following exerts its effects by depressing the reabsorption of sodium in the kidney tubules, thereby increasing sodium and water excretion?
    a. Furosemide (Lasix)
    b. Hydrochlorothiazide (Microzide)
    c. Acetazolamide (Diamox)
    d. Triamterene (Dyrenium)

15. Which of the following exerts its diuretic effect by inhibiting the reabsorption of sodium and chloride ions in the ascending portion of the loop of Henle and the early distal tubule of the nephron?
    a. Hydrochlorothiazide (Microzide)
    b. Acetazolamide (Diamox)
    c. Furosemide (Lasix)
    d. Spironolactone (Aldactone)

CHAPTER 49

Urinary Tract Anti-Infectives, Antispasmodics, and Other Urinary Drugs

Learning Objectives

- Discuss the uses, general drug actions, adverse reactions, contraindications, precautions, and interactions of the drugs used to treat infections and symptoms associated with urinary tract infections or an overactive bladder
- Discuss important preadministration and ongoing assessment activities the nurse should perform with the patient taking a drug for a urinary tract infection or an overactive bladder
- List nursing diagnoses particular to a patient taking a drug for a urinary tract infection or an overactive bladder
- Discuss ways to promote an optimal response to therapy, how to manage adverse reactions, and important points to keep in mind when educating patients about the use of drugs used to treat a urinary tract infection or symptoms associated with an overactive bladder

SECTION I: ASSESSING YOUR UNDERSTANDING

Activity A MATCHING

1. *Match the urinary drugs in Column A with their uses in Column B.*

Column A	Column B
1. Amoxicillin	a. Acute bacterial UTIs
2. Nitrofurantoin	b. Acute bacterial urinary tract infections (UTIs), other bacterial infections
3. Oxybutynin	c. Relief of pain associated with irritation of the lower genitourinary tract
4. Phenazopyridine	d. Overactive bladder, neurogenic bladder

2. *Match the anti-infectives with the interactant drugs in Column A with their effects on the anti-infective drugs in Column B.*

Column A

1. Anti-infective + anticholinergics
2. Anti-infective + metoclopramide
3. Anti-infective + oral anticoagulants
4. Anti-infective + magnesium trisilicate or magaldrate

Column B

a. Lowers plasma concentration and urinary tract excretion of fosfomycin
b. Decreased absorption of anti-infective
c. Delay in gastric emptying
d. Increased risk for bleeding

Activity B FILL IN THE BLANKS

1. Clinical manifestations of _____ include urgency, frequency, pressure, burning, and pain on urination.

2. _____ drugs counteract the smooth muscle spasm of the urinary tract by relaxing the detrusor and other muscles through action at the parasympathetic nerve receptors.

3. _____ bladder is an impaired bladder function caused by a nervous system abnormality, typically an injury to the spinal cord.

4. Excessive urination caused during the night is called _____.

5. _____ incontinence is characterized by involuntary urination after sudden sensation to void.

Activity C SHORT ANSWERS

A nurse's role in managing patients who are being administered urinary tract anti-infectives, antispasmodics, and other urinary drugs involves monitoring the patients and implementing interventions that aid in their recovery. Answer the following questions, which involve the nurse's role in the management of such situations.

1. A nurse has been caring for a patient with UTI. Post treatment, the nurse has to evaluate the effectiveness of the treatment plan. What factors should the nurse consider to determine the success of the treatment plan?

_____

_____

_____

2. A patient with UTI is undergoing an anti-infective drug therapy. What instructions should the nurse offer the patient and the patient's family to ensure compliance with the medication regimen?

_____

_____

_____

Activity D DOSAGE CALCULATIONS

1. A patient with acute bacterial urinary tract infections has been prescribed 500 mg of amoxicillin to be administered every 8 hours. On-hand availability of the drug is 500-mg tablets. How many tablets should the nurse administer the patient daily?

_____

_____

2. A patient with acute cystitis has been prescribed 6 g of fosfomycin to be taken with food daily. The drug therapy has to continue for 5 days. The drug is available in 3-g tablets. How many tablets should the nurse administer to the patient in 5 days?

_____

_____

3. A patient has been prescribed 1 g of methenamine to be administered orally twice in a day. The treatment has to be continued for 4 days. On-hand availability of the drug is 1-g tablets. How many tablets should the nurse administer in 4 days?

_____

_____

4. A patient has been prescribed nitrofurantoin for acute bacterial UTI. The physician has prescribed 200 mg of the drug to taken 4 times a day. The drug is available as 100-mg capsules in the pharmacy. How many capsules should the nurse administer the patient in a day?

_____

_____

SECTION II: APPLYING YOUR KNOWLEDGE

Activity E CASE STUDY

Stacey Anthony is a Caucasian female, 30 years of age. She presents to the physician's office with complaints of dysuria, oliguria, and increased frequency. After examining Ms. Anthony and interpreting her urinalysis, the physician diagnoses her with a urinary tract infection. The physician gives her a prescription for nitrofurantoin (Macrobid) 50 mg × 7 days.

1. Prior to leaving the office what adverse reactions should the nurse discuss with Ms. Anthony?

_____

_____

_____

2. What nonpharmacological measures should the nurse discuss with Ms. Anthony?

_____

_____

_____

SECTION III: PRACTICING FOR NCLEX

Activity F NCLEX-STYLE

Answer the following questions.

1. A nurse is caring for a patient with an overactive bladder who has been prescribed darifenacin HCl (Enablex) drug. The drug is known to cause dry mouth. What instructions should the nurse offer the patient to get relief from dry mouth?
   a. Suck on sugarless lozenges
   b. Refrain from consuming hard candy
   c. Consume foods rich in fiber
   d. Always take the drug with milk

2. A nurse is caring for a patient receiving solifenacin drug therapy for the treatment of an overactive bladder. What adverse reaction to the drug should the nurse monitor for in the patient?
   a. Headache
   b. Dry eyes
   c. Pruritus
   d. Rash

3. A patient with acute bacterial urinary tract infections is undergoing sulfamethoxazole drug therapy. The patient is also receiving an oral anticoagulant as a blood thinner. What condition should the nurse monitor in this patient as a result of the interaction of the two drugs?
   a. Increased risk of bleeding
   b. Urinary tract excretion of the anti-infective
   c. Delay in gastric emptying
   d. Decreased effect of sulfamethoxazole

4. A nurse is required to initiate antispasmodic drug therapy. For which of the following patients is the use of antispasmodics contraindicated?
   a. A patient with convulsive disorders
   b. A patient with cerebral arteriosclerosis
   c. A patient with myasthenia gravis
   d. A patient with a hepatic impairment

5. A nurse is caring for a patient who has been prescribed a urinary anti-infective. What interventions should the nurse perform when administering the drug to decrease the pain experienced by the patient on voiding?
   a. Administer the drug strictly with milk
   b. Administer the drug after meals
   c. Administer the drug with prune juice
   d. Ensure drug administration with warm water

6. A nurse is caring for a patient receiving a phenazopyridine drug for the treatment of irritation of the lower genitourinary tract. The patient is also receiving an antibacterial drug for UTI. What intervention should the nurse perform when administering phenazopyridine in combination with an antibacterial drug?
   a. Encourage patient to drink at least 2000 ml of fluid daily
   b. Administer the drug with cranberry or prune juice
   c. Avoid administering phenazopyridine for more than 2 days
   d. Administer phenazopyridine 2 hours before giving the antibacterial drug

7. A nurse is caring for a patient receiving flavoxate for the treatment of urinary problems. During assessment, the patient complains of constipation. What intervention should the nurse perform when caring for this patient?
   a. Increase the patient's intake of fluids
   b. Increase the patient's intake of citrus fruits
   c. Decrease the patient's consumption of milk products
   d. Administer the drug to the patient with warm water

8. A nurse is caring for a patient receiving nitrofurantoin urinary tract anti-infective at a health care facility. What nursing intervention should the nurse perform to prevent irritation in the stomach?
   a. Administer the drug with apple juice
   b. Administer the drug with milk
   c. Administer the drug at bedtime
   d. Administer the drug 1 hour before meals

9. A nurse is caring for a patient who has been prescribed a urinary tract anti-infective for the treatment of UTI. What preadministration assessments should the nurse perform when caring for the patient? Select all that apply.
   a. Question the patient regarding symptoms of infection
   b. Assess the patient for urinary frequency and bladder distention
   c. Take and record the vital signs of the patient
   d. Constantly monitor the patient's body temperature
   e. Assist in performing periodic urinalysis and culture test

10. A nurse at a health care facility is caring for a patient who has been prescribed anti-infective drug therapy for acute otitis media. For which of the following patients should the nurse use the prescribed drug cautiously?
   a. A patient with GI infections
   b. A patient with urinary retention
   c. A patient with renal impairment
   d. A patient with hypertension

11. Which of the following exerts a topical analgesic effect on the lining of the urinary tract?
   a. Phenazopyridine (Pyridium)
   b. Flavoxate (Urispas)
   c. Amoxicillin (Amoxil)
   d. Methenamine (Urex)

12. The use of nitrofurantoin (Macrobid) has been known to cause acute and chronic reactions in which of the following systems?
   a. Cardiovascular
   b. Digestive
   c. Respiratory
   d. Nervous

13. The nurse should advise patients taking phenazopyridine (Pyridium) that their urine may become discolored. Which of the following colors might it become?
   a. Brown
   b. Blue
   c. Purple
   d. Green

14. The nurse should not administer nalidixic (NegGram) to patients with which of the following?

   a. Convulsion disorders

   b. Rheumatoid arthritis

   c. Depression

   d. Asthma

15. It is important for the nurse to obtain an allergy history before administering an anti-infective because patients who are allergic to tartrazine should not take which of the following?

   a. Amoxicillin (Amoxil)

   b. Methenamine (Hiprex)

   c. Ciprofloxacin (Cipro)

   d. Nitrofurantoin (Macrobid)

CHAPTER 50

Immunologic Agents

Learning Objectives

- Discuss humoral immunity and cell-mediated immunity
- Distinguish between and define the different types of immunity
- Discuss the use of vaccines, toxoids, immune globulins, and antivenins to provide immunity against disease
- Discuss preadministration and ongoing assessments the nurse should perform with the patient receiving an immunologic agent
- Identify nursing diagnoses particular to a patient receiving an immunologic agent
- Discuss ways to promote an optimal response, management of common adverse reactions, special considerations, and important points to keep in mind when educating a patient taking an immunologic agent

SECTION I: ASSESSING YOUR UNDERSTANDING

Activity A MATCHING

1. *Match the generic name of immune globulins in Column A with their trade name in Column B.*

Column A	Column B
1. Botulism immune globulin	a. CytoGam
2. Cytomegalo virus immune globulin	b. Atgam
3. Immune globulin intravenous	c. BabyBIG
4. Lymphocyte immune globulin	d. Gamimune N
5. Rabies immune globulin	e. Bay Rab

2. *Match the terms associated with immunity in Column A with their definitions in Column B.*

Column A

1. Active immunity
2. Passive immunity
3. Toxin
4. Vaccine
5. Globulins

Column B

a. Injection of ready-made antibodies
b. Attenuated or killed antigen
c. Protein present in blood serum or plasma
d. Poisonous substance produced by some bacteria
e. Use of agents to stimulate antibody formation

Activity B FILL IN THE BLANKS

1. When salicylates are administered with varicella vaccine, there is an increased risk of developing _____ syndrome.

2. _____ acquired active immunity occurs when an individual is given a weakened antigen which stimulates the formation of antibodies.

3. _____ injection is administered as an additional dose of vaccine, to enhance the production of antibodies so that the desired level of immunity is maintained.

4. _____ refers to the ability of the body to identify and resist microorganisms that are potentially harmful.

5. _____ mediated immunity depends on the actions of the T lymphocytes.

Activity C SHORT ANSWERS

A nurse's role in managing patients receiving an immunologic agent involves diagnosis, planning and implementation. Answer the following questions, which involve the nurse's role in the management of such cases.

1. What information should the nurse document when preparing the patient's chart or form provided by the institution?

2. What information should the nurse include in the teaching plan when educating the parents of a child receiving a vaccination?

Activity D DOSAGE CALCULATIONS

1. A doctor prescribes an immunizing dose of 0.5 mL of meningococcal vaccine to a patient as part of a routine immunization program. After reconstitution, the solution becomes 8 mL. What amount of reconstituted solution is left in the vial after injecting the prescribed dose to the patient?

2. A single vial of PNEUMOVAX 23 contains 3 mL of the vaccine solution. The nurse administers 0.5 mL of the solution subcutaneously to each patient. How many patients can be vaccinated using a single vial?

3. The diluent for a single dose of *Haemophilus influenzae* vaccine is available as 0.6 mL per ampoule. How many mL of diluent are necessary to prepare 5 doses of *Haemophilus influenzae* vaccine?

4. A nurse has been advised to inject 0.5 mL of reconstituted hepatitis B vaccine solution. The diluent supplied is 0.6 mL and the vaccine in the vial is 0.25 mL. How many mL of the reconstituted solution are left in the syringe after injecting the prescribed dose?

_____

_____

5. A doctor prescribes 0.5 mL of a single-dose poliovirus vaccine for each patient to be given IM. The available vaccine solution after reconstitution is 4 mL. For how many patients can the vial be used?

_____

_____

6. A patient has been prescribed 250 units of tetanus immune globulin. The available 7.5 mL ampoule contains 3750 units of tetanus immune globulin. What volume of the solution should the nurse administer to the patient?

_____

_____

SECTION II: APPLYING YOUR KNOWLEDGE

Activity E CASE STUDY

Susan Surles is a Caucasian female, 11 years of age. She presents to the physician's office for her yearly sports physical. Her mother asked the physician if Susan can receive the human papillomavirus vaccine (Gardasil) today. The physician agrees and asks the nurse to administer the vaccine to Susan.

1. Immunization is what form of immunity?

_____

_____

2. What information does the nurse need to document in Susan's chart after administering the human papillomavirus vaccine (Gardasil)?

_____

_____

SECTION III: PRACTICING FOR NCLEX

Activity F NCLEX-STYLE

Answer the following questions.

1. In Japan, lentinan, a derivative of the shiitake mushroom, is used by health care providers for general health maintenance. Which of the following are possible health benefits of this herb? Select all that apply.

a. Boosts the body's immune system

b. Helps in lowering blood cholesterol levels

c. Prolongs the survival time of patients with cancer

d. Reduces the risks of heart diseases

e. Helps in lowering blood pressure

2. A nurse is educating a group of nursing students about the health benefits of the shiitake mushroom. Which of the following is the recommended dose of the shiitake mushroom?

a. 1 to 5 capsules daily

b. 10 fresh shiitake mushrooms

c. 1 dropper 8 times a day

d. 12 cups of shiitake juice per day

3. When educating patients on immunologic agents, the nurse identifies which of the following white blood cells that plays a major role in maintaining humoral immunity?

a. Neutrophil

b. Eosinophil

c. Lymphocyte

d. Basophil

4. When educating nursing students about vaccines, the nurse explains that in which of the following cases can vaccines and toxoids be administered to humans? Select all that apply.

a. Routine immunization of infants and children

b. Adults at high risk for certain diseases

c. Immunization of pregnant women against rubella

d. Immunization of adults against tetanus

e. Immunization of children and adults with leukemia

5. A patient was rushed to a hospital following a rattlesnake bite. The nurse was advised to inject antivenins. Antivenin injections should be administered within which of the following time periods to yield the most effective response?

   a. Within 7 hours
   b. Within 6 hours
   c. Within 5 hours
   d. Within 4 hours

6. A nurse is caring for a patient with chickenpox. Which of the following is a late complication of chickenpox about which a nurse should alert the patient?

   a. Reye syndrome
   b. Acute renal failure
   c. Herpes zoster
   d. Hepatitis

7. A patient traveling to South Africa and India is concerned about endemic diseases and is eager to know about any vaccination to prevent such diseases. Which of the following diseases are preventable by vaccination before traveling to endemic areas? Select all that apply.

   a. Typhoid
   b. Cholera diphtheria
   c. Tetanus
   d. Yellow fever
   e. Rubella

8. A child complains of pain at the injection site following the administration of the measles vaccine. Which of the following interventions should a nurse implement for pain management following vaccine administration? Select all that apply.

   a. Administer acetaminophen
   b. Massage the injection site
   c. Decrease fluid intake
   d. Encourage adequate rest
   e. Apply warm or cool compresses

9. When educating a group of nursing students on vaccines, the nurse identifies which of the following conditions as requiring vaccines to be administered with caution?

   a. Lactation
   b. Lymphoma
   c. Non-localized cancer
   d. Leukemia

10. A patient is advised to stay in the clinic for observation for about 30 minutes after administering an immunologic agent. Which of the following signs should a nurse assess to identify hypersensitivity reaction? Select all that apply.

    a. Pruritus
    b. Laryngeal edema
    c. Dyspnea
    d. Renal failure
    e. Convulsions

11. Cell-mediated immunity depends on which of the following?

    a. The action of B lymphocytes
    b. Antigen-antibody response
    c. The action of T lymphocytes
    d. Globulin production

12. Which of the following is responsible for a delayed-type immune response?

    a. B lymphocytes
    b. Macrophages
    c. Antibodies
    d. T lymphocytes

13. The administration of immunizations to a patient is a form of what type of immunity?

    a. Artificial active immunity
    b. Naturally active immunity
    c. Passive active immunity
    d. Attenuated active immunity

14. The administration of immune globulins or antivenins to a patient is a form of what type of immunity?

    a. Artificial immunity
    b. Natural immunity
    c. Passive immunity
    d. Attenuated immunity

15. The nurse must administer which of the following to a patient prior to exposure to the disease-causing organism in order for the patient to be protected against the disease?

    a. Toxoids
    b. Immune globulins
    c. Antivenins
    d. Antibodies

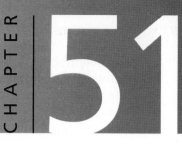

Antineoplastic Drugs

Learning Objectives

- List the types of drugs used in the treatment of neoplastic diseases
- Discuss the uses, general drug actions, general adverse reactions, contraindications, precautions, and interactions of the antineoplastic drugs
- Discuss important preadministration and ongoing assessment activities the nurse should perform with the patient taking antineoplastic drugs
- List nursing diagnoses particular to a patient taking antineoplastic drugs
- Discuss ways to promote an optimal response to therapy, how to manage common adverse reactions, and important points to keep in mind when educating patients about the use of an antineoplastic drug

SECTION I: ASSESSING YOUR UNDERSTANDING

Activity A MATCHING

1. *Match the terms in Column A with their corresponding meaning in Column B.*

Column A	Column B
1. Alopecia	a. Relief of symptoms at the end of life
2. Metastasis	b. Loss of hair
3. Palliation	c. Capable of soft tissue necrosis
4. Vesicant	d. Inflammation of the mouth
5. Stomatitis	e. Spread of cancer to other sites

2. *Match the phases of cell growth in Column A with their corresponding characteristics in Column B.*

Column A	Column B
1. G_1	a. DNA is prepared
2. S	b. Mitotic cell division
3. G_2	c. RNA and proteins are built
4. M	d. Dormant or resting phase
5. G_0	e. Preparing for cell division

Activity B FILL IN THE BLANKS

1. _____ cells appear to be more suscepti-ble to the effects of alkylating drugs than normal cells.

2. Interference with the bone marrow's ability to make new cells is called _____.

3. Patients with _____ have a decreased resistance to infection.

4. _____ consists of a red, warm, and sometimes painful area on the skin.

5. _____ refers to therapy with antineo-plastic drugs.

Activity C SHORT ANSWERS

A nurse's role in managing patients undergoing antineoplastic drug therapy involves not just the treatment or the cause for treatment, but also managing the effects produced by a partic-ular adverse reaction due to the treatment. Answer the following questions, which involve the nurse's role in caring for a patient undergo-ing antineoplastic drug therapy.

1. A nurse is caring for a patient who has been undergoing chemotherapy. What factors determine the nursing care in a patient receiving antineoplastic drugs?

2. A nurse is assigned to care for patients to be administered chemotherapy in a health care facility. What guidelines should the nurse fol-low when caring for patients receiving chemotherapeutic drugs?

Activity D DOSAGE CALCULATIONS

1. A patient has been prescribed vincristine sul-fate IV for treatment of acute leukemia. The dosage indicated is 4 mg. The drug is avail-able as Vincristine Sulfate Injection (Oncovin) in 2-mL vials and each mL contains vin-cristine sulfate 1 mg. How many vials should the nurse administer to the patient?

2. A patient is to receive 50 mg vinorelbine tartrate IV for the treatment of non–small-cell lung cancer (NSCLC). The drug is available as Navelbine Injection in 1 mL vials containing 10 mg vinorelbine tartare in water for injec-tion. How many vials should the nurse administer to the patient?

3. 60 mg of docetaxel IV is to be administered to a patient being treated for solid prostate tumor. The drug is available as Taxotere (doc-etaxel) Injection Concentrate in single-dose vials containing 20 mg (0.5 mL) docetaxel (anhydrous). Each mL contains 40 mg doc-etaxel (anhydrous). How many vials should the nurse administer to the patient?

4. A patient has been prescribed etoposide for the treatment of small-cell lung cancer (SCLC). The dosage indicated is 100 mg. The drug is available as VePesid 50-mg pink capsules. How many capsules should the nurse administer to the patient?

5. A patient is to receive 80 mg irinotecan hydrochloride IV for the treatment of a rectal tumor. The drug is available as Camptosar Injection in 2 mL vials containing 40 mg irinotecan. Each mL of solution contains 20 mg of irinotecan hydrochloride. How many vials should the nurse administer to the patient?

6. Thirty mg of methotrexate is to be adminis-tered to a patient being treated for severe psoriasis. The drug is available as Trexall (methotrexate) tablets for oral administration. Each tablet contains methotrexate sodium in an amount equivalent to 7.5-mg strength. How many tablets should the nurse adminis-ter to the patient?

SECTION II: APPLYING YOUR KNOWLEDGE

Activity E CASE STUDY

Antonia Lopez is an Hispanic female, 43 years of age. Mrs. Lopez was recently diagnosed with carcinoma of the breast. She is receiving chemotherapy with vincristine (Oncovin).

1. What class of antineoplastics is vincristine (Oncovin) in and what is its mechanism of action?

   _____

   _____

   _____

2. Following the administration of vincristine (Oncovin) to Mrs. Lopez, on what factors does the nurse base the ongoing assessment?

   _____

   _____

   _____

SECTION III: PRACTICING FOR NCLEX

Activity F NCLEX-STYLE

Answer the following questions.

1. A nurse is caring for a patient who has been receiving chemotherapy for breast cancer. The patient wants to know why chemotherapy is administered in a series of cycles. Which of the following should the nurse tell the patient? Select all that apply.
   a. To allow for recovery of the normal cells
   b. To release antioxidants into the system
   c. To release polyphenols and flavonoids
   d. To destroy more of the malignant cells
   e. To affect cells that rapidly divide and reproduce

2. A nurse is caring for a patient with hypertension. The patient asks the nurse if drinking green tea will be beneficial. Which of the following reasons should the nurse state for drinking green tea with caution? Select all that apply.
   a. Nervousness
   b. Insomnia
   c. Mouth ulcers
   d. GI upset
   e. Stomatitis

3. A nurse is caring for a patient who is prescribed Velban for leukemia. The nurse explains to the patient that Velban is a cell cycle–specific drug. Which of the following is a characteristic of a cell cycle–specific drug?
   a. Targets the cells at any phase of the cycle
   b. Targets only the cells that are malignant
   c. Targets the cells in various stages of cell division
   d. Targets the cells in one of the phases of cell division

4. The nurse is caring for a patient with osteosarcoma. The patient is prescribed Trexall, which is an antimetabolite drug. The patient asks the nurse to explain the action of the drug. Which of the following is the action of an antimetabolite?
   a. Changes the cell to a more alkaline environment
   b. Incorporates itself into the cellular components
   c. Interferes with amino acid production
   d. Interferes with the formation of microtubules

5. A nurse is assigned to care for an elderly patient who is receiving an antineoplastic drug. Which of the following factors should the nurse consider when preparing a nursing care plan for the ongoing assessment of the patient? Select all that apply.
   a. Guidelines established by the health care facility
   b. The patient's appetite
   c. The patient's general condition
   d. The patient's individual response to the drug
   e. The adequacy of health insurance coverage

6. A nurse is caring for a patient who is to be administered an antineoplastic drug subcutaneously. Which of the following is applicable to the subcutaneous administration of an antineoplastic drug?

   a. The injection should contain no more than 1 mL
   b. Use an angiocath for administration
   c. Use the Z-track method for administration
   d. The injection should contain only 3 mL

7. A nurse is caring for a patient receiving antineoplastic drugs. The patient's dietary requirements are not met due to loss of appetite. What is the nurse's role in caring for a patient with imbalanced nutrition?

   a. Provide 3 large meals
   b. Provide food with less salt
   c. Provide frequent small meals
   d. Provide food rich in fats

8. A patient being treated with antineoplastic drugs is at a high risk for thrombocytopenia. Which of the following must the nurse consider with regard to injections and blood withdrawal for tests?

   a. Use the same site for all withdrawals and injections
   b. Apply pressure to the injection site for 3 to 5 minutes
   c. Use electric razors when shaving
   d. Use nail trimmers to keep the patient's nails short

9. A nurse is caring for a patient who is experiencing anxiety after being diagnosed with cancer. What is the nurse's role when caring for this patient?

   a. Assist in making critical decisions regarding treatment
   b. Emphasize safety requirements for chemotherapy
   c. Plan and institute therapy to control the disease
   d. Offer consistent and empathetic support to the patient and their family

10. A nurse is caring for a patient who was prescribed antineoplastic drugs for oral therapy. Which of the following should the nurse include in the teaching plan for the patient and family?

    a. Take the exact amount of the drug at any time of the day
    b. Take the drug as directed on the prescription container
    c. Do not inform the dentist of the therapy followed
    d. Decrease the dose as the symptoms of illness decrease

11. The part of cell growth that entails RNA and protein synthesis preparing for division is known as which of the following?

    a. G_1 phase
    b. S phase
    c. G_2 phase
    d. M phase

12. The purpose of antineoplastic drugs is to affect cells that rapidly divide and reproduce. However, the adverse effects produced by antineoplastic drugs are the result of their systemic use which exposes nonmalignant cells in the body that are rapidly dividing and reproducing. Which of the following is not an example of a rapidly dividing and reproducing cell in the body?

    a. Nerve cell
    b. Bone marrow cell
    c. Hair follicle cell
    d. Oral mucosal cell

13. Which of the following herbal products has the benefits of overall well-being, cancer prevention, dental health, and maintenance of heart and liver health as a result of being loaded with antioxidants?

    a. Licorice
    b. Kava
    c. Ma Huang
    d. Green tea

14. Which of the following is an example of an antineoplastic drug that interferes with amino acid production in the S phase and the formation of microtubules in the M phase?

    a. Etoposide (Toposar)

    b. Vinblastine (Velban)

    c. Teniposide (Vumon)

    d. Irinotecan (Camptosar)

15. Which of the following classes of antineoplastic drugs stop cells in the S and G$_2$ phase, thereby causing cell division to cease?

    a. Podophyllotoxins

    b. Taxanes

    c. Vinca alkaloids

    d. Camptothecin analogs

CHAPTER 52

Immunostimulant Drugs

Learning Objectives

- Describe the function of the different types of blood cells
- List the drugs used in the treatment of anemia, bleeding, and prevention of infection
- Discuss the actions, uses, general adverse reactions, contraindications, precautions, and interactions of the agents used to treat anemia, bleeding, and prevention of infection
- Discuss important preadministration and ongoing assessment activities the nurse should perform on a patient receiving an agent used to treat anemia, bleeding, and prevention of infection
- Identify nursing diagnoses particular to a patient receiving an agent used to treat anemia, bleeding, or prevention of infection
- Discuss ways to promote an optimal response to therapy and important points to keep in mind when educating patients about the use of an agent used to treat anemia, bleeding, and prevention of infection

SECTION I: ASSESSING YOUR UNDERSTANDING

Activity A MATCHING

1. **Match the types of anemia in Column A with their corresponding descriptions in Column B.**

Column A

1. Iron-deficiency anemia

2. Anemia in chronic renal failure

3. Pernicious anemia

4. Folic-acid-deficiency anemia

Column B

a. Anemia occurring because of a dietary lack of folic acid, a component necessary in the formation of RBCs

b. Anemia resulting from lack of secretions by the gastric mucosa of the intrinsic factor essential to the formation of RBCs and the absorption of vitamin B_{12}

c. Anemia resulting from a reduced production of erythropoietin, a hormone secreted by the kidney that stimulates the production of red blood cells (RBCs)

d. Anemia characterized by an inadequate amount of iron in the body to produce hemoglobin

2. *Match the drugs used for treating anemia in Column A with their corresponding adverse reactions in Column B.*

Column A

1. Ferrous fumarate

2. Darbepoetin alfa

3. Folic acid

4. Sodium ferric gluconate complex

Column B

a. Conjunctivitis

b. Allergic sensitization

c. Cardiac arrhythmias

d. GI irritation

Activity B FILL IN THE BLANKS

1. _____ is the process of making RBCs in the body.

2. _____ is a condition caused by an insufficient amount of hemoglobin delivering oxygen to the tissues.

3. The technique of administering _____ after a large dose of methotrexate is called *folinic acid rescue.*

4. _____ anemia is characterized by the presence of large, abnormal, immature erythrocytes circulating in the blood.

5. A deficiency of the intrinsic factor results in the abnormal formation of erythrocytes because of the body's failure to absorb vitamin B_{12}, leading to _____ anemia.

Activity C SHORT ANSWERS

A nurse's role in managing patients who are being administered drugs for the treatment of iron-deficiency anemia involves monitoring them and implementing interventions that aid in their recovery. Answer the following questions, which involve the nurse's role in the management of such situations.

1. A patient with iron-deficiency anemia has been recommended ferrous gluconate. What should a nurse assess for in the patient before administering the first dose of ferrous gluconate?

_____

_____

_____

2. A patient is administered sodium ferric gluconate complex for the treatment of iron-deficiency anemia. What adverse reactions should the nurse monitor in this patient?

_____

_____

_____

Activity D DOSAGE CALCULATIONS

1. A patient has been prescribed 75 mg of elemental iron for the treatment of iron-deficiency anemia. Elemental iron is administered intramuscularly with the help of an iron dextran injection. Each mL of the available iron dextran contains 50 mg of elemental iron. How many mL of iron dextran will the nurse have to administer to the patient?

_____

_____

2. A patient is prescribed 25 mg of folic acid over a period of 5 days for the treatment of megaloblastic anemia. The folic acid is to be administered intravenously. The on-hand availability of the drug is 5 mg/mL folic acid solution. How many mL of folic acid will the nurse have to administer to the patient per day?

_____

_____

3. A patient is prescribed 90 mg of oral Feosol in two equally divided doses per day. Feosol is available as tablets of 45 mg. How tablets would the patient require for a week?

_____

_____

4. A physician prescribes 6000 units of epoetin alfa per day for a patient with CRF-associated anemia. Each 1 mL of epoetin alfa solution contains 3000 units of epoetin alfa. How many mL of epoetin alfa solution will the nurse have to administer to the patient per day?

_____

_____

SECTION II: APPLYING YOUR KNOWLEDGE

Activity E CASE STUDY

Antonia Lopez is an Hispanic female, 43 years of age. Mrs. Lopez was recently diagnosed with carcinoma of the breast. She is receiving chemotherapy with vincristine (Oncovin). She is also receiving filgrastim (Neupogen) to treat neutropenia during chemotherapy.

1. What are the common adverse reactions seen with the use of filgrastim (Neupogen)?

   _____

   _____

   _____

2. The nurse should obtain a thorough medical history prior to the administration of filgrastim (Neupogen) as it should be used cautiously in patients with what medical conditions?

   _____

   _____

   _____

SECTION III: PRACTICING FOR NCLEX

Activity F NCLEX-STYLE

Answer the following questions.

1. A patient with folic acid–deficiency anemia is administered a Folvite injection. What adverse reactions should the nurse monitor in this patient?
   a. Anorexia
   b. Allergic hypersensitivity
   c. Arthralgia
   d. Adrenal hyperplasia

2. A patient is prescribed epoetin alfa for the treatment of anemia associated with chronic renal failure. In which of the following patients is epoetin alfa contraindicated?
   a. Patients with hypersensitivity to human albumin
   b. Patients with allergy to cyanocobalamin
   c. Patients undergoing treatment for pernicious anemia
   d. Patients with hemolytic anemia

3. A nurse administers oral doses of vitamin B_{12} to a patient with vitamin B_{12} deficiency. During assessment, the nurse observes a reduction in the absorption of vitamin B_{12} in the patient's body. Which of the following has contributed to the reduction in the absorption of vitamin B_{12} in the patient? Select all that apply.
   a. The patient must have consumed alcohol
   b. The patient must have consumed caffeine
   c. The patient must have consumed neomycin
   d. The patient must have consumed nicotine
   e. The patient must have consumed colchicine

4. A patient with iron-deficiency anemia is prescribed iron dextran. Which of the following is the most appropriate assessment that a nurse should perform when calculating the dosage of iron dextran to be administered to the patient?
   a. Obtain the patient's weight and hemoglobin level
   b. Obtain the patient's heart rate
   c. Obtain the patient's blood pressure
   d. Obtain the patient's body temperature

5. A nurse is caring for a patient who has to be administered iron supplements. The patient informs the nurse that he has been taking methyldopa. Which of the following conditions should the nurse monitor in the patient as a result of the interaction between the two drugs once the iron drug regimen begins?
   a. Decreased blood pressure
   b. Increased heart rate
   c. Decreased effect of Parkinson's medication
   d. Increased absorption of iron

6. A nurse is caring for a patient who is being administered cyanocobalamin for vitamin B_{12} deficiency. Which of the following food items should the nurse ask the patient to consume in order to fulfill the nutritional deficiency of Vitamin B_{12} through a balanced diet? Select all that apply.
   a. Seafood
   b. Meat
   c. Eggs
   d. Leafy vegetables
   e. Breads and cereals

7. A patient receiving ferrous fumarate for the treatment of anemia is to be shortly discharged. What should the nurse include in the patient teaching plan when providing care on an outpatient basis?
   a. Take antacids in case of acidity
   b. Take drugs with meals in case of gastrointestinal upset
   c. Drink the liquid iron preparation through a glass
   d. Avoid using multivitamin preparations

8. A nurse is caring for a patient receiving parenteral administration of iron for the treatment of anemia. Which of the following adverse reactions should the nurse monitor for when caring for the patient? Select all that apply.
   a. Urticaria
   b. Dyspnea
   c. Insomnia
   d. Diabetes
   e. Rashes

9. What information should the nurse offer the patient when performing ongoing assessments for a patient receiving oral iron supplements?
   a. Inform the patient that the color of the stools will be black
   b. Inform the patient that his palpitations will be high
   c. Inform the patient that his weight will increase
   d. Inform the patient that he may develop a rash

10. A nurse is caring for a patient receiving iron supplements. Which of the following instructions should the nurse provide to the patient to prevent interference with the absorption of iron?
    a. Avoid milk
    b. Avoid poultry
    c. Avoid meat
    d. Avoid fish

11. Which of the following types of cells supply our cells with oxygen from the lungs?
    a. Leukocytes
    b. Megakaryocytes
    c. Erythrocytes
    d. Neutrophils

12. Which of the following types of cells control the bleeding from microscopic to major tears in our tissues?
    a. Megakaryocytes
    b. Erythrocytes
    c. Leukocytes
    d. Neutrophils

13. Which of the following is likely to occur when a patient becomes neutropenic as a result of antineoplastic therapy?
    a. Vomiting
    b. GI bleeding
    c. Venous thromboembolism
    d. Infection

14. Anemia can result in which of the following?
    a. Increased platelet production
    b. Decreased neutrophil production
    c. Decreased platelet production
    d. Increased neutrophil production

15. The process by which the body is stimulated to make more of a specific type of blood cells is known as which of the following?
    a. Hematopoiesis
    b. Metabolism
    c. Neogenesis
    d. Regeneration

Topical Drugs Used in the Treatment of Skin Disorders

Learning Objectives

- List the types of drugs used in the treatment of skin disorders
- Discuss the general drug actions, uses, and reactions to and any contraindications, precautions, and interactions associated with drugs used in treating skin disorders
- Discuss important preadministration and ongoing assessment activities the nurse should perform on patients receiving a drug used to treat skin disorders
- List nursing diagnoses particular to a patient using a drug to treat a skin disorder
- Discuss ways to promote an optimal response to therapy and important points to keep in mind when educating the patient about a skin disorder

SECTION I: ASSESSING YOUR UNDERSTANDING

Activity A MATCHING

1. *Match the antibiotic drugs in Column A with their uses in Column B.*

Column A

1. Azelaic acid
2. Bacitracin
3. Gentamicin
4. Mupirocin

Column B

a. Relief of primary and secondary skin infections

b. Acne vulgaris, rosacea

c. Impetigo infections caused by *Staphylococcus aureus*

d. To help prevent infections in minor cuts and burns

2. *Match the drugs in Column A with their adverse reactions in Column B.*

Column A

1. Butenafine HCl

2. Loprox gel

3. Clotrimazole

4. Haloprogin

Column B

a. Alopecia, eye pain, facial edema

b. Burning, itching, erythema

c. Vesicle formation, scaling, pruritus

d. Contact dermatitis, erythema, irritation

Activity B FILL IN THE BLANKS

1. The prolonged use of topical antibiotic preparations may result in a superficial _____.

2. Acyclovir is used in treating herpes simplex virus infections in _____ patients.

3. Adverse reactions to topical antiinfectives may include rash, itching, urticaria (hives), or dermatitis which may indicate a _____ reaction to the drug.

4. A/An _____ is a drug that stops, slows, or prevents the growth of microorganisms.

5. A drug that kills bacteria is known as a/an _____.

6. Topical _____ are drugs used to treat psoriasis.

Activity C SHORT ANSWERS

A nurse's role in managing patients who are receiving a topical drug for a skin disorder involves assisting the patients for assessment. Answer the following questions, which involve the nurse's role in the management of patients receiving a topical drug for a skin disorder.

1. As a preadministration assessment, what are the required nursing interventions?

_____

_____

_____

2. What are the interventions required as a part of the ongoing assessment?

_____

_____

_____

Activity D DOSAGE CALCULATIONS

1. A patient has been prescribed acyclovir ointment for a herpes simplex virus infection to be applied every 3 hours, 8 times per day, for 7 days. How many total applications would the nurse administer for the entire treatment?

_____

_____

2. A patient with tinea corporis has been prescribed tolnaftate to be applied twice daily for 3 weeks. How many total applications would the nurse administer for the entire treatment?

_____

_____

SECTION II: APPLYING YOUR KNOWLEDGE

Activity E CASE STUDY

Berilo Vasquez is an Hispanic male, 24 years of age. He has a past medical history significant for plaque psoriasis. He presents to the physician's office seeking treatment for a psoriasis flare. The physician prescribes calcipotriene (Dovonex) applied to affected areas BID. Mr. Vasquez has no known drug allergies and takes no medications.

1. What are the common adverse reactions seen with the use of calcipotriene (Dovonex)?

_____

_____

2. How should the nurse advise Mr. Vasquez to apply the calcipotriene (Dovonex)?

_____

_____

SECTION III: PRACTICING FOR NCLEX

Activity F NCLEX-STYLE

Answer the following questions.

1. A nurse is caring for a patient who has been prescribed masoprocol. The nurse should know that for which of the following is the administration of masoprocol contraindicated?

   a. For use on moles, birthmarks, or warts
   b. As monotherapy for bacterial skin infections
   c. For use on the face, groin, or axilla
   d. As sole therapy in plaque psoriasis

2. A patient undergoing treatment has been prescribed alclometasone dipropionate. The nurse should know that for which of the following is the administration of alclometasone dipropionate contraindicated?

   a. For use on moles and birthmarks
   b. As sole therapy in plaque psoriasis
   c. For use on genital or facial warts
   d. For use on infected skin

3. The primary health care provider has prescribed benzocaine to be administered to a patient. In which of the following should the nurse use benzocaine cautiously?

   a. In patients who are undergoing pregnancy or lactation
   b. Immunocompromised patients with herpes simplex virus infections
   c. In patients receiving Class I antiarrhythmic drugs such as tocainide
   d. In patients with cutaneous candidiasis or tinea pedis

4. A nurse is caring for a patient being treated for psoriasis. The primary health care provider has prescribed anthralin. Which of the following should the nurse monitor in the patient as an adverse reaction to anthralin?

   a. Hypothalamic-pituitary-adrenal axis suppression
   b. Cushing's syndrome
   c. Hyperglycemia and glycosuria
   d. Temporary discoloration of the fingernails

5. The primary health care provider has prescribed alclometasone dipropionate for a patient being treated for eczema. The nurse caring for the patient should know that which of the following is a systemic adverse reaction to alclometasone dipropionate?

   a. Hyperglycemia and glycosuria
   b. Mild and transient pain
   c. Numbness and dermatitis
   d. Flu-like syndrome

6. A patient is undergoing treatment for debriding chronic dermal ulcers and the primary health care provider has prescribed collagenase. Which of the following should the nurse caring for the patient monitor as an adverse reaction to the application of collagenase?

   a. Flu-like syndrome
   b. Numbness and dermatitis
   c. Cushing's syndrome
   d. Hyperglycemia and glycosuria

7. A nurse is caring for a patient who has been prescribed salicylic acid for the treatment of hyperkeratotic skin disorders. Which of the following should the nurse monitor as an adverse reaction to salicylic acid?

   a. Mild and transient pains
   b. Temporary discoloration of the hair
   c. Flu-like syndrome
   d. Hyperglycemia and glycosuria

8. A nurse is caring for a patient who has been prescribed accuzyme for treatment by the primary health care provider. The nurse should know that accuzyme is used to treat which of the following?

   a. Psoriasis
   b. Eczema
   c. Insect bites
   d. Chronic dermal ulcers

9. A patient has been admitted to the health care facility with inflamed skin resulting from severe insect bites. The primary health care provider has prescribed topical corticosteroid therapy. The nurse caring for this patient should know that which of the following is the action of a topical corticosteroid?
   a. Reduces itching, redness, and swelling
   b. Reduces the number of bacteria on the skin
   c. Prevents infection in the bite wounds
   d. Cleanses the skin thoroughly

10. A nurse is caring for a patient with a chronic skin disease diagnosed as psoriasis. In order to avoid infections, which of the following should the nurse use to wash her hands before and after caring for the patient?
    a. Topical antipsoriatics
    b. Topical antiseptics and germicides
    c. Topical enzymes
    d. Topical antifungals

11. Which of the following might be used topically by a patient with acne vulgaris?
    a. Clindamycin (Clindagel)
    b. Ciclopirox (Loprox)
    c. Nystatin (Mycostatin)
    d. Imiquimod (Aldara)

12. Which of the following might a patient use to treat onychomycosis?
    a. Erythromycin (Erygel)
    b. Acyclovir (Zovirax)
    c. Ciclopirox (Penlac)
    d. Vidarabine (Ara-A)

13. Which of the following herbal products has antiviral properties against HSV?
    a. Foxglove
    b. Ginger
    c. Ginseng
    d. Lemon balm

14. Which of the following can a nurse recommend to a patient for the treatment of HSV that is available without a prescription?
    a. Docosanol (Abreva)
    b. Penciclovir (Denavir)
    c. Acyclovir (Zovirax)
    d. Imiquimod (Aldara)

15. Which of the following herbal products can be used topically to prevent infection and promote healing of minor burns and wounds?
    a. Lemon balm
    b. Aloe vera
    c. Sweet clove
    d. Ginger

CHAPTER 54

Otic and Ophthalmic Preparations

Learning Objectives

- Discuss the general actions, uses, adverse reactions, contraindications, precautions, and interactions of otic and ophthalmic preparations
- Discuss important preadministration and ongoing assessment activities the nurse should perform on a patient receiving otic and ophthalmic preparations
- List nursing diagnoses particular to a patient taking an otic or ophthalmic preparation
- Discuss ways to promote an optimal response to therapy, how to administer the preparations, and important points to keep in mind when educating patients about the use of otic or ophthalmic preparations

SECTION I: ASSESSING YOUR UNDERSTANDING

Activity A MATCHING

1. *Match the drugs in Column A with their uses in Column B.*

Column A

1. Brimonidine tartrate
2. Apraclonidine hydrochloride 1% solution
3. Dapiprazole hydrochloride
4. Metipranolol hydrochloride

Column B

a. Reverses the diagnostic mydriasis after ophthalmic examination

b. Lowers intraocular pressure (IOP) in patients with open-angle (chronic) glaucoma

c. Treatment of elevated IOP in patients with ocular hypertension or open-angle glaucoma

d. Control or prevention of postoperative elevations in IOP

2. *Match the drugs in Column A with their adverse reactions in Column B.*

Column A

1. 1% hydrocortisone, 5 mg neomycin sulfate, 10,000 units polymyxin B

2. Floxacin otic

3. Brimonidine tartrate

Column B

a. Local irritation, itching, burning, earache

b. Burning and stinging

c. Ear irritation, burning, or itching

Activity B FILL IN THE BLANKS

1. Prolonged use of otic preparations containing an antibiotic, such as ofloxacin, may result in a/an _____.

2. _____ is a condition of the eye in which there is an increase in the IOP, causing progressive atrophy of the optic nerve with deterioration of vision.

3. Dapiprazole acts by blocking the a-adrenergic receptor in the smooth muscles and produces _____ through an effect on the dilator muscle of the iris.

4. Silver possesses _____ activity against gram-positive and gram-negative microorganisms.

5. _____ is the only ophthalmic antifungal in use.

6. _____ is the paralysis of the ciliary muscle, resulting in an inability to focus the eye.

Activity C SHORT ANSWERS

A nurse's role in managing patients who are receiving an otic preparation involves assisting the patients for assessment. Answer the following questions, which involve the nurse's role in the management of patients receiving otic preparations.

1. Before administration of an otic preparation, the primary health care provider examines the ear and external structures surrounding the ear and prescribes the drug indicated to treat the disorder. As a preadministration assessment, the nurse may be responsible for examining which areas of the ear?

_____

_____

2. How should the nurse assess the patient's response to otic therapy, and what further examinations should be carried out?

_____

_____

Activity D DOSAGE CALCULATIONS

1. A patient has been prescribed an otic preparation of 1% hydrocortisone, 5 mg neomycin sulfate, 10,000 units polymyxin. The dosage instructed is 4 gtt instilled 4 times daily. How many drops would the nurse be administering in total in a day?

_____

_____

2. A patient with trachoma has been prescribed sulfacetamide sodium 2 gtt q2h. How many drops would the nurse administer in total in a day?

_____

_____

SECTION II: APPLYING YOUR KNOWLEDGE

Activity E CASE STUDY

Jason Owens is a Causasian male, 65 years of age. The physician has given him a prescription for brimonidine (Alphagan) 1 gtt OU TID for glaucoma.

1. What should the nurse tell Mr. Owens about brimonidine (Alphagan)?

_____

_____

2. How should the nurse advise Mr. Owens to administer brimonidine (Alphagan)?

_____

_____

SECTION III: PRACTICING FOR NCLEX

Activity F NCLEX-STYLE

Answer the following questions.

1. A nurse is caring for a patient who has been using ofloxacin for a prolonged time. Which of the following are the risks associated with the prolonged use of such otic antibiotics?

   a. Danger of superinfection in the ear

   b. Systemic effects of cholinesterase inhibitors

   c. Exacerbation of existing hypertension

   d. Additive CNS depressant effects

2. The nurse should know that ofloxacin is used with caution in which of the following?

   a. While taking monoamine oxidase inhibitors

   b. During pregnancy and lactation

   c. During activities requiring mental alertness

   d. While performing activities in dimly lit areas

3. A nurse is caring for a patient who is to be administered an antibiotic ear solution. Before instilling the otic solution, what should the nurse inform the patient?

   a. Local effects such as headache and visual blurring may be felt

   b. Fatigue and drowsiness may be experienced

   c. A feeling of fullness may be felt in the ear

   d. Hearing in the treated ear may temporarily improve

4. Prior to instillation of otic preparations, the nurse should hold the container in the hand for a few minutes. What is the reason for doing this?

   a. To observe the number of drops in the applicator

   b. To confirm if the drug was kept refrigerated

   c. To observe if the drug is in suspension form

   d. To prevent dizziness after being instilled

5. A nurse needs to administer otic drops to a patient. Which of the following should the nurse do to ensure correct administration of the otic drops?

   a. Have the patient lie on his or her side with the ear toward the ceiling

   b. In upright position, have the head tilted straight down towards the floor

   c. Gently pull the cartilaginous portion of the outer ear down and forward

   d. Properly insert the applicator tip or the dropper tip into the ear canal

6. A nurse is caring for a patient who is being administered cerumenex for softening the dried earwax inside the ear canal. When should the nurse discontinue the use of cerumenex?

   a. After using the medication for one week

   b. When absolutely no cerumen remains

   c. When drainage or discharge occurs

   d. When dizziness or other sensations occur

7. A nurse is caring for a patient who is being administered dipivefrin hydrochloride for the treatment of open-angle glaucoma. Which of the following should the nurse monitor in the patient as a transient local reaction to dipivefrin hydrochloride?

   a. Deposits in conjunctiva

   b. Brow ache or headache

   c. Ocular allergic reactions

   d. Foreign body sensation

8. A patient has undergone an ophthalmic examination, and is being administered dapiprazole hydrochloride to reverse the diagnostic mydriasis. The nurse should know that which of the following is a local effect of dapiprazole hydrochloride?

   a. Abnormal corneal staining

   b. Decreased night vision

   c. Frequent urge to urinate

   d. Drooping of the upper eyelid

9. A patient has been administered echothiophate iodide for the treatment of accommodative esotropia. Which of the following ophthalmic adverse reactions should the nurse monitor in the patient?

   a. Eyelid muscle twitching

   b. Abdominal cramps

   c. Cardiac irregularities

   d. Urinary incontinence

10. A patient with glaucoma who does not respond to other drugs has been administered travoprost for the reduction of increased intraocular pressure. The nurse should know that which of the following is the patient likely to exhibit as a local adverse reaction?

    a. Unpleasant taste

    b. Eyelid discomfort

    c. Asthma

    d. Cold/flu symptoms

11. Antipyrine is used in otic preparations as which of the following?

    a. Solvent

    b. Decongestant

    c. Analgesic

    d. Anesthetic

12. Which of the following can a nurse recommend to a patient to aid in removing cerumen?

    a. Carbamide peroxide

    b. Acetic acid

    c. Phenylephrine

    d. Hydrocortisone

13. If a nurse needs to administer otic preparations in both of the patient's ears, how long should the nurse wait to place drops in the second ear?

    a. At least 30 seconds

    b. At least 1 minute

    c. At least 5 minutes

    d. At least 3 minutes

14. The nurse may use Cerumenex to aid in the removal of wax cerumen from the patients ear canal, however Cerumenex is not allowed to stay in the ear canal more than how long before irrigation?

    a. 5 minutes

    b. 30 minutes

    c. 10 minutes

    d. 15 minutes

15. A patient should not use over-the-counter ear wax removal products for more than how long before consulting a physician?

    a. 4 days

    b. 7 days

    c. 2 days

    d. 10 days

CHAPTER 55

Fluids, Electrolytes, and Parenteral Therapy

- List the types and uses of solutions used in the parenteral management of bodily fluids
- List the types of intravenous administration of a solution or electrolyte used in the management of bodily fluids
- Describe the calculations used to establish intravenous flow rates
- List the types and uses of electrolytes used in the management of electrolyte imbalances
- Discuss the more common signs and symptoms of electrolyte imbalance
- Discuss preadministration and ongoing assessment activities the nurse should perform with the patient administered an electrolyte or an IV solution to manage bodily fluids
- List nursing diagnoses particular to a patient receiving an electrolyte or a solution to manage bodily fluids
- Discuss ways to promote an optimal response to therapy and important points to keep in mind when educating patients about the use of an electrolyte or a solution to manage bodily fluids

SECTION I: ASSESSING YOUR UNDERSTANDING

Activity A MATCHING

1. *Match the electrolytes in Column A with their common uses in Column B.*

Column A	Column B
1. Potassium C	a. Plays an important role in the transmission of nerve impulses. It is also important in the activity of many enzyme reactions such as carbohydrate metabolism
2. Magnesium A	
3. Sodium D	
4. Calcium B	
	b. Necessary for the functioning of nerves and muscles, clotting of blood, building of bones and teeth, and other physiologic processes
	c. Necessary for the transmission of impulses, the contraction of smooth, cardiac, and skeletal muscles, and other important physiologic processes
	d. Important in maintaining acid-base balance, normal heart action, and in the regulation of osmotic pressure in body cells

Activity B FILL IN THE BLANKS

1. An ~~Electrolyte~~ is an electrically charged substance essential to the normal functioning of all cells.

2. A low pH in the blood means the body is in an acidic condition and a high blood pH indicates an ~~Alkaline~~ condition.

3. The term *fluid* ~~overload~~ describes a condition when the body's fluid requirements are met and the administration of fluid occurs at a rate that is greater than the rate at which the body can use or eliminate the fluid.

4. Sodium as an electrolyte is administered for ~~hyponatremia~~ or low blood sodium.

5. Protein ~~substrates~~ are amino acid preparations that act to promote the production of proteins.

Activity C SHORT ANSWERS

A nurse's role in managing patients who are using fluids and electrolytes involves monitoring and managing interventions that aid in their recovery. Answer the following questions, which involve the nurse's role in the management of such situations.

1. A nurse has been caring for a patient who has been administered intravenous replacement solutions. What factors should the nurse consider when evaluating the therapy to determine its effectiveness?

   ~~The nurse needs to consider the pt's nutrition, response to therapy, understanding of treatment and procedure, adverse reactions and fluid volume.~~

2. A nurse has been caring for a patient who has been administered potassium. What instructions should the nurse offer related to the intake of this electrolyte as part of the patient teaching plan post-discharge?

   ~~Nurse should instruct to the pt the time of drug take it when it says, do not skip or take more or less than told. You need to take "K" with full glass of water, after meals. Oral "K" must not be crushed or chewed. Call physician if tingling to hands or feet, nausea, abdominal pain or black stools occur. If tablet has a coating swallow it whole. Also if a effervescent tablet are prescribed you place tablet in 4, 8 oz of water or juice wait for fizzing to stop before drinking. Drink the liquid between 5-10 mins.~~

Activity D DOSAGE CALCULATIONS

1. A patient has been prescribed 2 g of bicarbonate per day to be taken orally in 2 equally divided doses every 12 hours. The drug is available in the form of 0.5-g tablets. How many tablets should the patient be taking in a day?

   ~~4 tablets~~

2. A patient is prescribed 5 g of magnesium sulfate to be taken via the IV route every 3 hours. The drug is available in the form of 1 g/2 mL. How much magnesium sulfate in solution should the nurse prepare for the patient to take for 2 days?

   ~~160 mL of Magnesium~~

3. A patient is prescribed potassium 60 mEq/day to be taken orally. The drug is available in the form of 30 mEq. How many tablets should the patient be administered in a day?

   ~~2 tablets~~

4. A regular dose of tromethamine is 30 mg/50 kg. The patient weighs 120 kg. The dose is available in the form of 15 mg/mL. How much tromethamine in solution has the physician prescribed, which the nurse has to prepare in solution form?

   ~~4.8 mL~~

SECTION II: APPLYING YOUR KNOWLEDGE

Activity E CASE STUDY

Tyler James is a Caucasian male, 19 years of age. He presents to the ED with symptoms of dehydration after intractable vomiting. The ED has ordered normal saline IV.

1. Calculate the drip rate (drops/minute) if a 1000-mL bag of normal saline is to be infused over a period of 4 hours with a drop factor of 10.

   ~~42 gtts/min~~

   ~~$\dfrac{1000\,mL \times 10\,gtts}{240\,hrs} = 41.6$~~   ~~42 gtts/min~~

2. Fluid overload is commonly associated with solutions administered via the parenteral route. What symptoms might Mr. James exhibit that would indicate fluid overload?

Rapid breathing, headache, weakness, weight gain, distended neck veins, coughing, confusion, hyponatremia, and increase in blood pressure.

SECTION III: PRACTICING FOR NCLEX

Activity F NCLEX-STYLE

Answer the following questions.

1. A nurse is assigned to care for a patient who needs to be administered magnesium. What should the nurse determine from the patient's health history before administering magnesium to know that the use of the electrolyte is not contraindicated for the patient?

a. Patient does not experience fluid retention

(b.) Patient does not have a heart block

c. Patient does not have untreated Addison's disease

d. Patient is not taking digitalis

2. A nurse is caring for a patient who is being administered electrolytes orally. During assessment, the nurse observes that the patient is experiencing GI disturbances. What nursing interventions should the nurse perform when caring for this patient? Select all that apply.

(a.) Offer meals in smaller quantities and more frequently

(b.) Monitor the patient for any signs and symptoms of nausea

c. Encourage the patient to increase the intake of fruit juices

(d.) Ensure that the drug is taken by the patient only with meals

e. Administer antacids to the patient as prescribed for nausea

3. A nurse is assigned to care for a patient whose protein intake is significantly less than required by the body. Which of the following conditions is the patient likely to experience?

a. Metabolic acidosis

b. GI disturbances

(c.) Negative nitrogen balance

d. Hypotensive episodes

4. A nurse is caring for a patient who is being administered fat emulsions. What nursing interventions should the nurse perform when conducting ongoing assessments for the patient?

a. Ensure that the solution is below room temperature

b. Monitor the patient for signs of diarrhea

(c.) Monitor the patient's ability to eliminate infused fat

d. Monitor the patient for signs of hypernatremia

5. A nurse is caring for a patient who is being administered plasma proteins. Which of the following adverse reactions should the nurse monitor for in this patient?

(a.) Urticaria

b. Flushing of skin

c. Dyspnea

d. Wheezing

6. A nurse is caring for a patient who is being administered sodium electrolyte solution by the IV route. What interventions should the nurse perform as part of the ongoing assessment when caring for this patient? Select all that apply.

a. Ensure that a microscopic filter is attached to the IV line

(b.) Observe the rate of IV infusion every 15 to 30 minutes

(c.) Measure the patient's intake and output every 8 hours

d. Inform the PHCP if the patient voids less than 100 mL of urine every 4 hours

(e.) Monitor the patient's condition for signs of pulmonary edema

7. A nurse is caring for a patient who needs to be administered bicarbonate. What information should the nurse obtain from the patient's health history to know that bicarbonate should be administered cautiously in this patient?

   a. The patient has metabolic alkalosis

   b. The patient has congestive heart failure

   c. The patient has hypocalcemia

   d. The patient is on a sodium-restricted diet

8. A nurse is caring for a patient who is being administered potassium through IV. When assessing the patient's condition, the nurse observes that the patient's heart rate is irregular. What nursing intervention should the nurse perform when caring for this patient?

   a. Check the patient's pulse rate every 4 hours

   b. Discontinue the IV infusion immediately

   c. Monitor the patient for signs of nausea and vomiting

   d. Ensure a direct IV injection of potassium for the next dose

9. A nurse is caring for a 65-year-old patient who needs to be administered plasma proteins. What interventions should the nurse perform when caring for this patient when monitoring and managing patient needs?

   a. Carefully monitor the patient for signs and symptoms of fluid overload

   b. Carefully observe the patient for difficulty in breathing, headache, flushing

   c. Report any signs of hypercalcemic syndrome immediately to the PHCP

   d. Test the patient's knee-jerk reflex before each dose to be administered

10. A nurse is caring for a patient who is being administered ammonium chloride. The nurse knows that the patient has been taking spironolactone. Which of the following adverse reactions should the nurse monitor for in this patient due to the interaction of ammonium chloride and spironolactone?

    a. Systemic alkalosis

    b. Respiratory depression

    c. Heart block

    d. Systemic acidosis

11. Depending on clinical judgment, how many unsuccessful venipuncture attempts on the same patient warrants having a more skilled individual attempt the procedure?

    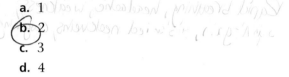

    a. 1

    b. 2

    c. 3

    d. 4

12. Which of the following is a major intracellular fluid electrolyte?

    a. Potassium

    b. Sodium

    c. Calcium

    d. Phosphate

13. Which of the following is a major extracellular fluid electrolyte?

    a. Potassium

    b. Magnesium

    c. Phosphate

    d. Sodium

14. Which of the following electrolytes is necessary for the contraction of smooth, cardiac, and skeletal muscles?

    a. Calcium

    b. Potassium

    c. Sodium

    d. Magnesium

15. The use of which of the following medications can lead to hypokalemia? (Choose one)

    a. Furosemide (Lasix)

    b. Spironolactone (Aldactone)

    c. Lisinopril (Prinivil)

    d. Losartan (Cozaar)

Answers

CHAPTER 1

SECTION I: ASSESSING YOUR UNDERSTANDING

Activity A MATCHING

1. 1. b   2. c   3. a
2. 1. c   2. d   3. a   4. b

Activity B FILL IN THE BLANKS

1. Absorption
2. Intravenous
3. Antagonistic
4. Synergism
5. Pharmacogenetic

Activity C SHORT ANSWERS

1. Physical and chemical changes occur due to changes in the cellular environment:
   - Physical changes in the cellular environment include changes in osmotic pressures, lubrication, absorption, or changes in the condition of the surface of the cell membrane.
   - Chemical changes in the cellular environment include inactivation of cellular functions or the alteration of the chemical components of bodily fluid, such as a change in the pH.
2. The United States Food and Drug Administration (FDA) is responsible for approving new drugs and monitoring drugs currently in use for adverse or toxic reactions. The process of drug development takes about 7 to 12 years and sometimes even more.

Activity D

1. The development of a new drug is divided into the pre-FDA phase and the FDA phase. During the pre-FDA phase, a manufacturer discovers a drug that looks promising. In vitro testing is performed using animal and human cells, followed by studies in live animals. The manufacturer then applies to the FDA for an Investigational New Drug (IND) status.
2. The nurse informs the patient that smoking or consumption of any type of alcoholic beverage carries risks to the fetus, such as low birth weight, premature birth, and fetal alcohol syndrome. Children born to mothers using addictive drugs, such as cocaine or heroin, are often born with an addiction to the drug abused by the mother.

SECTION II: APPLYING YOUR KNOWLEDGE

Activity E CASE STUDY

1. The patient should be informed that many botanicals have strong pharmacological activity, and some may interact with prescription drugs that the patient is taking. Botanicals may also produce toxic substances in the body.
2. The nurse should inquire if the patient is using any herbs, teas, vitamins, or other dietary supplements. The nurse should explain that herbal supplements are not necessarily safe or without side effects.

SECTION III: PRACTICING FOR NCLEX

Activity F NCLEX-STYLE

1. **Answer: d**
   RATIONALE: The nurse should refer to a drug by its generic name to avoid confusion. A generic name is the name given to a drug before it becomes official and can be used in many countries by all manufacturers. The official name is the name listed in *The United States Pharmacopeia–National Formulary*. The scientific name, also called the *chemical name*, gives

the molecular structure of that particular drug. The trade name is the name registered by the manufacturer and is followed by the trademark symbol. This name can be used only by the manufacturer.

2. **Answer: b, c, d**
RATIONALE: The purpose of the Controlled Substances Act of 1970 is to regulate the manufacture, distribution, and dispensing of drugs that have abuse potential. Adverse drug effects are reported by physicians through the FDA-established reporting program called *Med Watch*. The Orphan Drug Act of 1983 was passed to encourage development.

3. **Answer: b**
RATIONALE: During the pharmaceutic phase of drug activity, the liquid drug is absorbed into the bodily system. Solid tablets or capsules break into small pieces and dissolve into the bodily fluids in the gastrointestinal tract. Enteric-coated tablets disintegrate in the small intestine.

4. **Answers: c**
RATIONALE: The nurse should administer the drug intravenously, as the drug is rapidly absorbed by the system. Absorption occurs slowly when the drug is administered orally, intramuscularly, or subcutaneously. Because of the complex membranes of the gastrointestinal mucosal layers, muscle and skin delay the drug passage.

5. **Answers: a, c, e**
RATIONALE: The nurse should monitor physiologic functions such as blood pressure, urine output, and heart rate in altered cellular function. Impaired speech and slurred vision may be symptoms of altered cellular function in patients with drug allergies.

6. **Answers: a, c, e**
RATIONALE: Cancer drugs act on the cell membrane and the cell processes, eventually causing starvation and death of the cancer cells. Antacids cause chemical changes in the bodily fluids by changing the pH to neutralize the acidity.

7. **Answers: a, d, e**
RATIONALE: The patient is likely to exhibit drug toxicity. As the diseased kidney will not be able to eliminate excess drug, the drug levels in the blood will increase, causing a longer duration of drug action. A person who is addicted to certain drugs could be drug-

dependent and exhibit drug tolerance. As a result, higher dosages of the drug would have to be administered.

8. **Answers: a, b, c**
RATIONALE: The patient's age and weight are important in determining the drug dosage to be administered for effective action of the drug. If the patient has some disease, it could interfere with the drug action, so the dosage has to be adjusted accordingly. Patient's appetite and height do not influence the drug response.

9. **Answer: c**
RATIONALE: Patients with impaired liver function need to be monitored frequently during the drug administration, as impaired liver function influences the drug response. Impaired vision, speech, or hearing does not affect the drug response.

10. **Answer: a**
RATIONALE: Administration of a drug is primarily the responsibility of the nurse.

11. **Answer: b**
RATIONALE: Pharmacology is the study of drugs and their action on the living.

12. **Answer: a**
RATIONALE: The Food and Drug Administration (FDA) is responsible for the approval of new drugs in the United State.

13. **Answer: c**
RATIONALE: Prescription drugs are also called *legend drugs*.

14. **Answer: a**
RATIONALE: The generic name of a drug is the name found in the *National Formulary* or the *U.S. Pharmacopeia*.

15. **Answer: a**
RATIONALE: Physical dependence is the habitual use of a drug, in which negative physical withdrawal symptoms result from abrupt discontinuation.

CHAPTER 2

SECTION I: ASSESSING YOUR UNDERSTANDING

Activity A MATCHING

1.	1. c	2. d	3. a	4. b
2.	1. c	2. d	3. b	4. a

Activity B FILL IN THE BLANKS

1. Controllers
2. Subcutaneous
3. Unit
4. Sublingual
5. Buccal
6. Extravasation

Activity C SHORT ANSWERS

1. There are two methods to ensure that the right patient is administered the medication:
   - Check the patient's wristband containing the patient's name. If there is no written identification verifying the patient's name, the nurse can obtain a wristband or other form of identification before administering the drug.
   - Ask the patient to identify himself/herself and state his/her DOB prior to administering the drug.
2. It is important to report drug errors so that:
   - Any necessary steps to counteract the action of the drug can be taken.
   - Any observation can be made as soon as possible.

Activity D

1. The nurse's responsibilities with regard to the administration of a transdermal drug include:
   - Applying transdermal patches to clean, dry, nonhairy areas of intact skin
   - Removing the old patch when the next dose is applied in a new site
   - Rotating sites for transdermal patches to prevent skin irritation
   - Removing paper and tape and cleaning skin before next dose of ointment
   - Writing the nurse's initials, date, and time of application on the patch

SECTION II: APPLYING YOUR KNOWLEDGE

Activity E CASE STUDY

1. The nurse should compare medication, container label, and medication record to ensure that the right drug is administered to the right patient.
2. Immediate documentation is particularly important when drugs are given on an as-needed (PRN) basis. Immediate documentation prevents accidental administration of a drug by another individual. Proper documentation is essential to the process of administering drugs correctly.

SECTION III: PRACTICING FOR NCLEX

Activity F NCLEX-STYLE

1. **Answer: a**
   RATIONALE: After administering an as-needed (PRN) basis drug, the nurse should immediately record the fact. Evaluating the patient's response to the drug or recording the site used for parenteral administration should be done after the documentation of the administration of the drug. The nurse should inform the physician only if there are any adverse reactions.

2. **Answer: d**
   RATIONALE: The nurse should remove the old patch when the next dose is applied to a new site. The nurse should rotate sites for transdermal patches to prevent skin irritation and not place the new patch in the same location as the old patch. The nurse should not shave the area to apply the patch; shaving may cause skin irritation. The area where the transdermal patch is to be applied should be dry, not moist.

3. **Answer: b**
   RATIONALE: The nurse should obtain special instructions for application of the drug from the primary health care provider. The instructions may include whether to apply the drug in a thin or even layer or whether to cover the area after application of the drug to the skin or not. It is not essential to obtain information about the cause of skin infection, reasons for selecting the drug, and composition of the drug before administering the prescribed drug.

4. **Answer: c**
   RATIONALE: The inner part of the forearm is ideal for administering intradermal injection. The nurse should not administer the drug near moles, areas with hair cover, or pigmented skin. The thigh and the upper arm are ideal sites for intramuscular injections, but not for intradermal injections.

5. **Answer: b**
   RATIONALE: A venipuncture is a difficult procedure; after three unsuccessful attempts, the nurse should ask for assistance from a more skilled nurse. It is not advisable for the nurse to repeatedly attempt a venipuncture; this may cause the patient great discomfort. The nurse should not change the administration route even if it is getting difficult to administer a drug in a particular manner. Shifting the patient to a more conducive position is unlikely to help significantly.

6. Answer: a

RATIONALE: If an intramuscular injection volume is more than 3 mL, the nurse should divide the drug and give it as 2 separate injections, as volumes larger than 3 mL will not be absorbed properly. The nurse should use a one and a half-inch needle, for the injection, not half an inch. The upper back is not an ideal site for intramuscular injections. When giving a drug by the intramuscular route, the nurse should insert the needle at a 90-degree angle.

7. Answer: c

RATIONALE: In thin or cachectic patients, there usually is less subcutaneous tissue. For such patients, the upper abdomen is the most appropriate site for injection. The thigh or the upper arm is an administration site for intramuscular injections, not subcutaneous injections. The upper, not the lower, back is a site for subcutaneous injections.

8. Answers: a, c, e

RATIONALE: The nurse should crush the tablets and ensure that they are completely dissolved before administering to the patient. The nurse should check the tube for placement and flush the tube with water to clear it. The nurse should not put the tablets in water without crushing them, as the drug may not dissolve properly. The tube should be fixed after the drug has been mixed.

9. Answer: a

RATIONALE: A nurse should use 2 methods to identify the client before administering the medication.

10. Answer: c

RATIONALE: This order is represents a PRN order.

11. Answer: a, b

RATIONALE: Two drugs often associated with errors are insulin and heparin.

12. Answer: b

RATIONALE: The Joint Commission updates the NPSG on a yearly basis.

13. Answer: a

RATIONALE: The Institute for Safe Medication Practices is responsible for the Medication Errors Reporting Program.

14. Answer: d

RATIONALE: The nurse is responsible for the administration part of the drug distribution process. Primary and specialty providers are responsible for ordering and pharmacists are responsible for dispensing.

15. Answer: a

RATIONALE: A Pyxis machine is an example of an automated medication management system.

CHAPTER 3

SECTION I: ASSESSING YOUR UNDERSTANDING

Activity A MATCHING

| 1. | 1. bB | 2. d | 3. a | 4. c |
| 2. | 1. d | 2. a | 3. b | 4. c |

Activity B FILL IN THE BLANKS

1. Denominators
2. Lowest
3. Fractions
4. Numerator
5. Larger
6. Mixed
7. Improper
8. Proper
9. Ratio
10. Equality

Activity C SHORT ANSWERS

Think about the rationale for the redundancy system. Is that removed by the computer system?

Activity D DOSAGE CALCULATION

Five milliliters in each dose. Instead of labeling the drug in 1 unit of measure (tablet or capsule), the drug is written as a specific amount in a specific *quantity* of solution. For example, if the label states that there is 125 mg/5 mL, 5 mL is the *quantity* (or volume) in which there is 125 mg of this drug.

SECTION II: APPLYING YOUR KNOWLEDGE

Activity E CASE STUDY

a. Mr. Jones weighs 97.7 kg (215 lb × 1 kg/2.2lb = 97.7kg)
b. 36°C is 98.6°F (9/5 × 37=66.6; 66.6 + 32=98.6)

SECTION III: PRACTICING FOR NCLEX
Activity F NCLEX-STYLE

1. **Answer: a**
   RATIONALE: The best method of error detection is the manual redundancy system.

2. **Answer: c**
   RATIONALE: Problems can arise if a patient recognizes the brand name of the drug but does not recognize the generic name and refuses the medication. The nurse should know both the generic and trade name of each drug by reviewing the label and drug information carefully.

3. **Answer: a, b, e**
   RATIONALE: There are three systems of measurement associated with drug dosing: the metric system, the apothecary system, and household measurements.

4. **Answer: a**
   RATIONALE: When there is no number to the left of the decimal, a zero is written, for example 0.75 shows correct placement of the zero in a decimal.

5. **Answer: c**
   RATIONALE: There are 2.2 lb in 1 kg.

6. **Answer: b**
   RATIONALE: The correct expression of the ratio 3:100 in a fraction is 3/100.

7. **Answer: a, b**
   RATIONALE: 75/100 or 3/4 is the correct expression of 75 % in the form of a fraction.

8. **Answer: d**
   RATIONALE: There are 3 teaspoons in 1 tablespoon.

9. **Answer: a**
   RATIONALE: 37.5% represents 3/8 in percentage form.

10. **Answer: c**
    RATIONALE: There are 1000 milligrams in 1 gram.

11. **Answer: c**
    RATIONALE: When using dimensional analysis to calculate dosage problems, the identified unit of measure to be calculated is written followed by an equal sign. Then the dosage strength is written with the numerator always expressed in the same unit that was identified before the equal sign. Expressing the dosage strength as a fraction with the numerator having the same unit, writing the next fraction with the numerator having the same unit of measure as the denominator, and expanding the equation by filling in the missing numbers using the appropriate equivalent, are the steps associated with performing metric conversion using dimensional analysis.

12. **Answer: a**
    RATIONALE: Specific dosage strength may not be available for parenteral drugs in disposable syringes, and, it may therefore be necessary to administer less than the amount contained in the syringe to meet the dosage requirements. Parenteral drugs in dry form are available as a crystal or a powder, as ampoules or vials in dry form, and must be made a liquid before administration.

13. **Answer: b**
    RATIONALE: Ounces are the units of weight in the apothecary system. In the metric system, grams, meters, and liters are the units of weight, length, and volume, respectively.

14. **Answer: d**
    RATIONALE: The generic name is written in smaller print and is usually located under the trade name. The trade name is capitalized, written first on the label, and identified by the registration symbol.

15. **Answer: c**
    RATIONALE: A gram represents a unit of weight; a liter represents a unit of volume; a meter represents a unit of length. A deciliter represents one-tenth of a liter (unit of volume).

CHAPTER 4

SECTION I: ASSESSING YOUR UNDERSTANDING
Activity A MATCHING

1. 1. c 2. e 3. a 4. b 5. d
2. 1. e 2. a 3. c 4. b 5. d

Activity B FILL IN THE BLANKS

1. Objective
2. Ongoing
3. Diagnosis
4. Implementation
5. Individual

Activity C SHORT ANSWERS

1. Nursing process is a framework for nursing action consisting of problem-solving steps that help members of the health care team provide effective patient care. It is both a specific and an orderly plan used to gather data, identify patient problems from the data, develop and implement a plan of action, and then evaluate the results of nursing activities, including the administration of drugs. The five phases of the nursing process are:
   - Assessment
   - Nursing diagnosis (analysis)
   - Planning
   - Implementation
   - Evaluation
2. An initial assessment is made based on objective and subjective data collected when the patient is first seen in a hospital, outpatient clinic, health care provider's office, or other type of health care facility. The initial assessment is usually more thorough and provides a database from which later data can be compared and decisions made. An ongoing assessment is one that is made at the time of each patient contact and may include the collection of objective data, subjective data, or both. The scope of an ongoing assessment depends on many factors, such as the patient's diagnosis, the severity of illness, the response to treatment, and the prescribed medical or surgical treatment.

Activity D

Check Display 4.1 for some reasons that patients have problems staying on medications. Over which factors does the patient have control or no control when taking medications? What does the nurse need to know about patient habits to be sure they take the prescribed medications?

SECTION II: APPLYING YOUR KNOWLEDGE
Activity E CASE STUDY

1. During the assessment, the nurse must obtain a set of vital signs, record Mrs. Black's weight, review recent lab results, and ask how she is getting along with her current regimen. Note any signs of edema in the extremities. Obtain a list of all prescription and over the counter medications Mrs. Black is currently taking. Ask about any specific complaints or questions she may have.

2. The nurse should emphasize the following: proper use of the glucometer, proper clean procedure for obtaining the blood specimen, timetable for conducting finger sticks, how to properly log them, and when to contact the physician. Develop a trusting and comfortable relationship with the client. Assess the client's educational level, knowledge of the disease and testing procedure, ability to understand written versus verbal instructions, and interest level.

SECTION III: PRACTICING FOR NCLEX
Activity F NCLEX-STYLE

1. **Answer: a**
   RATIONALE: To obtain subjective data from the patient, the nurse should inquire about the number of cigarettes smoked in a day. Subjective data include facts which are supplied to the nurse and other health care professionals by the patient and patient's family. Monitoring the patient's body temperature, blood pressure, and pulse rate and rhythm are objective data which the nurse should obtain. Objective data include facts which the nurse obtains through physical assessment or physical examination.

2. **Answer: c**
   RATIONALE: When caring for a patient of childbearing age, the nurse needs to determine and assess the patient's pregnancy status before administering a drug, as the drug may be contraindicated or may require cautious use during pregnancy. Determining and assessing the patient for her relationship with her spouse, her menstrual history, or her family history are not appropriate interventions before administering a drug because they will not help in determining if the administration of the drug to the patient would be safe or not.

3. **Answer: d**
   RATIONALE: When developing an expected outcome, the nurse should focus on the patient's ability to recuperate. Expected outcome describes the maximum level of wellness that is reasonably attainable for the patient. The expected outcome defines the expected behavior of the patient or family that indicates the problem is being resolved or that progress toward resolution is occurring. When developing an expected outcome, the nurse need not focus on the type of drug administered, its dosage pattern, or the patient's ability to

recuperate, since these will not determine if the patient has the ability to achieve the maximum level of wellness.

4. **Answer: a**
RATIONALE: In her nursing diagnosis a nurse should include problems that can be solved by independent nursing actions; i.e., actions that do not require a physician's order and may be legally performed by a nurse. The nurse should not include problems that have a definite cure, or problems that cannot be prevented by nursing actions. Nursing diagnosis also does not include identification of the patient's condition or criticality.

5. **Answers: a, c, e**
RATIONALE: Planning for nursing actions specific for the drug to be administered promotes a greater accuracy in drug administration, patient understanding of the drug regimen, and improved patient compliance with the prescribed drug therapy after hospital discharge. The planning for nursing actions does not bring about a prevention of a relapse. Planning and implementing nursing actions does promote an optimal response to drug therapy, but it does not always promote an optimal response in minimum time.

6. **Answer: b**
RATIONALE: To combat the patient's non-compliant attitude, the nurse should try and find out the exact reason for noncompliance if possible so that it can be dealt with. Very often the non-compliant attitude develops due to fear and anxiety related to the drug regimen on the part of the patient. Preparing a fixed schedule for the patient to take the drug and teaching the patient the importance of the drug regimen are not appropriate interventions, since they will do little to deal with the problem encouraging the non-compliant attitude. If the attitude stems from anxiety, then these interventions will do little to reduce anxiety in the patient. Though the nurse should monitor for a relapse due to non-compliance with the drug regimen, doing so will not promote the patient to follow the regimen strictly.

7. **Answer: c, a, d, b, e**
RATIONALE: The nursing process is a framework for nursing action consisting of problem-solving steps that help members of the health care team to provide effective patient care. It is both a specific and an orderly plan used to gather data, identify patient problems from the data, develop and implement a plan of action, and then evaluate the results of nursing activities.

8. **Answer: a**
RATIONALE: Facts obtained by means of a physical assessment or physical examination are considered objective data.

9. **Answer: c**
RATIONALE: Facts supplied by the client or the client's family are considered subjective data.

10. **Answer: a**
RATIONALE: Assessment is the first step of the nursing process because none of the other steps can be accomplished without assessment.

11. **Answer: c**
RATIONALE: Assessment involves collecting objective and subjective data.

12. **Answer: a**
RATIONALE: A nursing diagnosis identifies problems that can be solved or prevented by independent nursing actions that do not require a physician's order.

13. **Answer: d**
RATIONALE: NANDA was formed to standardize the terminology used for nursing diagnoses and continues to define, explain, classify, and research summary statements about health problems related to nursing.

14. **Answer: a**
RATIONALE: Planning is the next step of the nursing process after the formulation of nursing diagnoses.

15. **Answer: b**
RATIONALE: When related to the administration of drugs, implementation refers to the preparation and administration of one or more drugs to a specific patient.

CHAPTER 5

SECTION I: ASSESSING YOUR UNDERSTANDING

Activity A MATCHING

1.	1. b	2. c	3. a
2.	1. c	2. a	3. b

Activity B FILL IN THE BLANKS

1. Physical
2. Affective
3. Chew
4. Sunlight
5. Scheduling

Activity C SHORT ANSWERS

1. To ensure that the patient perfectly remembers all the exercises taught, the nurse should supervise while the patient demonstrates the exercises.
2. To ensure that the patient's relative has understood the procedure of measuring the patient's temperature using an electronic thermometer, the nurse should:
   • Ask the relative to perform a return demonstration of the procedure;
   • Not pose questions such as "Do you understand? or "Is there anything you don't understand?" because the relative may be uncomfortable in admitting a lack of understanding.

Activity D

1. Since the patient is deficient in cognitive knowledge and psychomotor skills, the nursing diagnosis called *deficient knowledge* must be used to teach the patient administration of antimalarial drugs.
2. Learning how to perform breathing exercises involves the psychomotor domain which involves physical skills. Ineffective Therapeutic Regimen Management must be used to teach the client breathing exercises.
3. The affective domain of learning comes into picture when the patient implements the weight loss program.

SECTION II: APPLYING YOUR KNOWLEDGE
Activity E CASE STUDY

1. The nurse should pay particular attention to all three learning domains (cognitive, affective, and psychomotor) when developing a teaching plan for Mrs. Sanchez.
2. Barriers or obstacles the nurse faces in educating Mrs. Sanchez about her glucometer and her disease state include language, culture beliefs about food, decreased motor ability and possible problems with recall as a result of her past CVA.

SECTION III: PRACTICING FOR NCLEX
Activity F NCLEX-STYLE

1. **Answer: a, b, c**
   RATIONALE: Ineffective Therapeutic Regimen Management helps in discharge teaching, in managing complicated medication regimen, and in providing positive results to patients. It also describes patients who successfully manage drug regimens. Effective Individual Therapeutic Regimen Management gives information about drug reactions and teaches management of adverse reactions. Effective Individual Therapeutic Regimen Management generally describes a patient who is successfully managing the medication regime.

2. **Answer: a, b, d**
   RATIONALE: The teaching plan should be implemented a day or two before the patient's discharge. Care should be taken to see that the patient is alone, alert, and not sedated. Dividing the teaching material into sessions will make it easy for the patient to learn. The implementation of the teaching plan should not begin as soon as the patient is admitted to the hospital. Also, teaching everything at a single stretch may make learning difficult for the patient.

3. **Answer: a, d, e**
   RATIONALE: Carrying out a patient assessment before formulating a teaching plan helps a nurse to determine barriers and obstacles that the patient could face in the learning process, to choose the best teaching methods, and to develop an effective teaching plan. An effective teaching plan can help improve patient motivation or participation.

4. **Answer: a**
   RATIONALE: The psychomotor domain involves the learning of physical skills. The cognitive domain involves the patient's or the caregiver's attitudes, feelings, beliefs, and opinions. The cognitive domain involves intellectual activities or intellectual domain such as thought, recall, decision making, and drawing conclusions.

5. **Answers: a**
   RATIONALE: Implementation of the teaching plan means actually performing the interventions identified in the teaching plan. Determining the effectiveness of patient teaching comes under evaluation. Planning involves beginning with expected outcomes.

Using patient experiences is an aspect of adult learning.

6. **Answer: c, d, e**
   RATIONALE: The three domains of learning are psychomotor, which involves the learning of physical skills; cognitive, which involves the patient's or caregiver's attitudes, feelings, beliefs, and opinions; and affective, which involves decision making and drawing conclusions. Intellectual domain and the intuitive domain are not defined domains of learning.

7. **Answer: c**
   RATIONALE: Different literacy levels can pose a major obstacle in the process of learning. Low grasping power, patient's nervousness in using the inhaler, and lack of awareness can be overcome if the literacy levels are matched.

8. **Answer: a**
   RATIONALE: The affective domain includes the patient's or caregiver's attitudes, feelings, beliefs, and opinions. Here, the affective domain is involved in teaching the patient. The cognitive domain involves intellectual domain such as thought, recall, decision making and drawing conclusions. The psychomotor domain involves learning physical skills.

9. **Answer: a**
   RATIONALE: Patient teaching is an ongoing process.

10. **Answer: c**
    RATIONALE: A patient must have motivation to learn.

11. **Answer: a, b**
    RATIONALE: When learning occurs, the patient's behavior, thinking, or both can change.

12. **Answer: a**
    RATIONALE: Making sure the patient is not in pain is vital to the teaching/learning process.

13. **Answer: a**
    RATIONALE: The affective domain is often ignored by health care providers when teaching.

14. **Answer: b**
    RATIONALE: Preprinted material such as checklists are useful for helping a nurse remember important teaching points, but do not take into account a patient's affective domain.

15. **Answer: a**
    RATIONALE: Development of a therapeutic relationship with the patient is the most important prerequisite to learning about a patient's affective behavior.

CHAPTER 6

SECTION I: ASSESSING YOUR UNDERSTANDING
Activity A MATCHING

1. 1. c   2. d   3. a   4. b
2. 1. d   2. a   3. b   4. c

Activity B FILL IN THE BLANKS

1. 2
2. Bacteriostatic
3. Photosensitivity
4. Cranberry
5. Thrombocytopenia

Activity C SHORT ANSWERS

1. As part of the preadministration assessment, a nurse is required to perform the following:
   - Assess the patient's general appearance, general health history (surgeries, medical conditions, and medications) and allergies.
   - Take and record vital signs.
   - Obtain description of signs and symptoms of infection from the patient or family.
   - Review results of tests.
2. A nurse's teaching plan should include the following:
   - Take the drug as prescribed.
   - Keep all follow-up appointments to ensure the infection is controlled.
   - Complete the full course of therapy.
   - Drink at least eight to ten 8-oz glasses of fluid every day.
   - Take the drug on an empty stomach either 1 hour before or 2 hours after a meal.
   - Prolonged exposure to sunlight may result in skin reactions similar to severe sunburn.

Activity D DOSAGE CALCULATION

1. 6 tablets
2. 1 tablet
3. 20 mL
4. 3 tablets
5. 5 tablets

SECTION II: APPLYING YOUR KNOWLEDGE
Activity E CASE STUDY

1. When triaging a client who may have an infection, the nurse should assess the client's general appearance; take and record vital signs; obtain information regarding symptoms experienced by the client and the length of the symptoms; ask client about self-remedies used; and review the results of labs and tests. The nurse should also obtain a list of current medications and medical conditions and ask client about allergies to food, drugs, or environmental factors.

2. The nurse should discuss the possible side effects of sulfonamides with Mr. Williams (nausea, vomiting, anorexia, stomatitis, chills, fever, crystalluria, and photosensitivity). The client should be advised to take the medication with a full glass of water and to increase daily fluid intake. The client should be instructed to call the physician's office if an allergic reaction occurs, if he experiences any unusual bruising, or if worsening of his condition occurs. Mr. Williams should be instructed to take the Bactrim DS until it is gone even if he is feeling better and to keep all follow-up appointments with his physician.

SECTION III: PRACTICING FOR NCLEX
Activity F NCLEX-STYLE

1. **Answer: a**
   RATIONALE: The nurse should clean and remove the debris present on the surface of the patient's burnt skin before the application of cream. The nurse should not apply a thick layer of cream on the burned area. The drug is normally applied 1/16 inch thick; thicker application is not recommended. Applying drugs with a bare hand involves a risk of passing infection. It is advisable to use sterilized gloves while applying cream. The nurse should remove debris present on the surface of the skin before each application of the drug.

2. **Answer: d**
   RATIONALE: The nurse should inspect the patient's skin daily to assess the extent of bruising and evidence of exacerbation of existing ecchymotic areas. The patient can be shifted if required, but care should be taken to prevent bruising. There is no need to avoid brushing teeth as long as a soft-bristled toothbrush is used. While it is necessary to examine the patient's skin for trauma, palpating the patient's body can create unnecessary pain and may trigger bleeding.

3. **Answer: b**
   RATIONALE: The nurse should instruct the patient to wear protective clothing while outdoors. Applying sunscreen on exposed body parts is not enough to protect from photosensitivity and the patient should wear protective clothing even after applying sunscreen. Sulfasalazine, not sulfadiazine, causes a yellow stain on contact lenses. There is no need to avoid indoor lights as the effects of photosensitivity are caused by sunlight.

4. **Answer: a, c, e**
   RATIONALE: The nurse should inform the patient that the chief reason for increasing fluid intake during sulfonamide therapy is to remove microorganisms from the urinary tract and prevent crystalluria and stone formation in the genitourinary tract. Sulfonamides are easily absorbed by the gastrointestinal system and also easily excreted by the kidneys. Increasing the fluid intake will not have any significant impact on the absorption and excretion of sulfonamides.

5. **Answer: c**
   RATIONALE: Edema is one of the possible allergic reactions that may occur due to the application of mafenide, and the nurse should monitor the patient for edema. Urine turning orange-yellow is one of the symptoms of sulfasalazine, not mafenide. Crystalluria does not occur during mafenide therapy. A burning sensation while applying the drug to the skin is a normal reaction.

6. **Answer: c**
   RATIONALE: The nurse should inform the patient that using soft contact lenses during the sulfonamide therapy may result in a permanent yellow stain on the lenses. Wearing lenses will not, however, cause a burning sensation in eyes, headache and dizziness, or impaired vision.

7. **Answer: a, b, d**
   RATIONALE: While caring for patients with ulcerative colitis, the nurse should inspect the stool samples, record their appearance, and monitor for evidence of the relief or intensification of the symptoms. The nurse should also ensure that sulfasalazine is administered during meals or immediately afterwards. There is no need to measure urine output as the

patient does not have impaired urinary elimination. Loss of appetite is a mild adverse effect of sulfonamides.

8. **Answer: a**
   RATIONALE: The nurse should inform the patient that using cranberries with antibiotics prevents bacteria from attaching to the walls of the urinary tract. Crystalluria or the formation of crystals in urine can be prevented by increasing fluid intake. Specifically consuming cranberry juice will not have any significant effect in preventing crystalluria. The effects of photosensitivity can be reduced by wearing protective clothing or sunscreen when traveling outside and consumption of cranberry juice will not have any effect. Clots can be prevented by using oral anticoagulants with sulfonamides.

9. **Answer: a**
   RATIONALE: The nurse should inform the patient that sulfonamide is used in the treatment of urinary tract infection because it is easily absorbed by the gastrointestinal system. Sulfonamides don't kill bacterial cells directly. They inhibit the activity of folic acid in bacterial cell metabolism, which are then subsequently destroyed by the body's defense mechanisms. Decrease in the number of white blood cells is caused by leucopenia, which is also an adverse effect of sulfonamides. Sulfonamides may have life-threatening complications such as Stevens-Johnson syndrome.

10. **Answer: b**
    RATIONALE: The nurse should assess for lesions on the mucous membranes to determine whether the patient is showing signs of SJS. Inflammation of the mouth (stomatitis), crystals in the urine (crystalluria), and diarrhea are some of the common adverse reactions of sulfonamides and do not necessarily indicate that the patient has SJS.

11. **Answer: a, b, c, d**
    RATIONALE: The body is equipped with a natural defense system that includes our skin and bodily secretions.

12. **Answer: a, b, c, d**
    RATIONALE: Microbes enter the body in different ways, such as through a break in the skin or by ingestion, breathing, or contact with the mucous membranes of the body.

13. **Answer: a**
    RATIONALE: Sulfonamides treat bacterial infection and are considered antibiotics.

14. **Answer: b**
    RATIONALE: Drugs that slow or retard the multiplication of bacteria are known as bacteriostatic.

15. **Answer: a**
    RATIONALE: Drugs that destroy bacteria are known as bacteriocidal.

CHAPTER 7

SECTION I: ASSESSING YOUR UNDERSTANDING

Activity A MATCHING

1. 1. c   2. d   3. a   4. b
2. 1. c   2. d   3. b   4. a

Activity B FILL IN THE BLANKS

1. Intravenous
2. Extended
3. Hematopoietic
4. Antihistamines
5. Penicillinase

Activity C SHORT ANSWERS

1. Before administering penicillin for the first time, a nurse should perform the following assessments:
   - Obtain patient's general health history including medical and surgical treatments, drug history, history of drug allergies to penicillin or cephalosporin, and present symptoms of infection.
   - Take and record vital signs.
   - Obtain description of signs and symptoms of infection from the patient or family.
   - Assess infected area and record findings on the patient's chart.
   - Describe signs and symptoms relating to the patient's infection accurately, such as color and type of drainage from a wound, pain, redness and inflammation, color of sputum, and presence of odor.
   - Note patient's general appearance.
   - Obtain results of the culture and sensitivity test before giving the first dose.
2. When caring for a patient receiving penicillin who has developed impaired oral mucous

membranes, a nurse should perform the following interventions:

- If diet permits, provide yogurt, buttermilk, or acidophilus capsules to reduce risk of fungal superinfection.
- Give frequent mouth care with a nonirritating solution.
- Use a soft-bristled toothbrush.
- Recommend a nonirritating soft diet.
- Monitor dietary intake to ensure adequate nutrition.
- If recommended, administer antifungal agents and/or local anesthetics to soothe the irritated membranes.

Activity D DOSAGE CALCULATION

1. 15 cc
2. 3 cc
3. 3 mL
4. 2 mL
5. 2 tablets
6. 2.5 mL

SECTION II: APPLYING YOUR KNOWLEDGE
Activity E CASE STUDY

1. The nurse should reassure Lori's mother that anaphylactic reactions occur more frequently with parenteral administration of the penicillins, but it is good to know the signs and symptoms of a hypersensitivity reaction. The nurse should advise Lori's mother to watch for skin rash, hives, sneezing, wheezing, itching, difficulty breathing, swelling of the skin and mucous membranes, especially around and in the mouth and throat, and signs resembling serum sickness (chills, fever, edema, joint and muscle pain, and malaise). If any of these are present in Lori during treatment, her mother should stop the medication immediately and seek medical attention.

2. The nurse should advise Lori's mother to keep the container refrigerated, shake the drug well before pouring, and return the drug to the refrigerator immediately after pouring the dose. Drugs that are kept refrigerated like amoxicillin lose their potency when kept at room temperature. A small amount of the drug may be left after the last dose is taken. Any remaining amoxicillin should be discarded, because the drug begins to lose its potency after a few weeks. Lori's mother should use a medicine spoon or a dropper to measure the dose accurately, as not all teaspoons are created equal.

SECTION III: PRACTICING FOR NCLEX
Activity F NCLEX-STYLE

1. **Answer: d**
   RATIONALE: In mild hypersensitivity cases, the drug may be continued with the nurse administering frequent skin care to provide relief to the patient. Reducing the dosage from the prescribed limit should not be done unless specifically instructed by the primary health care provider, as it would lead to a fall in the blood level. A patient can take baths as long as harsh soaps and perfumed lotions are avoided. Avoiding contact with clothing for the affected areas is not necessary as long as the clothing is not rough or irritating.

2. **Answer: a**
   RATIONALE: The nurse should instruct the patient to take the drug at the prescribed times of day to maintain the drug level. Stopping antibiotic therapy before finishing the prescribed course, even if the patient feels better, may allow the infection to return. Women who are prescribed ampicillin, bacampicillin, and penicillin V and who take birth control pills containing estrogen should use additional contraception measures, but they need not stop using birth control pills. Intramuscular or intravenous drugs may be administered without considering the food-intake time of the patient.

3. **Answer: b**
   RATIONALE: It is important to inform the primary health care provider if previously used areas for injection appear red or the patient reports pain in the area. Penicillin solutions are often thick or viscous, and it is natural for the patient to feel pain at the injection site. Mild nausea is a normal reaction to any antibiotic and is not a cause for concern. Decrease in temperature is a response to the therapy and is not required to be reported to the primary health care provider.

4. **Answer: e, b, a, d, c**
   RATIONALE: Before beginning the treatment, the nurse obtains or reviews the patient's general health history, inquiring especially about any allergies to penicillins. A culture and sensitivity test is ordered in most cases; these tests help identify the appropriate penicillin. The prescribed penicillin is then administered and any improvements are recorded in the patient's charts.

5. **Answers: c, d, e**
   RATIONALE: As part of the ongoing assessment, the nurse evaluates the patient's response to the therapy, such as a decrease in temperature, relief from pain or discomfort, increase in appetite, and a change in the appearance or in the amount of drainage. These evaluations are then recorded on the patient's chart to monitor progress. Additional culture and sensitivity tests may be performed to check if the microorganisms have become penicillin-resistant or if a superinfection has occurred. The patient's general health history is obtained before the appropriate penicillin therapy is determined, and the patient's stools are saved only if he or she shows signs of diarrhea and there are signs of blood and mucous in the stools.

6. **Answers: 3, 2, 4, 1**
   RATIONALE: In situations where diarrhea is suspected, the nurse first inspects all stools. The primary health provider has to be notified immediately if diarrhea occurs, because it may be necessary to stop the drug. If there are signs of blood and mucus in the stool, it is important to save a sample to test it for occult blood to confirm presence of blood. If the stool tests positive for blood, the nurse saves another sample for possible further laboratory analysis.

7. **Answers: a, c, d**
   RATIONALE: Some of the signs of an anaphylactic shock are severe hypotension, loss of consciousness, and acute respiratory distress. Pain at the injection site is normal for penicillins administered intramuscularly. Nausea and vomiting are signs of gastrointestinal disturbances that may or may not be serious.

8. **Answers: b, c, e**
   RATIONALE: In cases of impaired comfort or increased fever, the nurse should take vital signs every 4 hours or more. The nurse should report any rise in temperature to the primary health care provider, who may take additional treatment measures, such as administering an antipyretic drug or changing the drug or dosage to bring down the temperature. The nurse should not discontinue the dosage unless specifically instructed by the primary health provider. Changing the patient's diet to a soft, nonirritating diet is not necessary unless the patient shows signs of impaired oral mucous membranes.

9. **Answers: a, c, e**
   RATIONALE: Symptoms of bacterial superinfection of the bowel include diarrhea or bloody diarrhea, rectal bleeding, and abdominal cramping. Vomiting is a common adverse reaction to penicillins, and lesions may occur due to a hypersensitivity reaction.

10. **Answer: b, e, d, a, c**
    RATIONALE: The nurse should first read the manufacturer's directions on the drug label to find out details of reconstitution and the diluent to be used. The next step is to obtain the diluent mentioned in the manufacturer's directions. The nurse needs to reconstitute the drug in the vial before extracting. After reconstitution, the nurse extracts the penicillin from the vial and administers it to the patient.

11. **Answer: a**
    RATIONALE: Natural penicillins exert a bactericidal effect on bacteria.

12. **Answer: a**
    RATIONALE: Penicillinase is an enzyme produced by certain bacteria that inactivates the penicillin.

13. **Answer: b, d**
    RATIONALE: Chemical modification to slow excretion of penicillins from the kidney and addition of a chemical compound to inhibit beta-lactamase inhibitors are ways the penicillins can be modified to broaden their spectrum of action.

14. **Answer: a**
    RATIONALE: Extended spectrum penicillins are used to treat *Pseudomonas*.

15. **Answer: a, b, c**
    RATIONALE: Penicillins are utilized in the treatment of meningitis, syphilis, intra-abdominal infections, and upper respiratory infections caused by bacteria.

CHAPTER 8

SECTION I: ASSESSING YOUR UNDERSTANDING

Activity A   MATCHING

1.	1. d	2. c	3. b	4. a
2.	1. c	2. a	3. d	4. b

Activity B FILL IN THE BLANKS

1. Inflammation
2. Disulfiram
3. Thrombophlebitis
4. Penicillins
5. Extravasation

Activity C SHORT ANSWERS

1. The steps the nurse must follow before the first dose of cephalosporin is administered are:
   - Obtain the patient's general health history, including medical and surgical treatments, drug history, history of drug allergies to penicillin or cephalosporin, and present symptoms of infection.
   - The nurse should check for any cultural and sensitivity tests that are done before the first dose of the drug is administered.
   - The nurse should keep in mind that approximately 10% of the people allergic to a penicillin drug are also allergic to a cephalosporin drug.
2. When a patient is to be administered cephalosporin by IV, the following interventions are important:
   - The nurse should inspect the needle insertion site for signs of extravasation or infiltration.
   - The needle insertion site and the area above the site should be inspected several times a day for phlebitis or thrombophlebitis.
   - If problems occur, the nurse should contact the primary health care provider, and the IV must be discontinued and restarted in another vein.
3. When a patient is to be administered cephalosporin by IM, the following interventions are important:
   - The nurse should inject the drug into a large muscle mass, such as the gluteus muscle or lateral aspect of the thigh.
   - If the patient has been non-ambulatory for any length of time, the nurse should assess the muscle carefully because the large muscle may be atrophied.
   - The nurse should remember to rotate injection sites.
   - The nurse should warn the patient that at the time the drug is injected into the muscle, there may be a stinging or burning sensation, and the area may be sore for a short time.

- The nurse should inform the primary health care provider if previously used areas for injection appear red or if the patient reports continued pain in the area.

Activity D DOSAGE CALCULATION

1. 2
2. 2 capsules at 8 PM
3. 1 tablet twice daily
4. 22.2 mL
5. 0.5

SECTION II: APPLYING YOUR KNOWLEDGE
Activity E CASE STUDY

1. An allergy history, medical and surgical history, medication history, and current symptoms of the infection should be included in the nurse's preadministration assessment prior to Mr. Labra receiving the ceftriaxone.
2. Upset stomach after taking penicillin does not constitute a true penicillin allergy. Since Mr. Labra does not have a true allergy, then the ceftriaxone should be administered. Swelling of the face, lips, throat or tongue, itchy rash or hives, or anaphylactic reaction would constitute a true allergy. If any of these reactions occurred in the past, the ceftriaxone should not be administered and the physician should be notified.

SECTION III: PRACTICING FOR NCLEX
Activity F NCLEX-STYLE

1. **Answer: c**
   RATIONALE: The nurse should measure and record fluid intake and output and notify the primary health care provider when caring for a patient with renal impairment. In case of diarrhea or loose stools containing bloody mucus, the nurse should inspect each bowel movement and immediately report to the primary health care provider. An antipyretic drug is administered when there is an increase in the body temperature of a patient receiving cephalosporin. Administration of cephalosporin to a patient with renal impairment does not maximize the risk of excessive perspiration.

2. **Answer: a**
   RATIONALE: When cephalosporin is given IV, the nurse should monitor the needle insertion site and the area above the site several times a day for signs of redness, which may indicate

phlebitis or thrombophlebitis. The nurse should inspect the site for tenderness when the drug is administered to the patient intramuscularly. Administration of cephalosporin by IV does not cause fever or angina.

3. **Answer: a**

RATIONALE: The nurse should identify an increased risk for bleeding in the patient as an effect of interaction of oral anticoagulants administered with cephalosporin. The patient is at an increased risk for nephrotoxicity when aminoglycosides are administered with cephalosporin. Administration of cephalosporin with oral anticoagulants does not maximize the risk of hypertension or cause an increase in the number of WBCs.

4. **Answer: d**

RATIONALE: The nurse should instruct the patient to take the drug 1 hour before or 2 hours after the meal. The patient can take the medication with food or milk if GI upset occurs after administration. The patient need not avoid sunlight or lie down; the drug does not cause photosensitivity or dizziness. The patient should be instructed to avoid alcohol completely during the course of therapy.

5. **Answer: 600**

RATIONALE: The nurse should administer 600 mg of the drug after every 24 hours, instead of 300 mg every 12 hours, to meet the recommended dose.

6. **Answer: c**

RATIONALE: If the patient has been nonambulatory for any length of time or has paralysis, the nurse should assess the muscle carefully when administering cephalosporin intramuscularly because the large muscle may be atrophied. The patient does not face an increased risk for hypersensitive reactions. There is increased risk of phlebitis or thrombophlebitis when the drug is given IV. A stinging or burning sensation will occur when the drug is administered intramuscularly; the patient needs to be warned, but the nurse need not monitor the patient for this.

7. **Answer: b, c, e**

RATIONALE: The expected outcomes for a patient receiving cephalosporin are optimal responses to theory and understanding and compliance with treatment. Complete recovery and improved dietary patterns are not typical expected outcomes of drug therapy.

8. **Answer: c**

RATIONALE: The patient has aplastic anemia, which is an adverse effect of cephalosporin therapy. The tests do not indicate nephrotoxicity or toxic epidermal necrolysis, which are also adverse effects of cephalosporin. Nephrotoxicity is damage to the kidney by toxic substances; toxic epidermal necrolysis is the death of the epidermal layer of the skin; anorexia is an eating disorder.

9. **Answer: c, d, e**

RATIONALE: The nursing interventions for a patient who has developed diarrhea as a result of cephalosporin are discontinuing the drug, reporting to the primary health care provider, and instituting the treatment for diarrhea. An antipyretic drug is administered when there is an increase in the body temperature of a patient receiving cephalosporin. The nurse saves a stool sample and tests for occult blood if blood and mucus appear to be in the stool.

10. **Answer: 6**

RATIONALE: The patient has been prescribed cefditoven 200 mg orally TID, so the nurse will require two 100-mg tablets for each dosage. TID indicates that the medication should be administered 3 times daily, so the nurse will require a total of 6 tablets each day.

11. **Answer: d**

RATIONALE: Cephalosporins are structurally and chemically related to penicillins.

12. **Answer: a, b**

RATIONALE: Fourth-generation cephalosporins have a broader spectrum of action and a longer duration of resistance to beta-lactamase; however, they have no ability to treat viral infections.

13. **Answer: a**

RATIONALE: Approximately 10% of clients who are allergic to penicillins are also allergic to cephalosporins.

14. **Answer: b**

RATIONALE: A disulfiram-like reaction may occur if alcohol is consumed within 72 hours after administration of certain cephalosporins.

15. **Answer: a, b, d**

RATIONALE: Cefamandole, cefoperazone, and cefotetan have been implicated in disulfiram-like reactions with alcohol.

CHAPTER 9

SECTION I: ASSESSING YOUR UNDERSTANDING

Activity A MATCHING

1. 1. c   **2.** a   **3.** d   4.b
1. 1. b   **2.** c   **3.** a

Activity B FILL IN THE BLANKS

1. Macrolides
2. Myoneural
3. Lincosamides
4. Telithromycin
5. Tetracyclines

Activity C SHORT ANSWERS

1. Roles of a nurse in monitoring and managing patient's needs are:
   - Observe the patient at frequent intervals, especially during the first 48 hours of therapy.
   - Report to the primary health care provider the occurrence of any adverse reaction before the next dose of the drug is due.
   - Report serious adverse reactions, such as a severe hypersensitivity reaction, respiratory difficulty, severe diarrhea, or a decided drop in blood pressure, to the primary health care provider immediately, because a serious adverse reaction may require emergency intervention.

2. In the teaching plan, the nurse should include the following information:
   - Take the correct dose of the drug as pre-scribed .
   - Complete the entire course of treatment.
   - Take each dose on an empty stomach with a full glass of water.
   - Avoid dairy products, antacids, laxatives, or products containing iron during the course of treatment.
   - Notify the primary health care provider of any adverse reactions.
   - Avoid the use of alcoholic beverages during therapy unless use has been approved by the primary health care provider.

Activity D DOSAGE CALCULATION

1. 2
2. 3
3. 2
4. 2

5. 15 mL
6. 2 mL

SECTION II: APPLYING YOUR KNOWLEDGE

Activity E CASE STUDY

1. Tetracyclines such as Doryx can decrease the effectiveness of oral contraceptives, leading to breakthrough bleeding or pregnancy. The nurse should advise Ms. Lopez to use a back-up method of contraception while taking the Doryx.

2. The nurse should advise Ms. Lopez that Doryx can cause nausea, vomiting, dizziness, photosensitivity reaction (wear sunscreen and avoid tanning beds), pseudomembranous coli-tis (report diarrhea to the physician immedi-ately), and hematologic changes (which the physician will monitor with periodic blood work).

SECTION III: PRACTICING FOR NCLEX

Activity F NCLEX-STYLE

1. **Answer: a**
   RATIONALE: Lincosamides are contraindicated for patients with minor bacterial or viral infec-tions. Patients less than 9 years of age are con-traindicated for tetracyclines. Patients with liver disease are contraindicated for macrolides.

2. **Answer: b**
   RATIONALE: Increased action of a neuromuscular blocking drug may lead to severe and pro-found respiratory depression. Increased risk for bleeding is caused by the interaction of oral anticoagulants with tetracyclines. Decreased absorption of the lincosamide is caused by the interaction of kaolin- or aluminum-based antacids with lincosamides. Increased risk for digitalis toxicity is caused by the interaction of digoxin with tetracyclines.

3. **Answer: a, d, e**
   RATIONALE: General malaise, chills, fever, and redness are signs and symptoms of an infec-tion. Diabetes is not a cause of any infection. Blood dyscrasia is an abnormality of the blood cell structure or function, which is an adverse effect of lincosamides.

4. **Answer: b, d, e**
   RATIONALE: Tests that are done before the first dose of a drug is administered are culture and sensitivity tests, renal function tests, and

urinalysis. A stress test is done to monitor heart conditions. A glucose tolerance test is done to check for diabetes.

5. **Answer: a, c, e**
   RATIONALE: The nurse must notify the primary health care provider if there is a significant drop in blood pressure, an increase in the pulse or respiratory rate, or a sudden increase in temperature. Regular urine output and normal blood sugar levels need not be immediately reported to the primary health care provider.

6. **Answer: b**
   RATIONALE: The nurse should instruct the patient not to perform any hazardous activities such as driving or operating machinery, as Ketek (telithromycin) can cause the patient's eyes to have difficulty focusing and adjusting to light. Esophagitis, photosensitivity, and skin rashes are adverse effects of clindamycin.

7. **Answer: a**
   RATIONALE: The teaching plan should instruct the patient to take the drug on an empty stomach with a full glass of water. Tetracyclines are not absorbed effectively if taken just before a meal or with dairy products. The dosage has to be distributed around the clock, not just at bedtime, to increase effectiveness.

8. **Answer: a**
   RATIONALE: Dirithromycin can cause anorexia, constipation, dry mouth, hypersensitivity reactions, photosensitivity reactions, pseudomembranous colitis, and electrolyte imbalance. Visual disturbance, headache, or dizziness is caused by telithromycin. Abdominal pain, esophagitis, skin rash, or blood dyscrasias is caused by clindamycin. Photosensitivity reactions, hematologic changes, or discoloration of teeth is caused by demeclocycline.

9. **Answer: d**
   RATIONALE: An immediate nursing intervention should be to save a sample of the stool for an occult blood test. Urine samples, measuring and recording of vital signs, and checking blood pressure are not immediately required; these may follow at a later stage and as required.

10. **Answer: b**
    RATIONALE: The patient should take nothing by mouth (except water) for 1 to 2 hours before and after taking lincomycin because food impairs its absorption. The patient can have food 1 to 2 hours before the administration; he/she should not be administered the drug on an empty stomach. The drug is to be administered only with water.

11. **Answer: b**
    RATIONALE: Using cephalosporins with aminoglycosides increases the risk of nephrotoxicity. There is an increased risk of ototoxicity when loop diuretics are administered along with aminoglycosides. Neuromuscular blockage occurs due to the interaction of Pavulon with aminoglycosides. Increased serum theophylline level occurs due to the interaction of theophylline with fluoroquinolones.

12. **Answer: a, d, e**
    RATIONALE: As part of the preadministration assessment, the nurse should obtain patient's urinalysis. The nurse should also ensure that the patient's hepatic and renal functions tests are conducted, and that patient's complete blood count is obtained. Monitoring patient's vital signs every 4 hours, and recording observations in patient's chart are interventions related to the patient's ongoing assessment, not preadministration assessment.

13. **Answer: a**
    RATIONALE: The nurse is most likely to observe signs of lethargy in a patient who is administered kanamycin. Numbness and muscle twitching are seen as symptoms of neurotoxicity caused by amikacin. Abdominal pain is an adverse effect seen in patients who are administered fluoroquinolones.

14. **Answer: a**
    RATIONALE: The nurse should know that the client has developed neuromuscular blockage. Neuromuscular blockage is characterized by apnea and acute muscular paralysis. Ototoxicity is not marked by apnea and muscular paralysis. Nephrotoxicity is marked by proteinuria and hematuria, not by muscular paralysis and apnea. Pseudomembranous colitis is an adverse reaction to fluoroquinolones.

15. **Answer: a**
    RATIONALE: Tetracyclines treat infection by inhibiting bacterial protein synthesis.

CHAPTER 10

SECTION I: ASSESSING YOUR UNDERSTANDING

Activity A MATCHING

1. 1. c   2. d   3. a   4. a
2. 1. a   2. c   3. d   4. b
3. 1. d   2. c   3. b   4. a

Activity B FILL IN THE BLANKS

1. Oxazolidinone
2. Phenylketonuria
3. Ertapenem
4. Carbapenems
5. Vancomycin
6. Theophylline
7. Bactericidal

Activity C SHORT ANSWERS

1. A nurse should perform the following assessments for a patient who is being administered fluoroquinolones:
   - Inspect needle site and area around the needle every hour.
   - Perform the assessment frequently if the patient is found restless or uncooperative.
   - Check the rate of infusion every 15 minutes.
   - Inspect the vein used for IV infusion every 4 hour for signs of tenderness, pain, and redness.
   - In apparent situation, restart IV in another vein and notify the primary health care provider.
2. To determine the effectiveness of the treatment plan, the nurse should ensure:
   - The therapeutic drug effect is achieved, and the infection is controlled.
   - Adverse reactions are identified, reported to the primary health care provider, and managed successfully.
   - Pain or discomfort following IM or IV administration is relieved or eliminated.
   - Anxiety is reduced.
   - The patient and family demonstrate understanding of the drug regimen.

Activity D DOSAGE CALCULATION

1. 8 tablets
2. 5 tablets
3. 5.2 mL
4. 20 tablets
5. 6 tablets
6. 35 mL

SECTION II: APPLYING YOUR KNOWLEDGE

Activity E CASE STUDY

1. Before administering a fluoroquinolone like Cipro, the nurse identifies and records the signs and symptoms of the infections, takes a thorough allergy history, takes and records vital signs, and obtains cultures, if ordered.
2. The nurse should prepare 40 mL for one 400 mg dose of Cipro to be administered to Mrs. Moore.

SECTION III: PRACTICING FOR NCLEX

Activity F NCLEX-STYLE

1. **Answer: a**
   RATIONALE: The nurse should monitor for Thrombocytopenia and pseudomembranous colitis as the most serious adverse reaction occurring due to linezolid. Nephrotoxicity and ototoxicity are adverse reactions occurring due to the administration of vancomycin. Phlebitis occurs as a reaction when miscellaneous anti-infectives are administered through the IV route. It does not occur when anti-infectives are administered orally.

2. **Answer: a, c, d**
   RATIONALE: To maintain continuity in care, the nurse should instruct the patient and patient's family to complete full course of treatment, avoid drinking alcoholic beverages, and understand potential adverse reactions. The nurse should instruct the patient to administer the drug with or without food in the stomach, depending on what has been prescribed by the physician. All drugs need not be taken with food. The nurse should instruct the patient and patient's family to monitor for adverse symptoms for 5 to 7 days, after which if symptoms worsen, the physician should be contacted immediately.

3. **Answer: b**
   RATIONALE: The nurse should prepare and administer a dose of 10 mL of spectinomycin to the patient intravenously. The available strength of the drug dose is 5 mL/2 g. The prescribed dose is 4 g, so the nurse should prepare a dose of 10 mL. The nurse should not prepare a dose of 15 mL, 6 mL, or 2 mL.

4. **Answer: c**

   RATIONALE: When caring for a patient who has been administered spectinomycin, the nurse should monitor for urticaria as one of the adverse effects. Fever occurs as an adverse reaction of vancomycin when it is administered to patients. Throbbing neck pain occurs when vancomycin is administered intravenously to the patient. Headache occurs as an adverse effect of aztreonam when it is administered to patients.

5. **Answer: b**

   RATIONALE: When caring for a patient who has been administered quinupristin/dalfopristin, the nurse should monitor for secondary bacterial or fungal infections, which occur due to the disruption of the normal flora. The nurse has to monitor for cross-sensitivity with cephalosporin if the patient is administered Aztreonam and not quinupristin/dalfopristin. The nurse should monitor for bone marrow depression if the patient is administered linezolid and has had a history of bone marrow depression. The nurse should monitor for hearing and kidney problems if the patient is administered vancomycin along with ototoxic or nephrotoxic drugs.

6. **Answer: c**

   RATIONALE: The nurse should be alert for a sudden decrease in the patient's blood pressure when vancomycin is administered through the parenteral route to the patient. Hypotension and shock occur only when the rate of infusion of drug through the IV route in the patient is rapid. The nurse should remain alert for a ringing in the ears in the patient only if the patient has a disturbed sensory perception.

7. **Answer: b, c, d**

   RATIONALE: When conducting an ongoing assessment, the nurse should monitor vital signs of the patient every 4 hours, observe for a sudden increase in temperature in the patient, and observe the patient frequently during first 48 hours of therapy. Determining signs of infection in the patient is part of the nurse's preadministration assessment before the administration of the drug, not during ongoing assessment. The nurse should monitor for a sudden increase and not a decrease in the pulse and respiratory rate.

8. **Answer: d**

   RATIONALE: Aztreonam has to be administered cautiously if the patient is taking penicillin.

The interaction between aztreonam and penicillins could lead to cross-sensitivity. Linezolid has to be administered cautiously in case the patient takes antiplatelet drugs. Interaction between linezolid and antiplatelet drugs leads to increased risk of bleeding and thrombocytopenia. Vancomycin should be administered cautiously if the patient has been taking nephrotoxic drugs. Interaction between vancomycin and nephrotoxic drugs may not cause ototoxicity or nephrotoxicity, but two drugs together increase risk of these adverse effects. Daptomycin has to be administered cautiously if the patient has been taking warfarin.

9. **Answer: b, c, d**

   RATIONALE: When caring for a patient receiving an intramuscular anti-infective, the nurse should rotate and monitor the injection sites frequently, inspect previous injection sites, and assess the vein used for infusion for any signs of irritation. It is important for the nurse to adjust the rate of infusion every 15 minutes instead of 30, and check the infusion site once every 4 to 8 hours, not every 12.

10. **Answer: b**

    RATIONALE: Quinupristin/dalfopristin will help reduce the infection caused by *Enterococcus faecium*. Quinupristin/dalfopristin is a bacteriostatic agent used in the treatment of vancomycin-resistant *Enterococcus faecium* (VREF). Daptomycin is a new category of antibacterial agents called *cyclic lipopeptides*. This drug binds to the cell membrane depolarizing the wall, inhibiting protein DNA and RNA synthesis, which causes the bacteria cell to die. It does not help in the treatment of vancomycin-resistant *Enterococcus faecium*. Fosfomycin tromethamine (Monurol) is an anti-infective used to treat urinary tract infections. Spectinomycin exerts its action by interfering with bacterial protein synthesis. Spectinomycin is used for treating gonorrhea in patients who are allergic to penicillin, cephalosporins, or probenecid but it does not help in treating vancomycin-resistant *Enterococcus faecium*.

11. **Answer: a**

    RATIONALE: The nurse should know that fluoroquinolones have to be administered cautiously in patients with a history of seizures. Aminoglycosides and not fluoroquinolones are administered cautiously to elderly patients, patients who have neuromuscular disorders, and patients who have renal failure.

12. Answer: d

RATIONALE: The nurse should monitor the patient carefully for signs of dizziness when the patient is administered fluoroquinolones. The nurse should monitor the patient for anorexia, rash, and urticaria if the patient is administered aminoglycosides and not fluoroquinolones.

13. Answer: b, d, e

RATIONALE: When caring for a patient receiving fluoroquinolones, the nurse should inspect the vein used for infusion frequently, inform any observations made to the physician, and perform assessment frequently. The nurse should check the rate of infusion every 15 minutes and not every 2 hours. The nurse should change the vein used for infusion only in case of thrombophlebitis or phlebitis seen in the patient and not otherwise.

14. Answer: a

RATIONALE: The nurse should ensure that the patient is not younger than 18 years of age to be certain that fluoroquinolone is not contraindicated. The nurse should also check that the patient does not have preexisting hearing loss, myasthenia gravis, or Parkinsonism to ensure that aminoglycoside is not contraindicated.

15. Answer: a, b, d

RATIONALE: The nurse should instruct the client to wear long-sleeve clothing, sunscreen, and brimmed hats to assist in preventing photosensitive reactions. Wearing light makeup will not help the patient avoid a skin reaction. Venturing out on hazy and cloudy days cannot be considered safe. The nurse should inform the patient that the glare during hazy or cloudy days can cause skin reactions as much as when the sky is clear.

CHAPTER 11

SECTION I: ASSESSING YOUR UNDERSTANDING

Activity A MATCHING

1. 1. d   **2.** c   **3.** a   **4.** b

Activity B FILL IN THE BLANKS

1. Vancomycin
2. Immunodeficiency
3. Extrapulmonary
4. Tyramine
5. 2

Activity C SHORT ANSWERS

1. When caring for a patient with tuberculosis, the nurse should perform the following interventions as part of the preadministration assessment:
   • Administer the drug that is prescribed that will best control the spread of the disease.
   • Assist the physician in helping to make the patient noninfectious to others.
   • Perform laboratory and diagnostic tests before starting antitubercular therapy.
   • Depending on the severity of the disease, patients may be treated initially in the hospital and then discharged for supervised follow-up care.
   • Obtain a family history and history of contacts, if the patient has active TB.

2. To decrease the chance of non-compliance with the drug regimen, the nurse emphasizes the following points when any of these drugs are prescribed on an outpatient basis:
   • Take the drug at the prescribed time intervals. These time intervals are important because a certain amount of the drug must be in the body at all times for the infection to be controlled.
   • Take the drug with food or on an empty stomach as directed on the prescription bottle.
   • Do not increase or omit the dose unless advised to do so by the primary health care provider.
   • Complete the entire course of treatment. Do not stop taking the drug, except on the advice of a primary health care provider, before the course of treatment is completed even if symptoms have improved or have disappeared. Failure to complete the prescribed course of treatment may result in a return of the infection.
   • Notify the primary health care provider if symptoms of the infection become worse or there is no improvement in the original symptoms after about 5 to 7 days.
   • Contact the primary health care provider as soon as possible if a rash, fever, sore

throat, diarrhea, chills, extreme fatigue, easy bruising, ringing in the ears, difficulty hearing, or other problems occur.
- Avoid drinking alcoholic beverages unless use has been approved by the primary health care provider.
3. The nurse should keep the following things in mind when evaluating the treatment plan:
- The therapeutic drug effect is achieved and the infection is controlled.
- Adverse reactions are identified, reported to the primary health care provider, and managed successfully.
- Pain or discomfort following IM or IV administration is relieved or eliminated.
- Anxiety is reduced.
- The patient and family demonstrate understanding of the drug regimen.

Activity D DOSAGE CALCULATION

1. 3 tablets
2. 2 tablets
3. 16 splits

SECTION II: APPLYING YOUR KNOWLEDGE
Activity E CASE STUDY

1. Preadministration assessment of any antitubercular drug should include culture and sensitivity testing, complete blood count, radiographic studies, medication history, and a family and contacts history for those with active TB.
2. Ongoing assessment of clients taking antitubercular drug therapy should include monitoring for adverse reactions and vital signs daily for ambulatory clients and as frequently as every 4 hours for hospitalized clients.

SECTION IV: PRACTICING FOR NCLEX
Activity F NCLEX-STYLE

1. **Answer: a**
RATIONALE: When caring for a patient who has been administered rifampin, the nurse should monitor for reddish-orange discoloration of the bodily fluids as one of the drug's generalized adverse reactions. Myalgia is the generalized adverse reaction of pyrazinamide and not rifampin. Jaundice is the generalized adverse reaction of isoniazid. Dermatitis and pruritus are the generalized adverse reactions of ethambutol and not rifampin.

2. **Answer: a, b, c**
RATIONALE: The nurse should ensure that the patient is not under 13 years of age, does not have cataracts, and does not have a hypersensitivity to the drug. Any of these conditions in the patient contraindicate the use of ethambutol. The nurse should ensure that the patient does not have diabetes mellitus or acute gout only if the patient has to be administered pyrazinamide and not ethambutol.

3. **Answer: a**
RATIONALE: The nurse knows that an alternative regimen of twice weekly dosing promotes nutrition and decreases the incidence of gastric upset in the patient. It also promotes patient compliance to the drug regimen on an outpatient basis. An alternative dosing regimen of twice weekly does not promote fluid balance in the body or reduce the incidence of liver dysfunction. Taking vitamin B6 or Pyridozine prevents the occurrence of neuropathy and not following an alternative regimen of twice weekly dosing.

4. **Answers: b, c, e**
RATIONALE: Liver, kidneys and spleen can be affected by extrapulmonary tuberculosis. On the other hand, the heart and brain are not affected by extrapulmonary tuberculosis.

5. **Answers: a, b, c**
RATIONALE: The nurse should know if the patient is taking digoxin, oral anticoagulants, or oral contraceptives along with prescribed rifampin. Rifampin taken along with digoxin decreases the serum level. Rifampin when taken along with oral anticoagulants leads to decreased anticoagulant effectiveness and when taken with oral contraceptives leads to decreased contraceptive effectiveness. Colchicine and allopurinol more commonly interact with pyrazinamide, leading to decreased effectiveness.

6. **Answer: c**
RATIONALE: The nurse should monitor for severe hepatitis as the manifestation of a severe toxic reaction to isoniazid. Severe, sometimes fatal, hepatitis may occur after many months of treatment. Hepatotoxicity is the principal adverse reaction seen with pyrazinamide use, which is characterized by severe jaundice. Anaphylactoid reactions are more severe reactions seen in patients administered ethambutol. Epigastric distress is a generalized reaction and not a severe toxic reaction to isoniazid.

7. **Answer: a**

RATIONALE: The nurse should monitor for severe jaundice as a manifestation of a severe hepatotoxic reaction to pyrazinamide. Epigastric distress and hematologic changes are some of the generalized reactions of isoniazid. Severe hepatitis is a manifestation of a severe toxic reaction to isoniazid and not pyrazinamide.

8. **Answer: d**

RATIONALE: The nurse should instruct the patient to reduce alcohol consumption to prevent the risk of hepatitis. Administering pyridozine promotes nutrition and prevents neuropathy, but it does not reduce the risk of hepatitis. Using the DOT method to administer medication encourages compliance by the patient to the medication regimen, but does not prevent the risk of hepatitis. Administering antitubercular drugs in combination also promotes compliance to the drug regimen by the patient but does not prevent the risk of hepatitis.

9. **Answer: b**

RATIONALE: Rifampin is contraindicated in patients with hepatic or renal impairment. Pyrazinamide is contraindicated in patients with diabetes mellitus and those who have tested positive for HIV. Ethambutol is contraindicated in patients with diabetic retinopathy.

10. **Answer: a, b**

RATIONALE: Individuals living in crowded conditions, those with compromised immune systems (like those with HIV), and individuals with debilitative conditions are especially susceptible to tuberculosis.

11. **Answer: c**

RATIONALE: Tuberculosis is transmitted from one person to another by droplets dispersed in the air when an infected person coughs or sneezes.

12. **Answer: a, b, c, d, e**

RATIONALE: Tuberculosis primarily affects the lungs, but can affect other organs including the liver, kidneys, spleen, and uterus. Tuberculosis found to affect organs outside the lungs is known as *extrapulmonary* tuberculosis.

13. **Answer: a, b, c**

RATIONALE: Antitubercular drugs treat active tuberculosis infection and are used as prophylactic therapy to prevent the spreading of tuberculosis. Antitubercular drugs treat but do not cure tuberculosis; they simply render the patient noninfectious to others.

14. **Answer: a, c, e**

RATIONALE: X-ray studies, sputum analyses, and physical examinations can be used to determine if an HIV patient with a negative skin test has active TB.

15. **Answer: a**

RATIONALE: Optic neuritis is a dose-related adverse reaction that can occur during treatment with ethambutol. The symptoms of optic neuritis are a decrease in visual acuity and change in color perception.

CHAPTER 12

SECTION I: ASSESSING YOUR UNDERSTANDING

Activity A MATCHING

1. 1. c   2. a   3. d   4. b
2. 1. a   2. d   3. b   4. c

Activity B FILL IN THE BLANKS

1. Lemon
2. Cidofovir
3. Ritonavir
4. Indinavir
5. Antiretroviral

Activity C SHORT ANSWERS

1. Before administering an antiviral drug, a nurse should perform the following assessments: Preadministration assessment of the patient receiving an antiviral drug depends on the patient's symptoms or diagnosis. These patients may have a serious infection that causes a decrease in their natural defenses against disease. Before administering the antiviral drug, the nurse determines the patient's general state of health and resistance to infection. The nurse then records the patient's symptoms and complaints. In addition, the nurse takes and records the patient's vital signs. Additional assessments may be necessary in certain types of viral infections or in patients who are acutely ill. For example, before treatment of patients with HSV 1 or 2, the nurse inspects the areas of the body affected with the lesions (e.g., the

mouth, face, eyes, or genitalia) as a baseline for comparison during therapy.

2. During the administering of an antiviral drug, a nurse should perform the following assessments:

The ongoing assessment depends on the reason for giving the antiviral drug. It is important to make a daily assessment for improvement of the signs and symptoms identified in the initial assessment. The nurse monitors for and reports any adverse reactions from the antiviral drug. Additionally, the nurse inspects the IV site several times a day for redness, inflammation, or pain and reports any signs of phlebitis.

Activity D DOSAGE CALCULATION

1. 5 mL
2. 35 ml
3. 70 mL
4. 4 tablets
5. 4 mL
6. 120 mL

SECTION II: APPLYING YOUR KNOWLEDGE
Activity E CASE STUDY

1. The nurse needs to obtain Mr. Jones' vital signs, a medication history (prescription and nonprescription), his symptoms and complaints, and assess his general state of health.

2. The nurse should tell Mr. Jones to stop taking St. John's wort because it can reduce the effectiveness of his antiretroviral therapy. The nurse should remind Mr. Smith to disclose the use of all over the counter medications and supplements to his physician and not to begin taking any over the counter medications or supplement without consulting the physician first. The nurse should also encourage Mr. Jones to discuss his depressive symptoms with the physician.

SECTION III: PRACTICING FOR NCLEX
Activity F NCLEX-STYLE

1. Answer: a, b, d
   RATIONALE: While administering ribavirin, the nurse should use a small-particle aerosol generator and discard and replace the solution every 24 hours. Ribavirin can worsen the respiratory status and the nurse should monitor the patient's respiratory system for any signs of deterioration. Ribavirin does not induce anorexia or nephrotoxicity in the patient.

2. Answer: b
   RATIONALE: When clarithromycin is taken along with an antiretroviral drug, it results in increased serum level of both drugs. Increased serum level of the antiretroviral is the effect of the interaction of antifungals and antiretroviral drugs. There is no risk of toxicity associated with combining the two drugs. Combining the two drugs also does not significantly decrease the effectiveness of either of the drugs.

3. Answer: c
   RATIONALE: Before beginning the treatment of the patient with HSV 1, the nurse should inspect the areas of the body affected with the lesions as a baseline for comparison during therapy. Recording a patient's temperature and blood pressure are routine interventions that the nurse should follow and are not specific to the treatment of HSV 1. There is no need to save a sample of the patient's urine unless specifically instructed to do so by the health care provider.

4. Answer: b, c, e
   RATIONALE: The nurse should include soft, non-irritating foods in the client's diet, keep the atmosphere clean and free of odors, and provide good oral care before and after meals. The nurse should administer small, frequent meals to the client and not reduce the frequency of the meals. Frequent sips of carbonated beverages or hot tea may be helpful and should not be eliminated from the patient's diet.

5. Answer: c
   RATIONALE: Phlebitis refers to the inflammation of the veins of the patient. It commonly occurs when drugs are administered intravenously. Phlebitis does not occur in patients who are being administered drugs orally, intramuscularly, or transdermally.

6. Answer: d
   RATIONALE: The nurse should exercise caution while caring for patients who have been administered indinavir and have a history of bladder stone formation. Indinavir does not react significantly to exacerbate the condition of patients with cardiac disorders or renal impairment. The drugs fosamprenavir and amprenavir, and not indinavir, should be used cautiously in patients with sulfonamide allergy.

7. **Answer: c**

RATIONALE: The nurse should avoid generating dust while preparing to administer didanosine to the patient. Didanosine should be given on an empty stomach and not with meals. The drug should be dissolved in 4 oz of water and not 2 oz. The solution should be given immediately to the patient after preparation and not refrigerated.

8. **Answer: b**

RATIONALE: One mL of solution contains 24 mg of the drug. Therefore, required amount is 225 mL (5400/24).

9. **Answer: d**

RATIONALE: Required dosage is 800 mg. Available drug is 200 mg. Number of tablets required is 4 (800/200) per dosage.

10. **Answer: c**

RATIONALE: Required dosage is 200 mg. Available drug is 50 mg/5 mL. Therefore, solution of drug in 1 mL is 10 mg (50/5). Required quantity is 20 mL (200/10) per dosage.

11. **Answer: a, c, d, e**

RATIONALE: A virus can enter the body through various routes including being swallowed, inhaled, injected with a contaminated needle, or transmitted through the bite of an insect.

12. **Answer: a, c, d, e**

RATIONALE: Viruses can cause infections of the skin, eye, nose, throat, and respiratory system such as warts, the common cold, or influenza. Viruses can also cause systemic infections including West Nile, Hepatitis C, and HIV.

13. **Answer: a, b, e**

RATIONALE: Antiviral medications are limited in their ability to treat viral infections because viruses are tiny, replicate inside cells, and can develop resistance to antiviral drugs.

14. **Answer: a**

RATIONALE: HAART is multidrug therapy that is used to treat HIV.

15. **Answer: a, b, c**

RATIONALE: Retroviruses contain an enzyme called reverse transcriptase which is used to turn the primary component RNA into DNA. Human immunodeficiency virus is an example of a retrovirus.

CHAPTER 13

SECTION I: ASSESSING YOUR UNDERSTANDING

Activity A MATCHING

1. 1. b   2. d   3. a   4. e   5. c
2. 1. b   2. c   3. d   4. a

Activity B FILL IN THE BLANKS

1. Systemic
2. Superficial
3. Creatinine
4. Liver
5. Heart
6. Electrolyte
7. Lesions
8. Mebendazole
9. Chloroquine
10. Paromomycin
11. Iodoquinol
12. Retinal

Activity C SHORT ANSWERS

1. The nurse should perform the following preadministration assessments before administering an antifungal drug:
   - Assess patient for signs of infection before first dose of an antifungal drug.
   - Inspect superficial fungal infections such as skin or skin structures and provide baseline data.
   - Document observations such as skin lesions, rough itchy patches, cracks between the toes, and sore and reddened areas to obtain an accurate database.
   - Ask about pain; describe white plaques or sore areas on mucous membranes, oral or perineal areas, and inquire for any vaginal discharge.
   - Take and record vital signs.
   - Weigh patient scheduled to receive amphotericin or flucytosine dose.
2. When caring for a patient on antifungal drug therapy, the nurse's role is to:
   - Inspect application site for localized skin reactions.
   - Ask patient about discomfort or other sensations experienced after insertion of the antifungal preparation which is administered vaginally.
   - Note in the chart any improvement or deterioration of lesions of the skin, mucous membranes, or vaginal secretions.

- Evaluate and chart daily the patient's response to therapy.
3. Before administering anthelmintic drugs for the first time, a nurse should perform the following assessments:
   - Instruct the patient how to take a specimen from the perianal area with a cellophane tape–covered swab early in the morning before the patient gets out of bed.
   - The nurse also may need to weigh the patient if the drug's dosage is determined by weight or if the patient is acutely ill.
4. If a patient develops nausea, vomiting, or abdominal pain during treatment for anthelmintic drugs, the nurse should perform the following interventions:
   - Give the drug with food to alleviate nausea.
   - Provide small meals of easily digestible food.
   - Consider the patient's food preferences and encourage the patient to eat nutritious,
   - well-balanced meals.
   - If vomiting is present, prescribe an antiemetic or a different anthelmintic agent.

Activity D DOSAGE CALCULATIONS

1. 2 tablets
2. 4 tablets
3. 8 tablets
4. 5 mL
5. 12 capsules
6. 2 tablets
7. 2 tablets
8. 3 tablets

SECTION II: APPLYING YOUR KNOWLEDGE
Activity E CASE STUDY

1. Ms. Landry is at increased risk for fungal infections because she is immunocompromised for antirejection and is taking prednisone, Advair, and Ortho Novum 7/7/7. Ms. Landry should also be reminded to rinse her mouth out after each use of Advair to help prevent oral thrush.
2. The nurse should instruct Ms. Landry to swish and hold the solution in her mouth for several seconds (or as long as possible), gargle, and then swallow the solution.

SECTION III: PRACTICING FOR NCLEX
Activity F NCLEX-STYLE

1. **Answer: b**
   RATIONALE: The nurse should check the lungs for deep mycotic infections. Deep mycotic infections develop inside the body, such as in the lungs, brain, or gastrointestinal tract. The nurse need not check the liver, mouth, or heart since deep mycotic infections occur only in the lungs, brain, or gastrointestinal tract.

2. **Answer: c**
   RATIONALE: The nurse needs to observe for any redness or stinging reaction in a patient who is treated with topical administration of an antifungal drug. Topical administration is unlikely to cause nausea and diarrhea; these are adverse reactions that can be caused by systemic administration of an antifungal drug.

3. **Answer: c**
   RATIONALE: History of heart failure is a contraindication the nurse must consider when assessing a patient for itraconazole therapy. The drug is not contraindicated in patients with bone marrow suppression, severe liver disease, or history of asthma. Severe liver disease is a contraindication to be considered when assessing a patient for griseofulvin therapy.

4. **Answer: a**
   RATIONALE: When administering an IV solution of amphotericin B, the nurse should ensure that the IV solution is protected from light since it is light sensitive. The nurse should ensure that the solution is used within 8 hours after the drug is reconstituted, not 24, to prevent loss of drug activity. The nurse should not freeze the unused solution; it should be discarded. The solution should not be stored.

5. **Answer: a**
   RATIONALE: The nurse needs to monitor the patient for vomiting as it is an adverse reaction to intravenous administration of amphotericin B. Abdominal pain, muscle pain, and anorexia are not adverse reactions of intravenous administration of amphotericin B. Abdominal pain is a reaction of topical administration of an antifungal drug, while anorexia and muscle pain are reactions of systemic administration of an antifungal drug.

6. **Answer: b**

RATIONALE: The nurse should encourage the patient to verbalize feelings since it will help reduce the patient's anxiety. The nurse need not check the patient's blood pressure, provide the client with a blanket, or keep the patient away from light since those won't help reduce the patient's anxiety. A patient's blood pressure needs to be taken during the administration of an antifungal drug. Providing warm blankets will only provide comfort to the patient and not reduce anxiety.

7. **Answer: d**

RATIONALE: In the teaching plan, the nurse should include informing the patient about keeping towels and face cloths separate from those of other family members to avoid the spread of the infection. It is important to keep the affected area clean and dry. Antifungal drugs neither cause photosensitivity nor do they affect mental status, so the patient does not need to avoid sunlight or activities. Sexual contact will not spread the infection unless it is in the vagina.

8. **Answer: c**

RATIONALE: The nurse should instruct the patient taking ketoconazole to expect headache, dizziness, and drowsiness. The patient is unlikely to experience unusual fatigue, yellow skin, darkened urine, fever, sore throat, skin rash, nausea, vomiting, or diarrhea, since these are not the adverse reactions caused by ketoconazole. Unusual fatigue, yellow skin, and darkened urine are reactions caused by itraconazole, while fever, soar throat, or skin rash are reactions caused by griseofulvin. Nausea, vomiting, or diarrhea is caused by flucytosine.

9. **Answer: d**

RATIONALE: As the patient is acutely ill, the nurse should carefully measure and record the fluid intake and output. The nurse should record the vital signs of the patient every 4 hours, not 12 hours, and observe the patient every 2 hours, not 4 hours, for malaria symptoms. There is no need to collect urine samples of the patient for testing.

10. **Answer: a**

RATIONALE: Quinine is contraindicated in patients with myasthenia gravis as it may cause respiratory distress and dysphagia. Quinine, however, is not contraindicated in patients with thyroid disease, blood dyscrasias, or diabetes.

11. **Answer: a, b, d**

RATIONALE: Drowsiness, dizziness, nausea, vomiting, abdominal pain, and cramps are some of the adverse reactions associated with anthelmintic drugs. Visual disturbances and tinnitus or a ringing sound in the ears are not generally associated with anthelmintic drugs.

12. **Answer: b**

RATIONALE: The nurse should follow hospital procedure for transporting the stool sample to the laboratory. Unless ordered otherwise, the nurse should save all stools that are passed after the drug is given. The nurse should visually inspect all stools and not just when the patient reports something unusual. Specimens should be taken by swabbing the perianal area with a cellophane tape-covered swab, not any container.

13. **Answer: a, d, e**

RATIONALE: The primary health care provider should be notified immediately if the patient experiences unusual muscle weakness, ringing in the ears and visual changes after the chloroquine drug has been administered. Yellow or brownish discoloration of urine is a natural and harmless side effect of chloroquine and need not be reported. Peripheral neuropathy is an adverse effect of metronidazole and is not associated with chloroquine.

14. **Answer: a**

RATIONALE: The nurse should caution the patient that Albendazole can cause serious harm to a developing fetus. Albendazole does not, however, cause miscarriage, decrease the chances of conception, or reduce estrogen levels.

15. **Answer: c**

RATIONALE: The nurse should educate the patient to use chlorine bleach to disinfect toilet facilities or the shower stall after bathing. The nurse should recommend the barrier method and not birth control pills for contraception. The dosage regimen should be adhered to even if the symptoms of affected condition have disappeared. Chloroquine should be taken with water and not milk.

16. **Answer: b**

RATIONALE: Nephrotoxicity and ototoxicity are adverse reactions associated with paromomycin. Peripheral neuropathy may occur with metronidazole use but not paromomycin. Thrombocytopenia is associated with anthelmintic medications, and vertigo and hypotension are the adverse effects of chloroquine.

17. **Answer: a**
RATIONALE: The nurse should instruct the patient to take metronidazole with meals or immediately afterwards. Alcohol should be avoided for the duration of the treatment and not just for the first week. Cimetidine should not be taken as it decreases the metabolism of metronidazole. Metronidazole does not cause photosensitity so there is no need to wear additional clothing to protect the skin from the sun.

18. **Answer: a**
RATIONALE: The nurse should caution the patient against exposure to sunlight as the skin becomes photosensitive during the administration of doxycycline. Skin eruptions, cinchonism, and thrombocytopenia are not adverse effects caused by doxycycline.

CHAPTER 14

SECTION I: ASSESSING YOUR UNDERSTANDING

Activity A MATCHING

1. **1.** b   **2.** d   **3.** a   **4.** c
2. **1.** c   **2.** a   **3.** d   **4.** b

Activity B FILL IN THE BLANKS

1. Prostaglandins
2. Platelets
3. Pancytopenia
4. Reye
5. Tinnitus

Activity C SHORT ANSWERS

1. The nurse can assess the patient's pain in the following ways:
   - The patient is taught to rate the pain on a scale of 0 to 10, with 0 being "no pain" and 10 being the "most severe pain imagined" by the patient.
   - Other methods such as scales of colors or facial expressions such as the Wong-Baker FACES Pain Rating Scale may be used.
2. The nurse can monitor and manage the discomfort of the patient receiving a salicylate or a nonsalicylate in the following ways:

- Notify primary health care provider if there has been no relief from pain or discomfort.
- Assess for bleeding or inflammation.
- To minimize GI distress, administer drug with food, milk, or give antacids.
- Check color of stools (bright red or black indicating bleeding) and report.

Activity D DOSAGE CALCULATION

1. 12 tablets
2. 6 tablets
3. 6 tablets
4. Half a tablet
5. 4 tablets
6. 2 tablets

SECTION II: APPLYING YOUR KNOWLEDGE

Activity E CASE STUDY

1. The nurse should advise Mrs. Matthews that the use of Ecotrin (a salicylate analgesic) with warfarin can increase her risk for bleeding because Ecotrin, like warfarin, increases the time it takes for blood to clot.
2. The nurse should advise Mrs. Matthews to try Tylenol (acetaminophen) to relieve her headaches because Tylenol does not interfere with blood clotting.

SECTION III: PRACTICING FOR NCLEX

Activity F NCLEX-STYLE

1. **Answer: b**
RATIONALE: The nurse needs to monitor the patient for GI bleeding, as it is an adverse reaction caused by the administration of salicylates. Skin eruptions, jaundice, and bleeding disorders are not adverse reactions of the administration of salicylates. Skin eruptions and jaundice are the adverse reactions of administration of acetaminophen. Incidence of a bleeding disorder contraindicates the administration of salicylates, but salicylates do not cause bleeding disorders.

2. **Answer: a, c, d**
RATIONALE: For patients with influenza, viral illness, or bleeding disorders, salicylate use is contraindicated. Salicylates are also contraindicated for patients with a known history of hypersensitivity to the salicylates. Salicylates are not known to be contraindicated in patients with a heart disease. Salicylates are administered with caution in patients with hepatic or renal disorders, but incidence of

these conditions does not contraindicate the administration of salicylates.

3. Answer: c
RATIONALE: Unlike aspirin, acetaminophen does not inhibit platelet aggregation; therefore, it is the analgesic of choice when bleeding tendencies are an issue. Acetaminophen and aspirin are both used to treat high fever or severe pain, and there is no reason why acetaminophen is preferred over aspirin for treating pain or fever. Acetaminophen is not used to treat inflammatory disorders.

4. Answer: d
RATIONALE: The nurse should assess for a decrease in inflammation and greater mobility as part of the ongoing assessment. The nurse should reassess the patient's pain rating 30 to 60 minutes, not 2 hours, following administration of the drug, and monitor the vital signs every 4, not 8, hours. There is no need to send a sample for testing immediately if the stools are dark as long as the nurse informs the primary care provider.

5. Answer: a
RATIONALE: Nausea is one of the symptoms that can be observed in a patient with salicylate levels between 150–250 micrograms/mL. Respiratory alkalosis, hemorrhage, and asterixis are associated with salicylate levels in excess of 400 micrograms/mL.

6. Answer: d
RATIONALE: Combining loop diuretics with acetaminophen may result in decreased effectiveness of the diuretic. Combining loop diuretics with acetaminophen does not increase the possibility of toxicity or bleeding, nor does it decrease the effectiveness of acetaminophen.

7. Answer: a, d, e
RATIONALE: The nurse should instruct the patient to avoid OTC drugs that may contain aspirin in the label. The patient should purchase the drug in small quantities when used on an occasional basis to prevent deterioration. If a surgery or a dental procedure is anticipated, the patient should notify the primary health care provider or dentist. The patient should avoid eating foods such as paprika, licorice, prunes, and raisins in diet as they are rich in salicylates. Salicylates should be stored in tightly closed containers and not in ventilated locations.

8. Answer: a
RATIONALE: One of the adverse reactions that the nurse should monitor for in a patient who has been administered salicylates such as salsalate is GI bleeding. Hypoglycemia, pancytopenia, or hemolytic anemia are symptoms associated with acetaminophen and not salsalate.

9. Answer: b
RATIONALE: Aspirin can be used to treat inflammatory conditions such as rheumatoid arthritis. Since aspirin increases bleeding tendencies, it is contraindicated in patients with hemophilia, patients who have just undergone surgical operations, or patients taking anticoagulants.

10. Answer: a
RATIONALE: Malaise is one of the symptoms associated with acetaminophen toxicity when a patient has been prescribed acetaminophen. Increased anxiety, hyperglycemia, and bradycardia are not symptoms generally associated with acetaminophen toxicity.

11. Answer: a
RATIONALE: The nervous system is the agent involved in the recognition and perception of pain.

12. Answer: a, c
RATIONALE: The two basic types of pain are acute pain and chronic pain.

13. Answer: a, b
RATIONALE: Acute pain is brief and lasts less than 3 to 6 months. Postoperative pain and procedural pain represent acute pain.

14. Answer: d
RATIONALE: Chronic pain lasts more than 6 months.

15. Answer: a, d, e
RATIONALE: Chronic pain lasts more than 6 months and is often associated with specific diseases, such as fibromyalgia, rheumatoid arthritis, and osteoarthritis.

CHAPTER 15

SECTION I: ASSESSING YOUR UNDERSTANDING

Activity A MATCHING

1. 1. c   **2.** a   **3.** b
2. 1. d   **2.** c   **3.** a   **4.** b

Activity B FILL IN THE BLANKS

1. Cyclooxygenase
2. Celecoxib
3. Ibuprofen
4. Reye
5. Inflammation

Activity C SHORT ANSWERS

1. NSAIDs are used for the treatment of:
   - Pain associated with osteoarthritis, rheumatoid arthritis, and other musculoskeletal disorders
   - Mild to moderate pain
   - Primary dysmenorrhea (menstrual cramps)
   - Fever reduction
2. The nurse should monitor the patient for the following adverse reactions of NSAIDs on the sensory organs:
   - Visual disturbances, blurred or diminished vision, diplopia (double vision), swollen or irritated eyes, photophobia (sensitivity to light), reversible loss of color vision
   - Tinnitus (ringing in the ears)
   - Taste change
   - Rhinitis (runny nose)

Activity D DOSAGE CALCULATION

1. 3 tablets
2. 5 tablets
3. 1.5 tablets
4. 2 tablets
5. 4 tablets

SECTION II: APPLYING YOUR KNOWLEDGE
Activity E CASE STUDY

1. The nurse should tell Mr. Smith that ibuprofen works in a way similar to his aspirin (inhibition of prostaglandin synthesis), and he may experience easy bruising and bleeding with the combination. He should also notify the other health care providers, including the dentist, that he is taking ibuprofen. The nurse should also relay that prolonged use of ibuprofen can increase blood pressure and that home monitoring is recommended to ensure his dose of lisinopril continues to be appropriate.
2. The nurse should tell Mr. Smith the following about the administration of his medication:
   - Take the medication every 8 hours as needed for pain,
   - Do not increase the dose without discussing it with the physician first.
   - Take the medication with food or milk and a full glass of water.

SECTION III: PRACTICING FOR NCLEX
Activity F NCLEX-STYLE

1. **Answer: a, c, e**
   RATIONALE: The nurse should inform the patient that epigastric pain, abdominal distress, and intestinal ulceration are the adverse reactions of NSAIDs on the gastrointestinal system. Appendicitis is the inflammation of the vermiform appendix. Appendicitis and indigestion are not adverse reactions of NSAIDs.

2. **Answer: c**
   RATIONALE: Celecoxib is not used to relieve postoperative pain for a patient who has undergone coronary artery bypass graft (CABG) surgery, as it causes an increased risk of myocardial infarction in the patient. Duodenal ulcer, gastric bleeding, and diarrhea are adverse reactions of Ketoprofen in the treatment of rheumatoid disorder.

3. **Answer: b**
   RATIONALE: The nurse should identify that patients with peptic ulceration are contraindicated for treatment with ibuprofen. Celecoxib is contraindicated in patients with allergy to sulphonamides, history of cardiac disease, or stroke.

4. **Answer: d**
   RATIONALE: Before administering an NSAID to the patient, the nurse should assess the patient for bleeding disorders. Visual disturbances, allergic skin, and dizziness are monitored during ongoing assessments.

5. **Answer: a**
   RATIONALE: The nurse should document limitations in mobility before administration of the prescribed NSAID. Examining the level of consciousness, checking level of mental stability, and examining the body temperature are not relevant assessments for a patient with osteoarthritis.

6. **Answer: c**
   RATIONALE: The nurse should suggest that the patient take medication with food. This will promote an optimal response to therapy. Avoiding exercise, restricting to a liquid diet, or restricting mobility will not promote an optimal response to therapy. Exercise and

mobility would be essential to maintain free movement of the joints. The patient undergoing therapy may be affected by acidity, hence the need to have a complete, nutritious diet, not just a liquid diet.

7. **Answer: d**

    RATIONALE: The nurse should monitor the patient for GI bleeding, which is an adverse reaction of indomethacin administration. Tinnitus, diarrhea, and rash are adverse reactions of etodolac administration.

8. **Answer: d**

    RATIONALE: NSAID treatment for patients above 65 years of age should begin with a reduced dosage, which is increased slowly because there is risk of serious ulcer diseases. Elderly patients are not at an increased risk for inflammation, erythema, or an increase in the number of RBCs due to NSAID.

9. **Answer: a**

    RATIONALE: The nurse should administer the patient 2 tablets of nabumetone 500 mg for the recommended dose of 1 g per day.

10. **Answer: b, d, e**

    RATIONALE: The nurse should suggest to the patient not to use the drugs on a regular basis unless notifying the PHCP, avoiding use of aspirin, and taking the drug with a full glass of water or with food in the patient's teaching plan. Avoiding physical activities during drug therapy and keeping towels separate from those of other family members are not points that the nurse should include in the plan.

11. **Answer: a**

    RATIONALE: Blocking cyclooxygenase-2 is responsible for the pain-relieving effects of NSAIDs.

12. **Answer: c**

    RATIONALE: Blocking cyclooxygenase-1 is responsible for the GI side effects caused by NSAIDS.

13. **Answer: a**

    RATIONALE: The most common side effects caused by the NSAIDs involve the GI tract, including the stomach.

14. **Answer: c**

    RATIONALE: A hypersensitivity to aspirin is a contraindication for all NSAIDs.

15. **Answer: a**

    RATIONALE: Celecoxib (Celebrex) is the NSAID that appears to work by specifically inhibiting cyclooxygenase-2, without inhibiting cyclooxygenase-1.

CHAPTER 16

SECTION I: ASSESSING YOUR UNDERSTANDING

Activity A MATCHING

1. 1. b   2. d   3. a   4. c
2. 1. c   2. a   3. d   4. b

Activity B FILL IN THE BLANKS

1. Morphine
2. Hypersensitivity
3. Opium
4. Heroin
5. Cachectic

Activity C SHORT ANSWERS

1. When a patient is receiving drugs through a PCA infusion pump, the nurse should educate the patient on the following points:
    - The location of the control button that activates the administration of the drug.
    - The difference between the control button and the button to call the nurse (when both are similar in appearance and feel).
    - The machine regulates the dose of the drug as well as the time interval between doses.
    - If the control button is used too soon after the last dose, the machine will not deliver the drug until the correct time.
    - Pain relief should occur shortly after pushing the button.
    - Call the nurse if pain relief does not occur after two successive doses.
2. The nurse should evaluate the following factors to confirm the success of an opioid treatment plan:
    - The therapeutic effect occurs and pain is relieved.
    - The patient demonstrates the ability to effectively use PCA.
    - Adverse reactions are identified, reported to the primary health care provider, and managed through appropriate nursing interventions.
    - No evidence of injury is seen.

- Body weight is maintained.
- Diet is adequate.
- The patient and family demonstrate understanding of the drug regimen.

Activity D DOSAGE CALCULATION

1. 2 tablets
2. 1 tablet
3. Physician has prescribed 6.3 mg of butorphanol. 18.9 mg of the drug should be taken a day
4. 1 mL
5. 12.5 mL
6. 2 tablets

SECTION II: APPLYING YOUR KNOWLEDGE
Activity E CASE STUDY

1. The nurse should include the following in the instruction of a PCA pump:
   How the pump works; location of the control button that activates the administration of the morphine; use machine to prevent pain; push button once; button does not need to be depressed to keep the morphine flowing in the IV; dose is ordered by the physician and set in the pump by the nurse; if more analgesia is necessary notify the nurse.
2. During ongoing assessment the nurse obtains the blood pressure, pulse, respiratory rate, and pain rating in 5 to 10 minutes because the morphine is being given IV. The pain assessment should include type, location, and intensity.

SECTION III: PRACTICING FOR NCLEX
Activity F NCLEX-STYLE

1. **Answer: b**
   RATIONALE: The nurse should monitor for urticaria as one of the allergic reactions of opioid analgesics in the patient. Other allergic reactions include rashes and pruritus. Although constipation, palpitations, and facial flushing are all adverse reactions to opioid analgesics, they are not allergic reactions specifically. Constipation is an adverse gastrointestinal reaction to opioid analgesics. Palpitations and facial flushing are specific cardiovascular system reactions to the administration of opioid analgesics.

2. **Answer: b**
   RATIONALE: The preadministration assessment conducted by the nurse before the administration of an opioid analgesic involves assessing and documenting the type, onset, intensity, and location of the pain. Other preadministration assessments include reviewing the patient's health history, allergy history, and past and current drug therapies. The nurse obtains the blood pressure, pulse and respiratory rate, and pain rating in 5 to 10 minutes if the drug is given intravenously (IV), 20 to 30 minutes after the drug is taken intramuscularly or subcutaneously, 30 or more minutes if the drug is given orally, but these interventions are a part of the ongoing assessment conducted while the patient is on the drug therapy and not before the administration of the drug.

3. **Answer: a**
   RATIONALE: The nurse should confirm that the patient is not taking monoamine oxidase inhibitors to ensure that the use of passion flower is not contraindicated in the patient. Use of passion flower is also contraindicated in patients who are pregnant. Administration of passion flower is not known to be contraindicated in patients taking opioid analgesics, patients with acute ulcerative colitis, or patients with a history of asthma, so the nurse need not ensure the absence of these conditions in patients.

4. **Answer: b**
   RATIONALE: The nurse should assess food intake after each meal when caring for a patient with imbalanced nutrition as a result of anorexia. It is important for the nurse to notify the primary health care provider of continued weight loss and anorexia. The nurse need not complement the patient's meal with additional protein supplements. Patient's bowel movements are recorded daily in case the patient has constipation and not nutritional imbalance. Ensuring an increase in the patient's fluid intake specifically is not a necessary intervention, since it will not help improve the patient's condition.

5. **Answers: a, b, c**
   RATIONALE: The nurse should look out for withdrawal symptoms such as excessive crying, vomiting, and yawning in the newborn of an opioid-dependent mother. Withdrawal symptoms in the newborn usually appear during the first few days of life. Other withdrawal symptoms in the infant include increased respiratory rate, tremors, fever, vomiting, and diarrhea. Coughing and sneezing are not

known to occur as withdrawal symptoms in the newborn of an opioid-dependent mother.

6. **Answers: a**

    RATIONALE: A nurse should administer naloxone with great caution to a patient who is prescribed an opioid for treatment for a decrease in respiratory rate. This is because naloxone removes all the pain-relieving effects of the opioid and leads to withdrawal symptoms or return of intense pain. Naloxone is not known to cause vomiting, dizziness, or headache.

7. **Answers: a, b, c**

    RATIONALE: The primary health care provider should be contacted immediately if the nurse observes a significant decrease in the respiratory rate or a respiratory rate of 10 breaths/min or below, a significant increase or decrease in the pulse rate or a change in the pulse quality, a significant decrease in blood pressure (systolic or diastolic), or a systolic pressure below 100 mm Hg. Opioid analgesics do not lead to an increase in body weight or an increase in body temperature; therefore the nurse is not likely to make these observations when caring for the patient.

8. **Answers: a, c, d**

    RATIONALE: The nurse should know that opioid analgesics are administered with caution in patients with undiagnosed abdominal pain, hepatic or renal impairment, and hypoxia. Other conditions that require cautious use of opioid analgesics include supraventricular tachycardia, prostatic hypertrophy, lactating patients, patients of an advanced age, opioid naïve patients, and patients undergoing biliary surgery. The drug need not be used cautiously with patients who are 13 years or younger or in patients with fungal infections.

9. **Answers: c**

    RATIONALE: Administration of barbiturates when the patient is on opioid therapy leads to respiratory depression, hypotension, and sedation. Barbiturates interacting with opioid analgesics are not known to cause bacterial infections, hypertension, or hypoxia.

10. **Answer: b**

    RATIONALE: The nurse should instruct the patient to avoid alcohol after being treated with opioid analgesics. Alcohol may intensify the action of the drug and cause extreme drowsiness or dizziness. In some instances, the use of alcohol and an opioid can have extremely serious and even life-threatening consequences that may require emergency medical treatment. The nurse need not instruct the patient to avoid traveling, avoid exercising, and avoid eating starchy food since they will not have a negative effect on the patient's health when the patient is on an opioid.

11. **Answer: a**

    RATIONALE: Morphine sulfate is considered the gold standard in pain management and is considered the prototype opioid.

12. **Answer: a**

    RATIONALE: The one bodily system that does not adapt and compensate for the secondary effects of opioids is the GI system.

13. **Answer: b**

    RATIONALE: A lactating female should wait at least 4 to 6 hours after taking an opioid analgesic to breastfeed the infant.

14. **Answer: a**

    RATIONALE: Passion flower has been used in medicine to treat pain, anxiety, and insomnia.

15. **Answer: c**

    RATIONALE: Passion flower contains coumarin, and the risk of bleeding may be increased in patients taking warfarin (Coumadin).

CHAPTER 17

SECTION I: ASSESSING YOUR UNDERSTANDING

Activity A MATCHING

1. **1.** a, b   **2.** a, b

Activity B FILL IN THE BLANKS

1. Antagonist
2. Opioid
3. Naloxone
4. Hypersensitivity
5. Postanesthesia
6. Respiratory
7. Narcan

Activity C SHORT ANSWERS

1. The nurse should perform the following preadministration assessments when caring for a patient who is prescribed opioid antagonists:
   - Awaken patient and instruct regarding the different breathing patterns.
   - Before administration of the antagonist, obtain blood pressure, pulse, and respiratory rate.
   - Review the record for the drug suspected of causing the symptoms of respiratory depression.
   - Review initial health history, allergy history, and current treatment modalities for the patient
2. The nurse should know that opioid antagonists are used in the following circumstances:
   - Postoperative acute respiratory depression
   - Reversal of opioid adverse effects
   - Suspected acute opioid overdosage

Activity D DOSAGE CALCULATION

1. 5 tablets
2. 6 mL
3. 5 mL

SECTION II: APPLYING YOUR KNOWLEDGE
Activity E CASE STUDY

1. The nurse's preadministration assessment should include taking and monitoring blood pressure, pulse, and respiratory rate.
2. After Mr. Smith vomits, the nurse should maintain a patent airway by turning and suctioning him as needed.

SECTION III: PRACTICING FOR NCLEX
Activity F NCLEX-STYLE

1. **Answer: b**
   RATIONALE: The nurse should know that an opioid antagonist reverses pain. An antagonist is given to reverse a specific adverse reaction; therefore the antagonist reverses all effects. A patient who receives an antagonist to reverse respiratory effects will also experience a reversal of pain relief— i.e., the pain will return. The opioid antagonist does not relieve or decrease pain, nor does it neutralize the effect of the opioid drug.

2. **Answer: a, c, d**
   RATIONALE: The critical factors that a nurse should evaluate in a patient receiving an opioid antagonist for respiratory depression are positive response to the therapeutic treatment, normal respiratory rate, and resumption of pain relief. The nurse need not evaluate normal blood pressure and normal heart rate in a patient who has received treatment for respiratory depression.

3. **Answer: c**
   RATIONALE: To promote an optimal response to naloxone in the patient, the nurse should balance the need for continued pain relief and the ability of the person to breathe independently. The nurse need not specifically monitor for an increase in the patient's body temperature because naloxone is not known to cause a rise in body temperature. Since administration of naloxone is not known to cause dehydration or any other form of water loss, the nurse need not monitor the patient for this condition. Naloxone is always given by slow IV push. The drug should not be administered through a rapid IV push because it is known to cause withdrawal and return of intense pain if administered with a rapid bolus.

4. **Answer: b, c, d**
   RATIONALE: In monitoring and managing the patient's needs during and after naloxone administration, the nurse should make suction equipment readily available for use because abrupt reversal of opioid respiratory depression causes vomiting. The nurse must maintain a patent airway and should turn and suction the patient as needed. Depending on the patient's condition, the nurse should use artificial ventilation and cardiac monitoring. Opioid antagonists are not known to cause hypotension or hematologic changes, and so the nurse need not monitor the patient for these conditions.

5. **Answer: b**
   RATIONALE: The nurse should know that opioid antagonists are administered very cautiously in patients who are lactating. Antagonists are also used cautiously in those who are pregnant (Pregnancy Category B), in infants of opioid-dependent mothers, and in patients with an opioid dependency and/or cardiovascular disease. Use of opioid antagonists is contraindicated in patients who are hypersensitive to the drug. Liver impairment

or renal failure is not known to enforce a cautious use of opioid antagonists in patients.

6. **Answer: a**
RATIONALE: The nurse should ensure adequate ventilation of the patient's body. The expected outcome for the patient with respiratory depression is an optimal response to therapy. This involves a return to normal respiratory rate, rhythm, and depth. The nurse meets the patient's needs by providing adequate ventilation of the body as well as continued pain relief. The nurse need not provide the patients with controlled analgesic pumps, administer prescribed IV sedatives, or provide an odor-free room, since these interventions will not help in bringing about an optimal response to the drug therapy.

7. **Answer: a**
RATIONALE: An antagonist is defined as a substance that counteracts the action of something else.

8. **Answer: c**
RATIONALE: Naltrexone is used primarily to treat alcohol dependence.

9. **Answer: a**
RATIONALE: Naloxone is capable of restoring respiratory function within 1 to 2 minutes of administration.

10. **Answer: b**
RATIONALE: The nonimprovement in patient symptoms may likely be due to the fact the patient is not experiencing an opioid overdose, but may have overdosed on a nonopioid substance, such as a benzodiazepine. If the patient has not taken or received an opioid, an opioid antagonist has no drug effect.

11. **Answer: a**
RATIONALE: Naloxone (Narcan) is an opioid antagonist, which means it will only reverse the effects of opioids like fentanyl (Duragesic).

12. **Answer: a**
RATIONALE: The use of opioid antagonists is contraindicated in those with a hypersensitivity to the opioid antagonists; therefore, a patient with a hypersensitivity to nalmefene (Revex) should not be given the drug.

13. **Answer: c**
RATIONALE: Opioid antagonists may produce withdrawal symptoms in patients physically dependent on opioids.

14. **Answer: a**
RATIONALE: Opioid naïve patients are defined as those that do not use opioids routinely.

15. **Answer: b**
RATIONALE: Opioid naïve patients are most at risk for respiratory depression after opioid administration.

CHAPTER 18

SECTION I: ASSESSING YOUR UNDERSTANDING
Activity A MATCHING
1. 1. c   2. d   3. a   4. b
2. 1.   2. c   3. b   4. a

Activity B FILL IN THE BLANKS
1. Conduction
2. General
3. Anesthesia
4. Anesthetist
5. Anesthesiologist
6. Volatile

Activity C SHORT ANSWERS
1. The nurse must ensure that the surgeon and the anesthesiologist are made aware of the abnormality. The nurse must attach a note to the front of the chart and also try to contact the surgeon or anesthesiologist via telephone.
2. After surgery, the nurse has the following responsibilities, which vary according to where the nurse first sees the postoperative patient:
   - Admit the patient to the unit according to hospital procedure or policy.
   - Check the airway for patency, assess the respiratory status, and give oxygen as needed.
   - Position the patient to prevent aspiration of vomitus and secretions.
   - Check blood pressure and pulse, IV lines, catheters, drainage tubes, surgical dressings, and casts.
   - Review the patient's surgical and anesthesia records.
   - Monitor the blood pressure, pulse, and respiratory rate every 5 to 15 minutes until the patient is discharged from the area.
   - Check the patient every 5 to 15 minutes for emergence from anesthesia. Suctioning is provided as needed.

- Exercise caution in administering opioids. The nurse must check the patient's respiratory rate, blood pressure, and pulse before these drugs are given, and 20 to 30 minutes after administration. The physician is contacted if the respiratory rate is below 10 before the drug is given or if the respiratory rate falls below 10 after the drug is given.
- Discharge the patient from the area to his or her room or other specified area. The nurse must record all drugs administered and nursing tasks performed before the patient leaves the PACU.
3. The administration of general anesthesia requires the use of one or more drugs. The choice of anesthetic drug depends on many factors, including:
   - The general physical condition of the patient
   - The area, organ, or system being operated on
   - The anticipated length of the surgical procedure

Activity D DOSAGE CALCULATION

1. 3 mL
2. 2 tablets
3. 5 doses in 5 days; 1 dose each day
4. 3 tablets
5. 45 min

SECTION II: APPLYING YOUR KNOWLEDGE
Activity E CASE STUDY

1. The preoperative nurse is responsible for describing the preparation for surgery ordered by the physician, assessing the physical status of the client, describing postoperative care, demonstrating postoperative client activities, and demonstrating the use of a PCA pump.
2. The nurse should administer 5 mL to the patient (5 mg × 1 mL/1 mg = 5 mL)

SECTION III: PRACTICING FOR NCLEX
Activity F NCLEX-STYLE

1. **Answer: c**
   RATIONALE: The nurse should know that methohexital is a barbiturate, and it depresses the CNS to produce hypnosis and anesthesia, but does not produce analgesia. Recovery after a small dose is rapid. Enflurane, which is a volatile anesthetic liquid, produces mild stimulation of respiratory and bronchial secretions

when used alone. Halothane, another volatile anesthetic liquid, causes moderate muscle relaxation. Cholinergic blocking drugs such as glycopyrrolate decrease secretions of the upper respiratory tract.

2. **Answer: a**
   RATIONALE: Stage 1 of anesthesia, known as the *induction* or analgesic stage of general anesthesia, begins with a loss of consciousness. Delirium, along with excitement, is marked in the second stage of anesthesia. Surgical analgesia and respiratory paralysis are noted in the third and fourth stages, respectively.

3. **Answer: b**
   RATIONALE: Topical anesthesia leads to desensitization of the skin and mucus membrane. Topical anesthesia does not bring about a decrease in anxiety and apprehension, or cardiovascular stimulation, or a loss of feeling in the lower extremities. Opioids, which are anesthetic drugs used for general anesthesia, bring about a decrease in anxiety and apprehension. Ketamine, a drug used for general anesthesia, causes cardiovascular and respiratory stimulation. Administration of spinal anesthesia causes a loss of feeling (anesthesia) and movement in the lower extremities.

4. **Answer: c**
   RATIONALE: As part of the postoperative interventions after the administration of anesthesia, the nurse should position the patient to prevent aspiration of vomitus and secretions. The nurse should review the patient's laboratory test records before the administration of anesthesia and not after. As part of the postoperative interventions done after the administration of anesthesia, the nurse should review the patient's surgical and anesthesia records. The nurse should also monitor the blood pressure, pulse, and respiratory rate every 5 to 15 minutes until the patient is discharged from the area, and not every 12 hours. The nurse should know that a hypnotic agent is administered to the patient before the administration of anesthesia and not after.

5. **Answers: b**
   RATIONALE: If a patient shows an increase in his respiratory secretions on the administration of the preanesthetic drug, the nurse should understand that the preanesthetic drug was not given to the patient on time. Preanesthetic drugs must be administered on time to produce their intended effects. Failure to give

the preanesthetic drug on time may result in such events as increased respiratory secretions caused by the irritating effect of anesthetic gases and the need for an increased dose of the induction drug because the preanesthetic drug has not had time to sedate the patient. Not assessing patient's IV lines well, not assessing patient's respiratory status, and not reviewing patient's anesthesia records do not cause an increase in the patient's respiratory secretions.

6. **Answers: a, b, c**
   RATIONALE: When caring for a patient receiving local anesthesia, the nurse should apply dressing to surgical areas and observe bleeding and oozing, if any, in the patient. Assessing the patient's pulse rate every 5 to 15 minutes and exercising caution when administering opioids to the patient are postoperative interventions, which a nurse has to perform. These interventions are not appropriate when caring for a patient about to undergo local anesthesia for the suturing of a wound.

7. **Answer: a**
   RATIONALE: The nurse should confirm that the patient is not over 60 years of age. Preanesthetic drugs may be omitted in patients aged 60 or older because many of the medical disorders for which these drugs are contraindicated are seen in older individuals. Epinephrine used with local anesthesia is contraindicated in cases when local anesthesia is to be applied to the extremities. Preanesthetic drugs are not contraindicated in cases of the application of anesthesia to the extremities. Preanesthetic drugs are not known to be contraindicated in patients who have a low body weight.

8. **Answer: a**
   RATIONALE: The nurse should administer a cholinergic blocking drug as it decreases the secretions of the upper respiratory tract. Scopolamine and glycopyrrolate are mild sedatives. Opioid is used to decrease the anxiety and apprehension of the patient before the surgery. Diazepam or valium are used as an anti-anxiety drug for preoperative sedation.

9. **Answer: a**
   RATIONALE: The nurse should know that the transsacral block is injected in epidural space at the level of the sacrococcygeal notch when administering a transsacral block as anesthesia

for a cesarean delivery. A transsacral block is often used in obstetrics. An epidural block is injected for anesthesia into the space surrounding the dura of the spinal cord. Spinal anesthesia is injected into the subarachnoid space of the spinal cord. A brachial plexus block involves the injection of a local anesthetic into the brachial plexus.

10. **Answer: d**
    RATIONALE: The nurse should confirm that the patient does not require anesthesia to be administered on the extremities to ensure that the use of epinephrine along with local anesthesia is not contraindicated in the patient. The anesthetic stays in the tissue longer when epinephrine is used. This is contraindicated, however, when the local anesthetic is used on an extremity. Epinephrine used with local anesthesia is not known to be contraindicated in patients who are anemic, patients who have a low blood pressure, or in patients who are over 60 years of age.

11. **Answer: a**
    RATIONALE: Regional anesthesia is a type of local anesthesia and includes spinal anesthesia and conduction block.

12. **Answer: c**
    RATIONALE: Topical anesthesia may be applied by the nurse with a cotton swab or sprayed on the area to be desensitized.

13. **Answer: a**
    RATIONALE: Local infiltration anesthesia is commonly used for dental procedures, the suturing of small wounds, or for making an incision into a small area.

14. **Answer: a**
    RATIONALE: Epinephrine can be mixed in certain situations with an injectable local anesthetic in order to cause local vasoconstriction.

15. **Answer: a**
    RATIONALE: A nurse may be asked to administer an antianxiety drug such as midazolam (Versed) prior to a colonoscopy to help the patient relax.

CHAPTER 19

SECTION I: ASSESSING YOUR UNDERSTANDING

Activity A MATCHING

1. **1.** b   **2.** c   **3.** a

Activity B FILL IN THE BLANKS

1. Carotid
2. Narcolepsy
3. Sympathomimetic
4. Medulla
5. Arrhythmias

Activity C SHORT ANSWERS

1. The nursing interventions while caring for a patient with ineffective breathing pattern who is being administered CNS stimulants are:
   - Record blood pressure, pulse, and respiratory rate.
   - Before administering drug, ensure patent airway.
   - Monitor respirations closely after administration.
   - Record the effects of therapy.
2. The interventions for a patient experiencing nausea and vomiting from an analeptic are:
   - Nurse should keep a suction machine nearby in case the patient vomits.
   - Nurse measures intake and output in case of urinary retention.
   - Nurse notifies the primary health care provider if the patient cannot void or if bladder appears distended on palpation.

Activity D DOSAGE CALCULATION

1. 4 tablets
2. 4 mL
3. 4 tablets
4. 3 tablets
5. 1 tablet

SECTION II: APPLYING YOUR KNOWLEDGE

Activity E CASE STUDY

1. The nurse's preadministration and ongoing assessment of a client receiving a CNS stimulant for the treatment of obesity should include blood pressure, pulse, respiratory rate, and weight.
2. The nurse should advise Ms. Johnson that the most common side effects of sibutramine (Meridia) are insomnia, headache, dry mouth, constipation, rhinitis, and pharyngitis.

SECTION III: PRACTICING FOR NCLEX

Activity F NCLEX-STYLE

1. **Answer: b**
   RATIONALE: Hyperactivity is one of the adverse reactions of CNS stimulants that a nurse should monitor for. Bradycardia, not tachycardia, is a reaction of CNS stimulants. Fever or high BP are not adverse effects generally associated with CNS stimulants.

2. **Answer: a**
   RATIONALE: The nurse should instruct the parents of the patient to give the drug in the morning 30 to 45 minutes before breakfast and before lunch. Specify that the drug should not be given in the late afternoon. The drug should be given with water, not milk, and should be consumed directly and not dissolved in water or milk first.

3. **Answer: c**
   RATIONALE: The CNS stimulants are contraindicated in patients with ventilation mechanism disorders (such as COPD). The drug is not contraindicated in patients with bone marrow suppression, severe liver disease, or ulcerative colitis.

4. **Answer: c**
   RATIONALE: Combining theophylline with CNS stimulants may result in increased risk of hyperactive behaviors. Combining the two does not lead to decreased effectiveness of the CNS stimulant or theophylline. When taken with CNS stimulants, anesthetics increase the risk for cardiac arrhythmias.

5. **Answer: c**
   RATIONALE: The nurse should monitor consciousness levels every 5 to 15 minutes. The nurse may send the blood sample for arterial blood gas analysis but not for a platelet count. Pulse rate and blood pressure should be monitored every 5 to 15 minutes, not every hour. The nurse should carefully monitor the respiratory rate until it returns to normal, and not just for 5 minutes after administration.

6. **Answer: a**
   RATIONALE: The nurse should encourage the patient to avoid napping during daytime. In patients with insomnia, the drug should be administered early in the day, not evening, whenever possible. Stimulants such as coffee

or tea should be avoided. The nurse should not administer any OTC sleeping pills.

7. Answer: a, b, e
RATIONALE: The nurse should instruct the parents to monitor the eating patterns of the child and check height and weight measurements to monitor growth. The nurse should also stress the importance of preparing nutritious meals and snacks. The child should be encouraged to have a substantial breakfast, as he or she may be in school during lunchtime and may not feel hungry. Sleeping pills should be avoided.

8. Answer: a, c, e
RATIONALE: When an amphetamine is used as part of obesity treatment, the nurse obtains and records the patient's blood pressure, pulse, respiratory rate, and weight before therapy is started. There is no need to observe the urinary output or measure blood glucose.

9. Answer: a, b
RATIONALE: The CNS is comprised of the brain and spinal cord.

10. Answer: a, d
RATIONALE: Analeptics are CNS stimulant drugs that stimulate the respiratory center of the brain and cardiovascular system.

11. Answer: b
RATIONALE: Anorexiants are drugs used to suppress the appetite.

12. Answer: a
RATIONALE: Provigil is used to treat narcolepsy and does not cause cardiac and other systemic stimulatory effects like other CNS stimulants.

13. Answer: d
RATIONALE: Most anorexiants are pregnancy category X and should not be used during pregnancy.

14. Answer: a
RATIONALE: Pediatric patients given atomoxetine (Strattera) should be monitored closely for suicidal ideations.

15. Answer: b, d
RATIONALE: Children taking CNS stimulants for the long-term treatment of ADHD should be monitored closely for weight loss and growth patterns.

CHAPTER 20

SECTION I: ASSESSING YOUR UNDERSTANDING

Activity A MATCHING

1. 1. b **2.** c **3.** d, **4.** a
2. 1. c **2.** a **3.** b

Activity B FILL IN THE BLANKS

1. Anxiolytics
2. Digoxin
3. Preanesthetic
4. Parenteral
5. Withdrawal

Activity C SHORT ANSWERS

1. Before administering alprazolam for the first time, a nurse should perform the following assessments:
   • Obtain patient's complete medical history, including mental status and anxiety level.
   • Obtain portions of the patient's history from a family member or friend.
   • Observe the patient for behavioral signs indicating anxiety.
   • Assess the blood pressure, pulse, respiratory rate, and weight.
   • Obtain a history of any past drug or alcohol use.

2. When caring for a patient receiving alprazolam who has developed constipation, a nurse should perform the following interventions:
   • Offer frequent sips of water to relieve dry mouth and to provide adequate hydration.
   • Administer oral antianxiety drugs with food or meals to decrease the possibility of gastrointestinal upset.
   • Meals should include fiber, fruits, and vegetables to prevent constipation.

Activity D DOSAGE CALCULATION

1. 1.5 tablets
2. Every 6 hours
3. 3 tablets
4. 10 tablets
5. 1.5 mg
6. 6 tablets

SECTION II: APPLYING YOUR KNOWLEDGE
Activity E CASE STUDY

1. Due to Mrs. Hinton's age, the lorazepam will be excreted more slowly leading to prolonged drug effects and an increase in adverse reactions. Therefore, the drug should be initiated at a low dose and titrated slowly. Mrs. Hinton should also be monitored closely for side effects and falls.

2. The nurse's ongoing assessment of Mrs. Hinton should include blood pressure check, mental status, anxiety level, and any side effects that may occur.

SECTION III: PRACTICING FOR NCLEX
Activity F NCLEX-STYLE

1. **Answer: b**
   RATIONALE: Diarrhea is an adverse reaction to the antianxiety drug in the patient, which is a cause of concern and should be immediately reported by the nurse to the primary health care provider. Seizures are not caused by antianxiety drugs. On the contrary, antianxiety drugs are used to control seizures or convulsions in patients. Abdominal cramps and bradycardia are not known to be adverse reactions to antianxiety drugs.

2. **Answer: c**
   RATIONALE: The nurse should assess for increased anxiety as the symptom of withdrawal of benzodiazepine. Increased RBC count and decreased pulse rate are not known to be observed in patients exhibiting benzodiazepine withdrawal symptoms. Benzodiazepine withdrawal symptoms are also marked by a decrease in appetite in patients bordering on anorexia. An increased appetite is not observed in patients with benzodiazepine withdrawal symptoms.

3. **Answer: d**
   RATIONALE: The nurse should monitor the patient for increased risk of digitalis toxicity due to the interaction of digoxin with diazepam. Increased risk for central nervous system depression is caused by the interaction of alcohol with diazepam. Increased risk for respiratory depression and sedation are caused by the interaction of tricyclic antidepressants or antipsychotics with diazepam.

4. **Answer Answer: a, c, e**
   RATIONALE: The nurse should take precautions when administering hydroxyzine drugs to patients with impaired liver function, impaired kidney function, and patients with debilitation. Patients with impaired pancreas function or bone marrow depression are not known to be contraindicated for administration of hydroxyzine.

5. **Answer: b**
   RATIONALE: Acute panic is an alcohol withdrawal symptom. Diarrhea, dry mouth, and lightheadedness are not known to be alcohol withdrawal symptoms. These are adverse reactions to chlordiazepoxide therapy, which is administered for acute alcohol withdrawal.

6. **Answer: b**
   RATIONALE: The nurse should ensure that the patient is not hypersensitive. When administering fluoroquinolones, the nurse should ensure that the patient is not under 18 years of age. When administering aminoglycosides the nurse should ensure that the patient does not have myasthenia gravis or Parkinsonism.

7. **Answer: c**
   RATIONALE: The nurse should provide the patient with a fiber-rich diet with plenty of fluids in order to prevent the occurrence of constipation. Providing vitamin supplements, or providing a diet of only fluids or vegetarian foods are ineffective measures to prevent constipation due to chlordiazepoxide.

8. **Answer: b**
   RATIONALE: The nurse should inform the patient to avoid alcohol. The patient with photosensitivity should be instructed to avoid sunlight. Photosensitivity is an adverse reaction to tricyclic antidepressants. The patient who is being treated with monoamine oxidase inhibitors should be instructed to avoid sour cream and yogurt, as these foods are rich in tyramine, which should be avoided when the patient is being treated with monoamine oxidase inhibitors.

9. **Answer: a**
   RATIONALE: The nurse should administer the drug intramuscularly in the gluteus muscle, which is a large muscle mass, and not on the arm, which has less muscle mass. The nurse should monitor for hearing and kidney problems if the patient is to be administered vancomycin along with ototoxic or nephrotoxic drugs. The nurse should monitor for secondary bacterial or fungal infections if the patient is administered quinupristin/dalfopristin.

10. Answer: c
RATIONALE: The nurse should monitor the patient for a metallic taste in the mouth, which is a withdrawal symptom of alprazolam. Diarrhea, dizziness, and dry mouth are adverse effects of the treatment.

11. Answer: a
RATIONALE: Antianxiety drugs are also referred to as anxiolytics.

12. Answer: a
RATIONALE: Benzodiazepines like lorazepam (Ativan) are classified as controlled substances by DEA regulations.

13. Answer: a
RATIONALE: Buspirone (BuSpar) exerts its anxiolytic effect by acting on the brain's serotonin receptors.

14. Answer: c
RATIONALE: Hydroxyzine (Atarax) exerts its anxiolytic effect by acting on the hypothalamus and brainstem reticular formation.

15. Answer: d
RATIONALE: Typically, benzodiazepine withdrawal symptoms are more likely to occur in patients taking the drug for 3 months or more, but can be seen when the drug is abruptly withdrawn after 4 to 6 weeks of treatment.

CHAPTER 21

SECTION I: ASSESSING YOUR UNDERSTANDING
Activity A MATCHING

1. 1. c   2. a   3. d   4. e   5. b
2. 1. b   2. c   3. a

Activity B FILL IN THE BLANKS

1. Healing
2. Insomnia
3. Valerian
4. Wakefulness
5. Melatonin
6. Barbiturates

Activity C SHORT ANSWERS

1. Before administering a sedative, the nurse takes and records the patient's blood pressure, pulse, and respiratory rate. The nurse also assesses the following patient needs by asking:
   - Is the patient uncomfortable with the idea of administering the sedative or hypnotic drug?
   - Is it too early for the patient to receive the drug? Is a later hour preferred?
   - Does the patient receive an opioid analgesic every 4 to 6 hours?
   - Are there disturbances in the environment that may keep the patient awake and decrease the effectiveness of the drug?
   - If the sedative is for a surgical procedure, then is its administration correctly timed?
   - Has a consent form been signed for the procedure before the drug is administered?
2. Nursing diagnoses particular to a patient taking a sedative or hypnotic are as follows:
   - Risk for injury related to drowsiness or impaired memory
   - Ineffective breathing pattern related to respiratory depression
   - Ineffective individual coping related to excessive use of medication

Activity D DOSAGE CALCULATION

1. 4 tablets
2. 3 tablets
3. 2 tablets
4. 2 tablets
5. 2 tablets

SECTION II: APPLYING YOUR KNOWLEDGE
Activity E CASE STUDY

1. Temazepam (Restoril) is a hypnotic drug.
2. A hypnotic is a drug that induces drowsiness or sleep, which allows the patient to fall asleep and stay asleep. A sedative is a drug that produces a relaxing, calming effect.

SECTION III: PRACTICING FOR NCLEX
Activity F NCLEX-STYLE

1. **Answer: a, c, d**
RATIONALE: Back rubs, a nightlight, and a darkened room can help to provide optimal response to sedative therapy. Bedtime coffee would promote wakefulness. Alcohol has an additive effect which, in combination with a sedative, can cause central nervous system depression and even result in death.

2. Answer: c
RATIONALE: The nurse can evaluate the effectiveness of the treatment being given to the patient from an improvement in the patient's sleep pattern. An improvement in the patient's consciousness level, a normalcy in the patient's respiration rate, and a decrease in the patient's restlessness do not indicate the effectiveness of the treatment.

3. Answer: b
RATIONALE: The nurse should record the patient's blood pressure before administering the sedative. Platelet count, hematocrit, and blood sugar are not altered by the sedative; hence these factors are not necessarily recorded before administration of the sedative.

4. Answer: a
RATIONALE: The nurse should monitor the patient for nausea, which is an adverse reaction of sedatives. Headache, restlessness, and anxiety are causes of insomnia for which a sedative may be prescribed.

5. Answer: d
RATIONALE: Sedatives must be administered cautiously to patients with renal impairment. Patients with hearing impairment, hyperglycemia, or glucose intolerance are not high-risk candidates for sedative administration.

6. Answer: b
RATIONALE: The interaction between antihistamines and sedatives causes increased sedation. Restlessness, headache, and chronic pain are symptoms of insomnia that may require treatment with sedatives.

7. Answer: b
RATIONALE: Respiratory depression is a symptom of acute toxicity due to barbiturates. Increased blood pressure, lowered blood sugar, and frequent micturition are not symptoms of toxicity. Instead, lowered blood pressure and oliguria are symptoms of toxicity. Blood sugar may not be affected by barbiturates.

8. Answer: c
RATIONALE: When barbiturates are administrated in the presence of pain, the patient could have delirium. Administration of barbiturates in the presence of pain does not cause an allergic reaction, increased body temperature, or increased blood sugar. Allergic reactions have been reported with the administration of melatonin. Lowered body temper

ature is an adverse effect of sedatives. Blood sugar may not be affected by barbiturates.

9. Answer: a, b, d
RATIONALE: Restlessness, euphoria, and confusion are withdrawal symptoms of barbiturates. Barbiturates may be used as a sedative for convulsions and seizures.

10. Answer: a, c, e
RATIONALE: The nurse should that mention relaxation, calming, and drowsiness are effects of sedatives. Nausea and dizziness are the adverse reactions of sedatives and hypnotics.

11. Answer: a
RATIONALE: Sedatives and hypnotics are used primarily to treat insomnia.

12. Answer: c
RATIONALE: A hypnotic is defined as a drug that induces drowsiness.

13. Answer: a
RATIONALE: Barbiturates like secobarbital cause more respiratory depression than the benzodiazepines or nonbenzodiazepine hypnotics.

14. Answer: d
RATIONALE: The nonbenzodiazepines have diminished hypnotic effects after approximately 2 weeks.

15. Answer: b
RATIONALE: Benzodiazepines are classified in pregnancy category X and their use is contraindicated in pregnancy.

CHAPTER 22

SECTION I: ASSESSING YOUR UNDERSTANDING

Activity A MATCHING

1. 1. d   2. c   3. b   4. a
2. 1. d   2. a   3. b   4. c

Activity B FILL IN THE BLANKS

1. Psychotherapy
2. Tyramine
3. Priapism
4. Tricyclic
5. Gluteus

Activity C SHORT ANSWERS

1. Clinical depression is treated with antidepressant drugs. Psychotherapy is used with antidepressants in treating major depressive episodes.

2. There are 4 types of antidepressants: tricyclic antidepressants, monoamine oxidase inhibitors, selective serotonin reuptake inhibitors, and miscellaneous unrelated drugs.

3. Treatment with antidepressants increases the sensitivity of postsynaptic α-adrenergic and serotonin receptors and decreases the sensitivity of the presynaptic receptor sites. This enhances recovery from the depressive episode by making neurotransmission activity more effective.

4. Tricyclic antidepressant drugs are used in the treatment of depressive episodes, bipolar disorder, obsessive-compulsive disorders, chronic neuropathic pain, depression accompanied by anxiety disorders, and enuresis. The unlabeled uses include peptic ulcer disease, sleep apnea, panic disorder, bulimia nervosa, premenstrual symptoms, and some dermatological problems. These drugs may be used with psychotherapy in severe cases.

Activity D DOSAGE CALCULATION

1. 3 tablets
2. 6 tablets
3. 2.5 tablets
4. 6 hours
5. 6 tablets
6. 2 tablets

SECTION II: APPLYING YOUR KNOWLEDGE

Activity E CASE STUDY

1. The following is a list of symptoms that may be present in patients who are depressed:
   - Feelings of hopelessness or helplessness
   - Diminished interest in activities of life
   - Significant weight loss or gain (without dieting)
   - Insomnia or hypersomnia
   - Agitation, restlessness, or irritability
   - Fatigue or loss of energy
   - Feelings of worthlessness
   - Excessive or inappropriate guilt
   - Diminished ability to think or concentrate, or indecisiveness
   - Recurrent thoughts of death or suicide (or suicide attempt)

2. The nurse should tell Mrs. Smith to take the escitaloprm (Lexapro) in the morning, as this will lessen the likelihood of insomnia and that it can take 2 to 4 weeks to see a difference in mood. The nurse should advise Mrs. Smith of the following adverse effects: headache, insomnia, somnolence, and nausea. The nurse should tell Mrs. Smith to avoid the use of cimetidine due to increased anticholinergic symptoms and NSAIDs due to the increased risk of GI bleeding.

SECTION III: PRACTICING FOR NCLEX

Activity F NCLEX-STYLE

1. **Answer: a**
   RATIONALE: Photosensitivity is one of the adverse reactions to tricyclic antidepressant drugs. Hypertensive episodes and severe convulsions are the effects observed when tricyclic antidepressants are administered along with MAOIs. Nervous system depression is the effect of the interaction of tricyclic antidepressants with sedatives, hypnotics, and analgesics.

2. **Answer: d**
   RATIONALE: The nurse should screen the patient for cerebrovascular diseases when administering monoamine oxidase inhibitors. Patients with seizure disorder and myocardial infarction are contraindicated in the use of maprotiline. Urinary retention is observed when cimetidine used for gastric upsets interacts with SSRI antidepressant drugs.

3. **Answer: a**
   RATIONALE: The nurse should monitor the patient for an increased risk of bleeding. Increased risk for hypotension is observed when antihypertensive drugs interact with antidepressants. Increased anticholinergic symptoms are observed when cimetidine used for GI upset interacts with antidepressants. Increased risk for nervous system depression is observed in patients when an analgesic interacts with antidepressants.

4. **Answer: c**
   RATIONALE: The nurse should monitor the patient for somnolence, a possible neuromuscular reaction of SSRIs. Vertigo and blurred vision are adverse reactions observed when monoamine oxidase inhibitors are administered. Tremor is an adverse reaction in other miscellaneous antidepressants.

5. Answer: a

RATIONALE: Extremely high blood pressure results in hypertensive crisis. The medical intervention involves lowering of the blood pressure. Blood sugar, temperature, and respiration rate are not causes of hypertensive crisis.

6. Answer: a

RATIONALE: The nurse should instruct the patient to report priapism or inappropriate penile erection, which is an adverse reaction observed in patients who are administered trazodone. Orthostatic hypotension or unsteadiness when changing position is observed in patients administered mirtazapine. Insomnia and diarrhea are observed in patients administered sertraline.

7. Answer: a, b, e

RATIONALE: The nurse should obtain a complete medical history, blood pressure measurements, pulse and respiratory rate as a part of preadministration assessment. Complete blood count and blood sugar levels are not adversely affected by antidepressant drugs.

8. Answer: b

RATIONALE: The nurse should closely monitor the patient for hypertensive crisis, a life-threatening adverse effect of tyramine interacting with MAOI antidepressants. Orthostatic hypotension and blurred vision are adverse effects of MAOIs. Photosensitivity is an adverse reaction of tricyclic antidepressants.

9. Answer: a

RATIONALE: The nurse should instruct the patient to change positions slowly and assist the patient if required. Instructing the patient to drink plenty of fluids, monitoring changes in vital signs, or monitoring for hyperglycemia will not help the patient overcome orthostatic hypotension.

10. Answer: c

RATIONALE: The nurse should administer fluoxetine in the morning, which is the best time for its administration. Most antidepressant drugs, except SSRIs, are best administered at night before bedtime, rather than with lunch or dinner, so that the sedative effects promote sleep, and the adverse reactions appear less troublesome.

11. Answer: a

RATIONALE: Anticholinergic side effects commonly occur with the use of the tricyclic class of antidepressants.

12. Answer: b

RATIONALE: Tricyclic antidepressants exert their effects by inhibiting reuptake of norepinephrine and serotonin.

13. Answer: a

RATIONALE: Selective serotonin reuptake inhibitors exert their effects by inhibiting reuptake of serotonin.

14. Answer: d

RATIONALE: Monoamine oxidase inhibitors such as phenelzine (Nardil) exert their effects by inhibiting the activity of monoamine oxidase.

15. Answer: a

RATIONALE: Atypical antidepressants like bupropion (Wellbutrin) exert their effects by affecting the neurotransmission of norepinephrine, serotonin, and dopamine.

CHAPTER 23

SECTION I: ASSESSING YOUR UNDERSTANDING

Activity A MATCHING

1. 1. b   2. d   3. a   4. c
2. 1. c   2. a   3. d   4. b

Activity B FILL IN THE BLANKS

1. Bipolar
2. Dopamine
3. Serotonin
4. Flattened
5. Extrapyramidal

Activity C SHORT ANSWERS

1. Before administering antipsychotics for the first time, a nurse should perform the following assessments:
   • Obtain a complete mental health, social, and medical history.
   • In the case of psychosis, obtain the mental health history from a family member or friend.
   • Observe the patient for any behavior patterns that appear to be deviations from normal.

- Obtainblood pressure, pulse, respiratory rate, and weight.
2. When caring for a patient who is being administered Risperdal and is showing signs of acute psychosis, a nurse should perform the following interventions:
   - Repeat parenteral administration every 1 to 4 hours until the desired effects are obtained.
   - Monitor the patient closely for cardiac arrhythmias, rhythm changes, or hypotension.

Activity D DOSAGE CALCULATION

1. 4 tablets
2. 2.5 mL
3. 4 tablets
4. 5 mL
5. 5 mL

SECTION II: APPLYING YOUR KNOWLEDGE
Activity E CASE STUDY

1. The nurse should relay the following to Mr. Jenkins regarding his new medication:
   - Take exactly as directed; do not change dosage without consulting prescriber.
   - Do not crush or chew extended- or slow-release tablets or capsules.
   - Maintain adequate hydration (2 to 3 L per day of fluids) unless instructed to restrict fluid intake (especially in summer).
   - Avoid changes in sodium content (e.g., low-sodium diets); reduction of sodium can increase lithium toxicity.
   - Limit caffeine intake;diuresis can increase lithium toxicity.
   - Frequent blood test and monitoring will be necessary.
   - Decreased appetite or altered taste sensation is normal; small frequent meals may help maintain nutrition.
   - Drowsiness or dizziness may also be experienced, especially during early therapy; use caution when driving or engaging in tasks requiring alertness until response to drug is known.
   - Immediately report unresolved diarrhea, abrupt changes in weight, muscular tremors, lack of coordination, fever, or changes in urinary volume.
2. Mr. Jenkins will need to have a serum lithium level drawn every 4 to 5 days during initial therapy until his clinical status stabilizes and his serum lithium level is 1 mEq/mL. His serum lithium level should be drawn as a trough level just prior to the next dose (8 hours after the last dose). Lab work should also be completed to analyze Mr. Jenkins' renal and thyroid functions, serum electrolytes, CBC with differential, and urine.

SECTION III: PRACTICING FOR NCLEX
Activity F NCLEX-STYLE

1. **Answer: b**
   RATIONALE: The nurse should ask the patient to avoid sunlight, as photosensitivity can result in severe sunburn when the patient is taking Haldol. Tanning beds should also be avoided. Minimizing alcohol use or drinking 5 glasses of water a day will not have a significant impact on photosensitivity.

2. **Answer: b**
   RATIONALE: The nurse should monitor the patient for polyuria or excessive urination. Rashes or dystonia are not symptoms generally associated with lithium carbonate. Lithium carbonate causes drowsiness, not insomnia.

3. **Answer: a**
   RATIONALE: The nurse observes the patient for any behavior patterns that appear to be deviations from normal such as poor eye contact. Inappropriate responses to questions, not brief replies, constitute deviations from normal behavior. The nurse should record instances of laughter only if inappropriate in the given situation. Shyness or timidity may be a personality trait and should not be considered as deviant behavior.

4. **Answer: d**
   RATIONALE: The nurse should ensure that assistance is available for securing the patient as the patient is displaying markedly violent behavior patterns. The drug should be given intramuscularly, not intravenously, and preferably in a large muscle mass. The nurse should keep the patient lying down, not upright, for about 30 minutes after administering the drug.

5. **Answer: c**
   RATIONALE: The nurse can mix the oral drugs in liquids such as fruit juices, tomato juice, or milk. The nurse can administer the drug in divided doses, and not just a single daily dose. To confirm whether the patient has swallowed

the drug, the nurse should inspect the patient's mouth, since the patient may lie when questioned. The nurse should not compel the patient to swallow the drug and should instead report this to the primary care provider.

6. **Answer: b**
RATIONALE: The nurse should immediately report rhythmic, involuntary movements of the tongue, face, mouth, jaw, or the extremities, as they may indicate that the patient has developed tardive dyskinesia. Dry mouth, orthostatic hypotension, and drowsiness are reactions commonly observed in patients who have been administered antipsychotics and need not be reported.

7. **Answer: d**
RATIONALE: The nurse should monitor the patient for bone marrow suppression and other adverse reactions. The patient should be informed that only a 1-week supply of this drug is dispensed at a time. WBC count tests should be scheduled every week, not every two weeks, and the testing should continue for 4 weeks, not 1 week, after therapy is discontinued.

8. **Answer: b**
RATIONALE: The nurse should continually monitor patients taking lithium for signs of toxicity, such as muscular weakness. The nurse should obtain the sample at least 8 to 12 hours after the last dose, not 5 hours. The nurse should also ensure that the sample is drawn immediately before the next dose, not 1 hour before. In the acute phase, serum lithium levels should be monitored twice every week, not once every 2 weeks.

9. **Answer: d**
RATIONALE: The nurse should administer the drug at bedtime to minimize risk of injury to the patient. Providing the drug with food, calcium supplement, or administering the drug every 8 hours won't help in minimizing the risk of injury to the patient.

10. **Answer: a, b, e**
RATIONALE: The nurse should include the following points in her education plan: Report any unusual changes or physical effects; inform the patient about the risks of EPS and TD; and avoid exposure to the sun. Altering dosage if the symptoms increase and taking the drug on an empty stomach are not the instructions provided in the nurse's

education plan for patients undergoing antipsychotic drug therapy.

11. **Answer: a**
RATIONALE: Anhedonia is a symptom of psychosis that is defined as finding no pleasure in activities that are normally pleasurable.

12. **Answer: a**
RATIONALE: Lithium is considered with the antipsychotic medications because of its use in regulating the severe fluctuations of the manic phase of bipolar disorder.

13. **Answer: b**
RATIONALE: Antipsychotic medications are thought to act by inhibiting the release of dopamine in the brain and possibly increasing the firing of nerve cells in certain areas of the brain.

14. **Answer: a**
RATIONALE: Chlorpromazine may be administered rectally to patients with nausea and vomiting.

15. **Answer: c**
RATIONALE: Toxic reaction may occur when serum lithium levels are greater than 1.5 mEq/mL.

CHAPTER 24

SECTION I: ASSESSING YOUR UNDERSTANDING

Activity A MATCHING

1.	1. b	2. c	3. d	4. a
2.	1. c	2. a	3. d	4. b

Activity B FILL IN THE BLANKS

1. Myocardial
2. Parasympathetic
3. Hypertension
4. C
5. Vasopressors

Activity C SHORT ANSWERS

1. Before administering metaraminol for the first time, a nurse should perform the following assessments:
   - Obtain patient's complete medical history, including mental status.
   - Obtain blood pressure, pulse rate and quality, and respiratory rate and rhythm.

- Assess patient's symptoms, problems, or needs.
- Record any subjective or objective data on the patient's chart.

2. The following nursing interventions are involved during the ongoing administration of metaraminol:
   - Observe the patient for the drug's effect.
   - Evaluate and document the drug's effect.
   - Obtain and document vital signs.
   - Compare assessments made before and after administration.
   - Report adverse drug reactions to the primary health care provider.

Activity D DOSAGE CALCULATION

1. 2 tablets
2. 3 tablets
3. 2 tablets
4. 1 mL
5. 2 tablets

SECTION II: APPLYING YOUR KNOWLEDGE
Activity E CASE STUDY

1. Ms. Lacy is most likely suffering from neurogenic shock, a type of distributive shock as a result of the head trauma and spinal cord injury from the motor vehicle accident.
2. Other symptoms of shock the nurse may observe in Ms. Lacy are decreased cardiac output, cool and clammy skin, pallor, cyanosis, sweating, decrease in urinary output, hypoxia, increased concentration of intravascular fluid, tachypnea, pulmonary edema, tachycardia, arrhythmias, wide pulse pressure, gallop rhythm, confusion, agitation, disorientation, and coma.

SECTION III: PRACTICING FOR NCLEX
Activity F NCLEX-STYLE

1. **Answer: c**
   RATIONALE: When caring for a patient who has been administered metaraminol and is taking digoxin, the nurse should monitor for cardiac arrhythmias. Epigastric distress or a decrease in blood pressure is not known to be caused due to the interaction of digoxin and metaraminol, though increase in blood pressure is an adverse reaction caused due to the action of adrenergic drugs. Dopamine, which is an adrenergic drug, is contraindicated in those with pheochromocytoma. Pheochromocytoma is not an adverse reaction caused by the interaction between digoxin and metaraminol.

2. **Answer: b**
   RATIONALE: Isoproterenol is contraindicated in patients with tachyarrhythmias, tachycardia, or heart block caused by digitalis toxicity, ventricular arrhythmias, and angina pectoris, but not in patients with narrow-angle glaucoma, hypotension, or pheochromocytoma. Dopamine is contraindicated in those with pheochromocytoma (adrenal gland tumor). Epinephrine is contraindicated in patients with narrow-angle glaucoma. Norepinephrine is contraindicated in patients who are hypotensive from blood volume deficits.

3. **Answer: b**
   RATIONALE: The nurse should immediately report any changes in the pulse rate or rhythm, as older adults are more likely to have preexisting cardiovascular disease that predisposes them to potentially serious cardiac arrhythmias. Nausea, headache, or urinary urgency are not known to occur in older clients due to the administration of adrenergic drugs and therefore need not be reported to the primary health care provider.

4. **Answer: a**
   RATIONALE: The nurse should monitor for supine hypertension while caring for a patient who is being administered midodrine. Midodrine causes bradycardia, not tachycardia. Orthostatic hypotension is not an adverse effect of midodrine; instead, the drug is taken to reduce orthostatic hypotension. Midodrine is not known to cause respiratory distress.

5. **Answer: a, c, e**
   RATIONALE: The nurse should perform the following interventions: Administer only via IV route; use an electronic infusion pump to administer these drugs; and inspect needle site and surrounding tissues at frequent intervals. The nurse should not mix dopamine with other drugs unless specifically instructed. The nurse should monitor blood pressure every 2 minutes, not every 30 minutes, from the beginning of therapy until the desired blood pressure is achieved.

6. **Answer: a**
   RATIONALE: The nurse should immediately report a consistent fall in the patient's blood pressure, especially if the systolic blood pressure is below 100 mm Hg. Decrease in gastric motility and increase in the heart rate are

desirable outcomes of administering metaraminol. Blood glucose levels are not known to increase with the administration of metaraminol.

7. **Answer: a, b, e**
   RATIONALE: The nurse should identify circumstances that disturb sleep and work towards minimizing their effect. Curtains can be drawn over windows to filter light. The nurse can also provide bedtime snacks to the patient. Caffeinated beverages such as tea and coffee should be avoided. Administering drugs only during daytime will not have a significant effect in restoring the patient's sleep pattern.

8. **Answer: a**
   RATIONALE: The nurse should immediately discontinue the old IV line and establish another IV line before calling the primary care provider. Moving the head of the bed to an elevated position will not help minimize the effect of tissue perfusion. Norepinephrine should not be diluted with alkaline solutions.

9. **Answer: b**
   RATIONALE: The sympathetic nervous system is also known as the adrenergic branch.

10. **Answer: a**
    RATIONALE: The sympathetic branch of the autonomic nervous system is stimulated during the body's fight-or-flight response to a stressful condition.

11. **Answer: a**
    RATIONALE: Norepinephrine is the primary neurotransmitter of the sympathetic nervous system.

12. **Answer: c**
    RATIONALE: Sympathomimetics are drugs that produce activity similar to the neurotransmitter norepinephrine.

13. **Answer: a**
    RATIONALE: Vasoconstriction of peripheral blood vessels occurs as the result of stimulation of α_1 receptors.

14. **Answer: d**
    RATIONALE: Increased heart rate and increased force of myocardial contraction are the result of stimulation of β_1 receptors.

15. **Answer: a**
    RATIONALE: Decreased tone, motility, and secretions of the GI tract are the result of stimulation of α_2 receptors.

CHAPTER 25

SECTION I: ASSESSING YOUR UNDERSTANDING

Activity A MATCHING

1. 1. b 2. d 3. a 4. c
2. 1. c 2. d 3. b 4. a

Activity B FILL IN THE BLANKS

1. Norephinerine
2. Sympatholytic
3. Phentolamine
4. Blockers
5. Glaucoma
6. Sotalol

Activity C SHORT ANSWERS

1. The nurse should perform the following preadministration assessments before administering an adrenergic blocking drug:
   - Establish database before adrenergic blocking drug is administered.
   - For peripheral vascular disease, record the symptoms of disorder.
   - For patient with hypertension. take blood pressure and pulse in both arms in sitting, standing, and supine positions before therapy.
   - For patients with cardiac arrhythmia, take pulse rate, determine the pulse rhythm, and note the patient's general appearance.
   - Obtain subjective data from patient (complaints,description).

2. When caring for a patient receiving adrenergic blocking drug therapy for hypertension, the nurse's role is to:
   - Take blood pressure before each dose.
   - Observe patient for unusual responses.
   - Take blood pressure on both arms and in sitting, standing and supine positions during the first week or more of therapy.
   - After blood pressure is stable, take blood pressure before each drug administration using the same arm and position for each reading.

Activity D DOSAGE CALCULATION

1. 4 tablets
2. 18 tablets
3. 9 tablets
4. 50 tablets
5. 2 tablets

SECTION I: APPLYING YOUR KNOWLEDGE
Activity E CASE STUDY

1. The nurse should include the following in the preadministration assessment of metoprolol to Mrs. Anderson: blood pressure on both arms, pulse rate and rhythm, general appearance, complaints or description of symptoms, and an electrocardiogram.

2. Mrs. Anderson's ongoing nursing assessment should include: blood pressure, pulse rate and rhythm; observation for the appearance of adverse reactions (orthostasis, bradycardia, dizziness, vertigo, headache, nausea, vomiting, diarrhea, dyspnea, weight gain, peripheral edema, confusion, and peripheral vascular insufficiency); and resolution of symptoms.

SECTION III: PRACTICING FOR NCLEX
Activity F NCLEX-STYLE

1. **Answer: b**
   RATIONALE: The nurse needs to monitor for orthostatic hypotension in a patient who is treated with phentolamine. Phentolamine is unlikely to cause nausea and diarrhea, bradycardia, or bronchospasm. Diarrhea, bradycardia, and bronchospasm are adverse reactions caused by betaxolol or HCL.

2. **Answer: c**
   RATIONALE: Coronary artery disease is a contradiction that the nurse must consider when assessing a patient for alpha-adrenergic blocking drug therapy. The drug is not contraindicated in patients with sinus bradycardia, heart failure, or emphysema. Sinus bradycardia, heart failure, or emphysema are contraindications to be considered when assessing a patient for beta-adrenergic blocking drug therapy.

3. **Answer: d**
   RATIONALE: The nurse should discontinue the drug when a patient receiving adrenergic blocking drugs shows a decrease in blood pressure. The nurse need not monitor for excessive perspiration or confusion, since these conditions do not occur with the administration of adrenergic blocking drugs. Shifting the patient into a more conducive position is not the most appropriate intervention, since it will not provide comfort to the patient or reduce the symptoms of a decreased blood pressure.

4. **Answer: a**
   RATIONALE: The nurse should monitor vascular insufficiency in the elderly patient when administering a beta-adrenergic blocking drug. The nurse need not monitor occipital headache, dizziness, and CNS depression in the elderly patient when administering a beta-adrenergic blocking drug, since these conditions are not known to occur in older patients on the administration of beta-adrenergic blocking drugs.

5. **Answer: b**
   RATIONALE: Interaction of lidocaine with beta-adrenergic blockers causes an increase in the serum level of the beta-blocker. Increased risk of hypotension is the result of the interaction between loop diuretics and beta-adrenergic blockers. Increased risk of paradoxical hypertensive effect is the result of interaction between clonidine and beta-adrenergic blockers. Similarly, increased effect of the beta-blocker is the result of the interaction of antidepressants with beta-adrenergic blockers.

6. **Answer: d**
   RATIONALE: The nurse should monitor light-headedness as the adverse reaction in a patient who is administered peripherally acting antiadrenergic drugs. The nurse need not monitor dry mouth, drowsiness, and malaise as the adverse reactions of peripherally acting antiadrenergic drugs. Dry mouth, drowsiness, and malaise are the generalized reactions that are associated with antiadrenergic drugs that are centrally acting when administered to patients.

7. **Answer: a**
   RATIONALE: The nurse should measure the apical pulse rate when the patient is administered a sympatholytic drug. If pulse is below 60 bpm, if there is any irregularity in the patient's heart rate or rhythm, or if systolic blood pressure is less than 90 mm Hg, the nurse should withhold the drug and contact the primary health care provider. The nurse need not measure the body temperature, heart rate, or the respiratory rate in the patient who is to be administered the sympatholytic drug, since these are not likely to be affected with the administration of a sympatholytic drug.

8. **Answer: c**
   RATIONALE: The nurse should include contacting the primary health care provider in the teaching plan of the patient who is prescribed

adrenergic blocking drugs for glaucoma if changes in vision occur. Informing the patient to monitor his/her own pulse and blood pressure, and to take drugs as directed with food or on an empty stomach are included in the teaching plan of a patient with hypertension, angina, or arrhythmia. The nurse need not instruct the patient who has been treated for glaucoma to ambulate often.

9. **Answer: a**
RATIONALE: The nurse should measure the intraocular pressure to determine the effectiveness of drug therapy. The nurse need not monitor the blood pressure, respiratory rate, or pulse rate of the patient who is administered beta-adrenergic blocking ophthalmic preparations such as timolol, since monitoring these will not determine the effectiveness of the therapy.

10. **Answer: b**
RATIONALE: The nurse should assess the patient for increased risk of psychotic behavior in the patient due to the interaction of antiadrenergic drug with haloperidol. Interaction of antiadrenergic drug with lithium causes increased risk of lithium toxicity. Increased risk of hypertension is the result of interaction between antiadrenergic drugs and beta blockers. Increased effect of anesthetic is a result of the interaction between antiadrenergic drugs and anesthetic agents.

11. **Answer: b**
RATIONALE: Alpha-blockers result in vasodilation when administered to patients.

12. **Answer: a**
RATIONALE: Phentolamine (Regitine) is an alpha-adrenergic blocker.

13. **Answer: a**
RATIONALE: The majority of beta-adrenergic receptors are found in the heart.

14. **Answer: c**
RATIONALE: Hypertension research studies demonstrate better patient outcomes for African Americans when beta-blockers (atenolol) are used in combination with diuretics (chlorthalidone) than other drugs to treat hypertension, such as ACE inhibitors.

15. **Answer: d**
RATIONALE: Carvedilol (Coreg) is an example of an alpha/beta-adrenergic drug.

CHAPTER 26

SECTION I: ASSESSING YOUR UNDERSTANDING
Activity A MATCHING

1. **1.** b **2.** c **3.** a
2. **1.** b **2.** c **3.** a

Activity B FILL IN THE BLANKS

1. Muscarinic
2. Parasympathetic
3. Acetylcholine
4. Anticholinesterases
5. Nicotinic

Activity C SHORT ANSWERS

1. Before administering ambenonium for the first time, a nurse should perform the following assessments:
   - Perform a complete neurologic assessment.
   - Assess for signs of muscle weakness, such as drooling, inability to chew and swallow, drooping of the eyelids, inability to perform repetitive movements, difficulty breathing, and extreme fatigue.
2. The nurse should explain that myasthenia gravis is a disease that involves rapid fatigue of skeletal muscles because of the lack of ACh released at the nerve endings of parasympathetic nerves. Cholinergic drugs that prolong the activity of ACh by inhibiting the release of AChE are called *indirect-acting cholinergics* or anticholinesterase muscle stimulants. Drugs used to treat this disorder act indirectly to inhibit the activity of AChE and promote muscle contraction.

Activity D DOSAGE CALCULATION

1. 7 tablets
2. 2 tablets
3. 1 vial
4. 2 tablets per dose
5. 0.5 mL

SECTION II: APPLYING YOUR KNOWLEDGE
Activity E CASE STUDY

1. Before the nurse gives abenonium (Mytelase) to Mr. Simms, the nurse should assesses for signs of muscle weakness, such as drooling, inability to chew or swallow, drooping of the eyelids, inability to perform repetitive

movements, difficulty breathing, and extreme fatigue.

2. The nurse should advise Mr. Simms of the following adverse effects that may result from the use of ambenonium (Mytelase): nausea, diarrhea, abdominal cramping, salivation, skin flushing, cardiac arrhythmias, and muscle weakness.

SECTION III: PRACTICING FOR NCLEX
Activity F NCLEX-STYLE

1. **Answer: a**
   RATIONALE: The nurse should observe for temporary reduction of visual acuity and headache as adverse reactions of the topical administration of cholinergic drugs. Increased ocular tension, decreased sweat production, and anaphylactic shock are not related adverse reactions. Increased ocular tension, decreased sweat production, and anaphylactic shock are adverse reactions of cholinergic blocking drugs.

2. **Answer: a**
   RATIONALE: The nurse should instruct the patient to remove and replace the system every 7 days. The nurse should also instruct the patient that replacement is best during bedtime and not daytime. The nurse should notify the primary health care provider if eye secretions are excessive or irritation occurs, and not instruct the patient to change the system every day if eye secretions are excessive. It is important for the patient to carry identification indicating that the patient has myasthenia gravis and not glaucoma.

3. **Answer: d**
   RATIONALE: The nurse should check the patient for mechanical obstruction of the GI or genitourinary tracts before administration of bethanecol. Tachyarrhythmias, myocardial infarction, and coronary occlusion are not related disorders that a nurse needs to check before the administration of bethanecol. Cholinergic drugs are used cautiously in patients with recent coronary occlusion and not particularly bethanecol.

4. **Answer: b**
   RATIONALE: The nurse should anticipate the decreased effect of the cholinergic as the effect of the interaction between ambenonium and corticosteroids. Increased neuromuscular blocking effect, increased absorption of the cholinergic, and decreased serum levels of corticosteroids are not related effects of the interactions between ambenonium and corticosteroids. Increased neuromuscular- blocking effect is the effect of the interaction of aminoglycoside antibiotics with cholinergic drugs.

5. **Answer: c**
   RATIONALE: The nurse should remove excessive secretions with a cotton ball or gauze soaked in normal saline or other cleansing solution recommended by the primary health care provider as part of the ongoing assessment for the patient. Assessing for signs of muscle weakness is the preadministration nursing assessment for a patient with myasthenia gravis. Drying of upper respiratory and oral secretions and measuring and recording fluid intake and output are not ongoing assessments for a patient with glaucoma. Measuring and recording the fluid intake and output is the ongoing assessment for a patient with urinary retention and not with glaucoma.

6. **Answer: c**
   RATIONALE: The nurse caring for a patient who is being administered a cholinergic drug should ensure that aminoglycoside antibiotics are administered cautiously, as it increases the risk of neuromuscular-blocking effects. Salicylates, analgesics, and antidiabetics need to be administered cautiously to the patient undergoing anticonvulsant drug therapy.

7. **Answer: a, b, c**
   RATIONALE: The nurse should instill the drug in the lower conjunctival sac, avoid the tip of the dropper touching the eye, and support the hand by holding the dropper against the patient's forehead while managing a patient who is being prescribed Miostat. The nurse need not advise the patient to wear or carry identification about glaucoma.

8. **Answer: c, d, e**
   RATIONALE: The nurse should observe for salivation, clenching of the jaw, and muscle rigidity and spasm as symptoms of drug overdose in the patient to make frequent dosage adjustments. Drooping of the eyelids and rapid fatigability of the muscles are symptoms of drug underdose.

9. **Answer: c**
   RATIONALE: The nurse should place call light and items that the patient might need within easy reach while managing the care of patient-administered cholinergic therapy for urinary retention. Instructing the patient to

void before the drug is administered, encouraging the patient to take the drug with milk to enhance absorption, and encouraging the patient to have 5 to 7 glasses of water after drug administration are not related nursing activities while caring for a patient administered cholinergic therapy.

10. **Answer: a, c, e**
    RATIONALE: The nurse should ensure that bedpan or bathroom is readily available, encourage the patient to ambulate to assist the passing of flatus, and keep a record of the number, consistency, and frequency of stools if the patient develops diarrhea after administering urecholine drug orally. Checking for blood stains in the stool and encouraging the patient to increase fibrous food intake are not related nursing activities.

11. **Answer: a**
    RATIONALE: Acetylcholine is the substance responsible for transmission of nerve impulses across the parasympathetic nervous system.

12. **Answer: a**
    RATIONALE: The stimulation of muscarinic receptors in the parasympathetic nervous system stimulates smooth muscle.

13. **Answer: b**
    RATIONALE: The stimulation of nicotinic receptors in the parasympathetic nervous system stimulates skeletal muscle.

14. **Answer: a**
    RATIONALE: Acetylcholinesterase is the enzyme responsible for activating acetylcholine, the primary neurotransmitter in the parasympathetic nervous system.

15. **Answer: a**
    RATIONALE: Bethanechol (urecholine) is an example of a direct-acting cholinergic that acts like the neurotransmitter acetylcholine.

CHAPTER 27

SECTION I: ASSESSING YOUR UNDERSTANDING
Activity A MATCHING

1. **1.** d **2.** c **3.** a **4.** b
2. **1.** c **2.** a **3.** d **4.** b

Activity B FILL IN THE BLANKS
1. Acetylcholine
2. Parasympathetic
3. Cycloplegia
4. Atropine
5. Idiosyncrasy

Activity C SHORT ANSWERS

1. The nurse should include the following when evaluating the patient's treatment plan:
   - Therapeutic effect is achieved.
   - Adverse reactions are identified, reported, and managed successfully.
   - Oral mucous membranes remain moist.
   - Patient complies with the prescribed drug regimen.
   - Patient and family demonstrate an understanding of the drug regimen.
   - Patient verbalizes the importance of complying with the prescribed therapeutic regimen.

2. The nurse should offer the following instructions to an elderly patient's family when caring for the patient receiving cholinergic blocking drugs for treatment:
   - The nurse should inform the family of possible visual and mental impairments (blurred vision, confusion, agitation) that may occur during therapy with these drugs. Objects or situations that may cause falls, such as throw rugs, footstools, and wet or newly waxed floors, should be removed or remedied whenever possible.
   - The nurse should instruct the family to place against the walls any items of furniture (e.g., footstools, chairs, stands) that obstruct walkways.
   - The nurse should alert the family to the dangers of heat prostration and explains the steps to take to avoid this problem.
   - The patient must be closely observed during the first few days of therapy, and the primary health care provider should be notified if mental changes occur.

Activity D DOSAGE CALCULATION

1. 3 tablets
2. 2 tablets
3. 1.25 mL
4. 3 tablets

SECTION II: APPLYING YOUR KNOWLEDGE
Activity E CASE STUDY

1. The following is a list of adverse reactions that should be included in the nurse's teaching plan for Mrs. Mason: photophobia, dry mouth, constipation, heat prostration, and drowsiness.

2. The nurse should observe elderly patients receiving a cholinergic drug such as tolterodine (Detrol) at frequent intervals for excitement, agitation, mental confusion, drowsiness, urinary retention, or other adverse effects. These effects may be seen even with small doses in the elderly. If any of these adverse effects occur, it is important to withhold the next dose and contact the physician.

SECTION III: PRACTICING FOR NCLEX
Activity F NCLEX-STYLE

1. **Answer: d**
   RATIONALE: A nurse should use atropine cautiously in patients with asthma. The nurse should not administer cholinergic blocking drugs for patients with tachyarrhythmias, myasthenia gravis, or glaucoma since the presence of these conditions contraindicates the use of these drugs.

2. **Answer: b**
   RATIONALE: When caring for a patient on cholinergic drugs complaining of constipation, the nurse should suggest that the patient increase his or her consumption of food rich in fiber. The nurse should also instruct the patient to increase fluid intake up to 2000 mL daily (if health conditions permit) and obtain adequate exercise. The nurse should instruct the patient to increase fluid intake, which will help minimize the adverse reactions of constipation and dry mouth, while the cholinergic blocking drug would help eliminate the sensations of urinary frequency and urgency. The nurse should not instruct the patient to take antacids in case of severe constipation, since antacids will not help relieve the patient's condition. The nurse need not instruct the patient to increase the consumption of citrus fruits, because this will not relieve the patient's constipation.

3. **Answer: d**
   RATIONALE: The nurse should monitor for a change in pulse rate or rhythm when caring for a patient receiving atropine for a third-degree heart block. The nurse should place the patient on a cardiac monitor during and after administration of the drug, and not before the drug administration. The nurse need not provide oxygen support to the patient every hour in this case. The nurse need not monitor for symptoms of mydriasis and cycloplegia, since these conditions are visual impairments and are not known to occur with the administration of atropine for a third-degree heart block.

4. **Answer: a, b, d**
   RATIONALE: The nurse should suggest that the patient wear loose clothes, sponge the skin with cool water, and use a fan to cool the body to lessen the intensity of heat prostration. The nurse need not suggest that the patient apply sunscreen to reduce the discomfort or symptoms of heat prostration. The nurse should instruct the patient with photophobia to wear sunglasses when moving outdoors and not when caring for a patient with heat prostration.

5. **Answer: c**
   RATIONALE: The nurse should assess for an increased effect of atropine as the effect of the interaction between atropine and the tricyclic antidepressant. The interaction of these two drugs is not known to cause a decrease in the effectiveness of the antidepressant, an increase in the respiratory rate, or a decrease in blood pressure.

6. **Answer: a, b, e**
   RATIONALE: The nurse should monitor for nausea, altered taste perceptions, and dysphagia when caring for a patient who is administered glycopyrrolate. Tachycardia and mydriasis are not known to occur due to the administration of glycopyrrolate. Tachycardia occurs with the administration of mepenzolate bromide. Mydriasis occurs with the administration of trihexyphenidyl.

7. **Answer: a**
   RATIONALE: The nurse should ensure that the cholinergic drug is not administered preoperatively for this 65-year-old patient, because cholinergic blocking drugs are usually not included in the preoperative drugs of patients older than 60 years due to their effects on the eyes and central nervous system. The nurse should monitor the patient's pulse rate or rhythm when caring for a patient receiving atropine for a third-degree heart block. The nurse need not position the patient in a

Fowler's position, but it is mandatory to instruct the patient to remain in bed with the side rails raised after the drug is administered. The nurse need not ensure if the patient has received antibiotics preoperatively or not.

8. **Answer: c**
RATIONALE: The nurse should administer the drug at the exact time prescribed by the physician in order to allow the drug to produce the greatest effect before the administration of anesthetic. The nurse need not administer the drug at the exact time to avoid abdominal cramping in the patient after the drug administration, to ensure the effectiveness of the drug after the administration of anesthetic, nor to avoid excessive salivation or make the patient feel comfortable.

9. **Answer: b**
RATIONALE: The nurse should monitor for signs of mouth dryness after the oxybutynin is administered to the patient. Mydriasis is an adverse reaction related to the administration of trihexyphenidyl. Blurred vision and hesitancy are the adverse reactions associated with the administration of atropine, belladonna alkaloids, glycopyrrolate, dicyclomine HCl, glycopyrrolate, mepenzolate bromide, methscopolamine, propantheline bromide, and scopolamine hydrobromide.

10. **Answer: d**
RATIONALE: The nurse should identify drowsiness as part of the desired response for the patient who has been administered atropine preoperatively. Vomiting, elevated temperature, and low pulse rate are not known to be the desired responses to the administration of atropine when it is administered preoperatively.

11. **Answer: a**
RATIONALE: Oxybutynin (Ditropan) is an example of a parasympatholytic drug.

12. **Answer: c**
RATIONALE: Oxybutynin (Ditropan) used for the treatment of overactive bladder exerts it effect by inhibiting the action of muscarinic receptors.

13. **Answer: b**
RATIONALE: The antispasmodic dicyclomine (Bentyl) used for the treatment of irritable bowel syndrome exerts its effect by inhibiting the action of nicotinic receptors.

14. **Answer: d**
RATIONALE: The cholinergic blocking drug glycopyrrolate (Robinul) is used in conjunction with anesthesia to reducte oral secretions.

15. **Answer: c**
RATIONALE: The nurse should observe patients receiving a cholinergic blocking drug during the hot summer months because these patients are at increased risk of heat prostration.

CHAPTER 28

SECTION I: ASSESSING YOUR UNDERSTANDING

Activity A MATCHING

1. 1. d   2. c   3. b   4. a
2. 1. b   2. c   3. a

Activity B FILL IN THE BLANKS

1. Alzheimer's
2. Cholinergic
3. Liver
4. Brain
5. Hepatotoxicity

Activity C SHORT ANSWERS

1. The nurse should assess the following in patients who are prescribed cholinesterase inhibitors:
   - Cognitive ability such as orientation, calculation, recall and language, and functional ability such as performance of daily activities and self-care
   - Agitation and impulsive behavior
   - Mental health and medical history, including history of Alzheimer's symptoms
   - Physical assessments such as blood pressure measurements (on both arms with patient in a sitting position), pulse, respiratory rate, and weight
   - Patient's vital signs and body weight
2. The nurse should perform the following interventions when caring for a patient receiving tacrine:
   - Monitor for liver damage by checking levels of alanine aminotransferase.
   - Obtain alanine aminotransferase levels weekly.
   - Monitor transaminase levels every 3 months from at least week 4 to week 16.

- Monitor for adverse reactions including nausea, vomiting, diarrhea, dizziness, and headache.

Activity D DOSAGE CALCULATION

1. 9 tablets
2. 2 tablets
3. 2 capsules
4. 3 capsules

SECTION II: APPLYING YOUR KNOWLEDGE
Activity E CASE STUDY

1. Mrs. Barnes is in the early stage of Alzheimer's disease, as she has displayed characteristics of memory difficulty, poor judgment, and withdrawal behaviors.
2. The most common adverse effect with the use of donepezil (Aricept) include: headache, nausea, diarrhea, insomnia, and muscle cramps.

SECTION III: PRACTICING FOR NCLEX
Activity F NCLEX-STYLE

1. **Answer: a**
   RATIONALE: The nurse should monitor diarrhea in the patient as an adverse reaction of cholinesterase inhibitors. High blood pressure, seizure disorders, and renal dysfunction are not adverse reactions of cholinesterase inhibitors.

2. **Answer: d**
   RATIONALE: Tacrine should be used cautiously in the case of patients with bladder obstruction. Tacrine need not be used cautiously in patients with vaginitis, diabetes mellitus, or cardiovascular problems.

3. **Answers: a, b, c**
   RATIONALE: When performing a physical assessment before administering cholinesterase inhibitors, the nurse should monitor pulse, respiratory rate, and weight of the patient. The nurse need not monitor brainwaves and hepatic function when performing a physical assessment of the patient before administering cholinesterase inhibitors.

4. **Answer: b**
   RATIONALE: The nurse should immediately report any elevated ALT level to the primary health care provider. The primary health care provider may want to continue monitoring the ALT level or discontinue use of the drug because of the danger of hepatotoxicity. How-

ever, abrupt discontinuation may cause a decline in cognitive functioning. The abrupt discontinuation of tacrine does not lead to a loss of functional ability, impulsive behavior, or nervous breakdown.

5. **Answer: c**
   RATIONALE: Increased risk of GI bleeding is the effect of the interaction of nonsteroidal anti-inflammatory drugs with cholinesterase inhibitors. Asthma, sick sinus syndrome, and increased risk of theophylline toxicity are not effects of the interaction of nonsteroidal anti-inflammatory drugs with cholinesterase inhibitors. Increased risk of theophylline toxicity is the effect of the interaction of theophylline with cholinesterase inhibitors. Asthma and sick sinus syndrome are contraindications in the use of tacrine.

6. **Answers: c**
   RATIONALE: The intervention that a nurse should perform when administering tacrine to a patient is to monitor the patient for liver damage. Cardiovascular disease, pulmonary disease, and goiter are not associated with the administration of tacrine.

7. **Answers: a, c, e**
   RATIONALE: When caring for a patient administering cholinesterase inhibitors, the nurse should use side rails, or keep the bed in a low position, or use nightlights in order to reduce the risk of injury in the patient. The nurse should monitor the patient frequently to reduce the risk of injury, instead of monitoring every 12 hours. The nurse need not use soft bedding, as it may not help reduce the risk of injury in the patient.

8. **Answer: b**
   RATIONALE: The nurse should administer tacrine to the patient on an empty stomach. The nurse need not administer this drug 30 minutes before meals, 1 hour after meals, or around the clock intravenously to the patient. Instead, the nurse should administer tacrine 1 hour before or 2 hours after meals and around the clock orally.

9. **Answer: a**
   RATIONALE: Ginkgo is contraindicated in patients receiving monoamine oxidase inhibitors (MAOIs) because of the risk of a toxic reaction. Ginkgo is not contraindicated in patients receiving sedatives and hypnotics, opioid analgesics, or anticholinergic drugs.

10. **Answer: a**
RATIONALE: It is important for the nurse to provide proper attention to the dosing of medication, as it helps to decrease the adverse GI reactions. The proper attention to the dosing of medication is not related to the patient's faster recovery, maintenance of the patient's normal body temperature, or decreased variations in the patient's pulse rate.

11. **Answer: b**
RATIONALE: Cholinesterase inhibitors are utilized for the treatment of Alzheimer's disease and Parkinson's disease.

12. **Answer: a**
RATIONALE: Tacrine is a cholinesterase inhibitor use to treat dementia which can cause hepatotoxicity

13. **Answer: a**
RATIONALE: Ginseng is an herbal product that has been used to improve mental performance.

14. **Answer: d**
RATIONALE: Early-stage Alzheimer's disease is characterized by difficulties with memory, poor judgment, and withdrawal behaviors.

15. **Answer: b**
RATIONALE: The middle stage of Alzheimer's disease is typically the longest.

CHAPTER 29

SECTION I: ASSESSING YOUR UNDERSTANDING
Activity A MATCHING
1. 1. b 2. d 3. a 4. c
2. 1. c 2. a 3. d 4. b

Activity B FILL IN THE BLANKS
1. Parkinson's
2. Achalasia
3. On-off
4. Choreiform
5. Pyridoxine

Activity C SHORT ANSWERS
1. The nurse should monitor the following for the neuromuscular evaluation of the patient:
   • Tremors of the hands or head while the patient is at rest

• A mask-like facial expression
• Changes (from the normal) in walking
• Type of speech pattern (halting, monotone)
• Postural deformities
• Muscular rigidity
• Drooling, difficulty in chewing or swallowing
• Changes in thought processes
• Patient's ability to carry out any or all of the activities of daily living (e.g., bathing, ambulating, dressing)

2. The nurse should keep the following factors in mind when evaluating the patient's treatment plan:
   • The therapeutic effect is achieved and the symptoms of Parkinsonism are controlled.
   • Adverse reactions are identified, reported to the primary health care provider, and managed successfully through appropriate nursing interventions.
   • No evidence of injury is seen.
   • The patient verbalizes an understanding of the treatment modalities, adverse reactions, and the importance of continued follow-up care.
   • The patient and family demonstrate an understanding of the drug regimen.

3. The nurse should not abruptly discontinue use of the antiparkinsonism drugs. Neuroleptic malignant-like syndrome may occur when the antiparkinsonism drugs are discontinued or the dosage of levodopa is reduced abruptly. The nurse should carefully observe the patient and report the symptoms of muscular rigidity, elevated body temperature, and mental changes when caring for a patient showing an on-off phenomenon on the administration of levodopa.

4. The nurse should perform the following interventions when caring for a patient taking antiparkinsonism drugs and experiencing GI disturbances:
   • Create a calm environment.
   • Serve small, frequent nutritious meals.
   • Monitor the patient's weight.
   • Discontinue the drug or change the antiparkinsonism drug in cases of severe nausea and vomiting.

5. The nurse should include the following information in the patient and family teaching plan:
   • Take the drug as prescribed. Increase, decrease, or omit a dose only as directed by the primary health care provider. If gastrointestinal upset occurs, take the drug with food.

- If dizziness, drowsiness, or blurred vision occurs, avoid driving or performing other tasks that require alertness.
- Avoid the use of alcohol unless use has been approved by the primary health care provider.
- Relieve dry mouth by sucking on hard candy (unless the patient has diabetes) or taking frequent sips of water. Consult a dentist if dryness of the mouth interferes with wearing, inserting, or removing dentures or causes other dental problems.
- Inform patients that orthostatic hypotension may develop with or without symptoms of dizziness, nausea, fainting, and sweating. Caution the patient against rising rapidly after sitting or lying down.
- Notify the primary health care provider if any of these problems occur: severe dry mouth, inability to chew or swallow food, inability to urinate, feelings of depression, severe dizziness or drowsiness, rapid or irregular heartbeat, abdominal pain, mood changes, and unusual movements of the head, eyes, tongue, neck, arms, legs, feet, mouth, or tongue.
- Keep all appointments with the primary health care provider or clinic personnel because close monitoring of therapy is necessary.
- When taking levodopa, avoid vitamin B_6 (pyridoxine) because this vitamin may interfere with the action of levodopa.

Activity D DOSAGE CALCULATION

1. 4 tablets
2. 62.5 mg of Lodosyn
3. 10 increments
4. 5 tablets

SECTION II: APPLYING YOUR KNOWLEDGE
Activity E CASE STUDY

1. It is hard to supplement dopamine because of the blood-brain barrier, the meshwork of tightly packed cells in the walls of the brain's capillaries that screen out certain substances. Dopamine is a large molecule that is prohibited from crossing the blood-brain barrier.
2. The nurse's ongoing assessment for Mr. Sanchez should include evaluating the patient's response to therapy by observing the patient for various neuromuscular signs (tremors of the head and hands at rest, mus-

cular rigidity, mask-like facial expression, and ambulation stability) and compare these observation with data obtained during the initial physical assessment.

SECTION III: PRACTICING FOR NCLEX
Activity F NCLEX-STYLE

1. **Answer: b**
   RATIONALE: When caring for a patient exhibiting choreiform and dystonic movement, the nurse should withhold the next dose of the drug and notify the primary health care provider because it may be necessary to reduce the dosage of levodopa or discontinue use of the drug. The nurse should offer frequent sips of water to the patient throughout the day when caring for a patient experiencing dry mouth. The nurse should monitor the patient for persistent nausea, fatigue, lethargy, and anorexia when caring for a patient experiencing constipation. The nurse need not monitor vital signs frequently when caring for a patient exhibiting choreiform and dystonic movement due to the use of carbidopa.

2. **Answer: b, c, d**
   RATIONALE: The nurse should instruct the patient to increase the intake of fiber and fluids and use a stool softener to help prevent constipation. The nurse need not suggest that the patient decrease the intake of carbohydrates or increase the intake of vitamin C, since these will not help reduce the patient's constipation or the discomfort caused by it.

3. **Answer: a, b, c**
   RATIONALE: The nurse should carefully monitor for muscular rigidity, elevated body temperature, and mental changes in the patient with neuroleptic malignant-like syndrome, which occurs when the antiparkinsonism drugs are discontinued or the dosage of levodopa is reduced abruptly. The nurse need not monitor for tachycardia or orthostatic hypotension, since these conditions are not known to occur with an abrupt reduction of levodopa. Tachycardia is an adverse reaction caused by cholinergic blocking drugs. Orthostatic hypotension is an adverse reaction associated with the use of COMT inhibitors.

4. **Answer: c**
   RATIONALE: The nurse should anticipate the increased effect of levodopa as the effect of the interaction between levodopa and

antacids. Increased risk of hypertension and dyskinesia are the effects of the interaction between levodopa and tricyclic antidepressants. Increased risk of cardiac symptoms is the effect of the interaction between COMT inhibitors and adrenergic drugs.

5. **Answer: a**
RATIONALE: The nurse should know that catechol-O-methyltransferase (COMT) inhibitors should be used with caution in patients with decreased renal function. The nurse should use cholinergic- blocking drugs with caution in patients with tachycardia, cardiac arrhythmias, and GI tract problems.

6. **Answer: a, b, c**
RATIONALE: When preparing a discharge care plan for a patient who has had antiparkinsonism drugs, the nurse should instruct the patient to avoid taking vitamin B_6 with levodopa. The nurse should instruct the patient to avoid consuming alcohol and to contact the PHCP in case the patient experiences any symptoms of dry mouth, chewing, urination, depression, dizziness, or unusual muscle movement. The nurse should instruct the patient to have small and frequent meals if the patient is experiencing constipation due to drug therapy. The nurse need not instruct the patient to increase their intake of vitamin C.

7. **Answer: a**
RATIONALE: When caring for a patient on antiparkinsonism drugs experiencing GI disturbances like nausea and vomiting, the nurse should discontinue the antiparkinsonism drug or change it. Severe nausea or vomiting may necessitate discontinuing the drug and changing to a different anti-Parkinsonism drug. Administering the drug before meals, administering antacids after meals, or refraining from giving liquids after meals are not very appropriate interventions when caring for a patient who is vomiting or experiencing other GI disturbances.

8. **Answer: c**
RATIONALE: When caring for a patient on antiparkinsonism drugs who is responding to therapy, the nurse should closely monitor the patient's behavior at frequent intervals. Antiparkinsonism drugs can exacerbate mental symptoms and precipitate a psychosis. If sudden behavioral changes are noted, the nurse withholds the next dose of the drug and

reports to the PHCP immediately. The nurse could observe a drug holiday in case the patient is experiencing an on-off phenomenon. The nurse should discontinue the antiparkinsonism drug or change it when the patient experiences GI disturbances.

9. **Answer: a**
RATIONALE: The nurse should observe for changes in facial expression that may indicate abdominal pain in the patient. The nurse observes the patient with Parkinsonism for outward changes that may indicate one or more adverse reactions, like a sudden change in the facial expression or changes in posture that may indicate abdominal pain or discomfort, which may be caused by urinary retention, paralytic ileus, or constipation. The nurse need not monitor for changes in the style of walking, diet intake, or sleeping patterns, since these are not known to indicate abdominal pain.

10. **Answer: d**
RATIONALE: The use of cholinergic blocking drugs is contraindicated in patients with prostatic hypertrophy. It is not known to be contraindicated in patients with bone marrow depression, cardiac disorders, and visual impairment.

11. **Answer: a**
RATIONALE: *Parkinsonism* is the term which refers to a group of symptoms involving motor movement characterized by tremors, rigidity, and bradykinesia.

12. **Answer: c**
RATIONALE: Carbidopa (Lodosyn) is classified as a dopaminergic agent that treats Parkinsonism by supplementing the amount of dopamine in the brain.

13. **Answer: a**
RATIONALE: Entacapone (Comtan) and tolcapone (Tasmar) are classified as catechol-O-methyltransferase (COMT) inhibitors.

14. **Answer: c**
RATIONALE: Apomorphine (Apokyn) and pramipexole (Mirapex) are classified as non-ergot dopamine receptor agonists.

15. **Answer: d**
RATIONALE: Benztropine (Cogentin) is classified as a cholinergic blocking drug used to treat Parkinsonism.

CHAPTER 30

SECTION I: ASSESSING YOUR UNDERSTANDING

Activity A MATCHING

1. 1. c   **2.** a   **3.** d   **4.** b
2. 1. c   **2.** d   **3.** b   **4.** a

Activity B FILL IN THE BLANKS

1. Convulsion
2. Hydantoins
3. Oxazolidinediones
4. Succinimides
5. Barbiturates

Activity C SHORT ANSWERS

1. The nurse should perform the following preadministration assessments before administering an anticonvulsant drug:
   - Check for abnormal behavior in the patient.
   - Check for the type of seizure disorder in the patient.
   - Document the type of seizure, frequency, length, description of aura, degree of impairment of consciousness, known triggers, family history of seizures, and recent drug therapy.
   - Obtain vital signs to provide baseline data for the patient.
   - Perform various types of laboratory and diagnostic tests to identify the cause of seizures and confirm diagnosis.
2. When caring for a patient on anticonvulsant drug therapy, the nurse's role is to:
   - Frequently adjust the dosage of anticonvulsants based on patient response to the therapy and the occurrence of adverse reactions during the initial treatment
   - Add a second anticonvulsant to the therapeutic regimen depending on the patient's response to therapy
   - Measure regular serum levels of anticonvulsants for toxicity
   - Document time of occurrence and duration of seizure, and psychic or motor activity occurring before, during, and after
   - Assist primary health care provider in their evaluation of drug therapy

Activity D DOSAGE CALCULATION

1. 24 capsules
2. 4 capsules
3. 2 tablets
4. 4 tablets
5. 2 tablets
6. 2 tablets

SECTION II: APPLYING YOUR KNOWLEDGE

Activity E CASE STUDY

1. The nurse should obtain the following information from those who observed the seizure: description of the seizures (the motor or psychic activity occurring during the seizure), frequency of the seizures (approximate number per day), average length of a seizure, description of an aura if any has occurred (a subjective sensation preceding a seizure), description of the degree of impairment of consciousness, description of what, if anything, appears to bring on the seizure.
2. Mr. Miller may be experiencing phenytoin toxicity. Signs of toxicity include slurred speech, ataxia, lethargy, dizziness, nausea, vomiting.

SECTION III: PRACTICING FOR NCLEX

Activity F NCLEX-STYLE

1. **Answer: a**
   RATIONALE: While administering trimethadione, the nurse should monitor for eye disorders in the patient. The nurse need not monitor for bone marrow depression, hypotension, and myocardial insufficiency in the patient while administering trimethadione. The nurse should monitor for hypotension and myocardial insufficiency while administering phenytoin. The nurse should monitor for bone marrow depression while administering succinimides.

2. **Answer: d**
   RATIONALE: The nurse should monitor for palpations in the patient who has been prescribed with tranxene anticonvulsant. The nurse need not monitor for dyspepsia, vomiting, and fatigue in the patient with tranxene anticonvulsant. Dyspepsia, vomiting, and fatigue are the adverse reactions that a nurse should monitor in a patient that has been prescribed Felbatol.

3. **Answer: b, c, e**
   RATIONALE: In the teaching plan of the patient undergoing hydantoins drug therapy, the nurse should include: brushing and flossing teeth after each meal, since long-term administration of the hydantoins can cause gingivitis and gingival hyperplasia (overgrowth of gum tissue); avoiding consumption of discolored capsules; and taking medication with food. Avoiding taking drugs during pregnancy is included in the teaching plan of the patient on anticonvulsant therapy with oxazolidinediones, and not in the teaching plan of the patient undergoing hydantoins drug therapy. Notifying the health care provider if blurred vision occurs is included in the teaching plan of the patient undergoing succinimides drug therapy, and not in the teaching plan of the patient undergoing hydantoins drug therapy.

4. **Answer: c**
   RATIONALE: The nurse should immediately report to the primary health care provider incidence of thrombocytopenia in the patient. The nurse need not report sinus bradycardia, sinoatrial block, or Adams-Stokes syndrome, as they are not the hematologic changes but contraindications for phenytoin.

5. **Answer: a, b, c**
   RATIONALE: The nurse should instruct the patient to stay out of the sun, apply sunscreen, and wear protective clothes. Wearing light-colored clothes and placing cotton pads soaked in rosewater on the eyes will not help in reducing symptoms or discomforts associated with disturbed sensory perception.

6. **Answer: c**
   RATIONALE: The nurse should know that phenytoin is contraindicated in a patient with hepatic abnormalities. The drug phenytoin is not contraindicated in patients with cardiac problems, history of asthma, and liver dysfunction.

7. **Answer: d**
   RATIONALE: The nurse should carefully observe for apnea and cardiac arrest in a patient undergoing diazepam therapy. The nurse should examine the mouth and gums of patient with impaired oral mucous membranes. The nurse should examine the affected areas of the skin in a patient with impaired skin integrity and not in the patient receiving diazepam.

Diazepam is not known to cause throat irritation, and therefore the nurse need not observe the patient for such symptoms.

8. **Answer: d**
   RATIONALE: The nurse should be aware that increasing the depressant effect of the analgesics is a possible effect of the interaction of analgesics with anticonvulsants. Administering protease inhibitors with anticonvulsants increases the carbamazepine levels. Administering antiseizure medications with anticonvulsants increases seizure activity. Administering antidiabetic medications with anticonvulsants increases blood glucose levels.

9. **Answer: b**
   RATIONALE: The nurse should identify that phenytoin plasma levels are greater than 20 micrograms/mL if the patient exhibits signs of drug toxicity. Patients with plasma levels greater than 20 micrograms/mL may exhibit nystagmus. Patients with plasma levels greater than 30 micrograms/mL may develop ataxia and mental changes. Phenytoin plasma levels between 10 and 20 micrograms/mL give the optimal anticonvulsant effect.

10. **Answer: b, d, e**
    RATIONALE: The nurse should document each seizure with regard to the time of occurrence and duration, and the psychic or motor activity occurring before, during, and after the seizure. The nurse should also measure serum plasma levels of the anticonvulsant for a patient on barbiturate therapy. The nurse need not document the vital signs of the patient every 4 hours and measure blood pressure every hour for patients undergoing barbiturate therapy.

11. **Answer: c**
    RATIONALE: Simple seizures, motor seizures, and somatosensory seizures are classified as partial seizures.

12. **Answer: a**
    RATIONALE: Tonic-clonic seizures and myoclonic seizures are classified generalized seizures.

13. **Answer: c**
    RATIONALE: Generalized seizures involve a loss of consciousness.

14. Answer: b

RATIONALE: Hydantoins like phenytoin (Dilantin) elicits their effects by stabilizing the hyperexcitability postsynaptically in the motor cortex of the brain.

15. Answer: a

RATIONALE: Carboxylic acid derivatives like valproic acid (Depakote) elicit their effects by increasing levels of gamma-aminobutyric acid (GABA), which stabilizes cell membranes.

CHAPTER 31

SECTION I: ASSESSING YOUR UNDERSTANDING

Activity A MATCHING

1. 1. c   2. d   3. a   4. b
2. 1. b   2. a   3. d   4. c

Activity B FILL IN THE BLANKS

1. Bisphosphonates
2. Allopurinol
3. Immunosuppression
4. Gout
5. Colchicine

Activity C SHORT ANSWERS

1. The preadministration assessments that the nurse should conduct before administration of a musculoskeletal drug are as follows:
   - Obtain patient's history of disorders, onset, symptoms, and current treatment or therapy.
   - Appraise the patient's physical condition and limitations.
   - Examine affected joints in extremities for appearance of skin over joint, evidence of joint deformity, and mobility of affected joint.
   - Assess for pain in upper and lower back or hip.
   - Document vital signs and weight.
   - Perform laboratory tests and bone scans to measure bone density as ordered by the primary health care provider.
2. The ongoing assessments that a nurse should perform when caring for a patient administered with a musculoskeletal drug are as follows:
   - Evaluate periodically for musculoskeletal disorders.
   - Inquire about pain relief and adverse reactions.
   - Evaluate daily or weekly depending on condition and drug.
   - Administer more toxic drugs if first-line treatments are not successful, as ordered by the primary health care provider.
   - Closely observe the patient for the development of adverse reactions and report these to the primary health care provider if they occur.

Activity D DOSAGE CALCULATION

1. 3 tablets
2. 4 tablets
3. 3 tablets
4. 2 tablets
5. 6 tablets

SECTION II: APPLYING YOUR KNOWLEDGE

Activity E CASE STUDY

1. The nurse examines the affected joints and notes the appearance of the skin over the joints and any joint enlargement prior to the physician examining the patient.
2. The nurse should inspect the joints involved every 1 to 2 hours to identify immediate response or nonresponse to therapy. The nurse should also question Mrs. Morgan regarding the relief of pain, as well as adverse drug reactions.

SECTION III: PRACTICING FOR NCLEX

Activity F NCLEX-STYLE

1. **Answer: a**
   RATIONALE: Dyspepsia is the adverse reaction that the nurse should monitor in the patient. Sleepiness, lethargy, and constipation are the adverse reactions of the skeletal muscle reactant diazepam.

2. **Answer: b**
   RATIONALE: The use of alendronate is contraindicated in hypocalcemia patients. The use of alendronate is not contraindicated in patients with hypertension, insomnia, or diabetes.

3. **Answer: c**
   RATIONALE: The nurse should monitor methotrexate toxicity in the patient as

an interaction of sulfa antibiotics with disease-modifying antirheumatic drugs. Theophylline toxicity occurs when theophylline interacts with the uric acid inhibitor allopurinol. Rash occurs when ampicillin interacts with allopurinol. Hepatotoxicity does not occur as an interaction when disease-modifying antirheumatic drugs are administered along with sulfa antibiotics.

4. **Answer: a, b, c**
RATIONALE: The nurse should monitor hematology, liver function, and renal function in patients administered methotrexate every 1 to 3 months. The primary care provider is notified of abnormal hematology, liver function, or kidney function findings. The nurse need not monitor pancreatic and cardiovascular function in patients administered methotrexate, since these conditions are not known to occur as adverse reactions to methotrexate.

5. **Answer: d**
RATIONALE: After administering DMARDs, the patient should notify the primary health care provider in the case of diarrhea. Administering drugs with food, drinking 10 glasses of water a day, and avoiding driving or hazardous tasks in case of drowsiness are the instructions that a patient should follow when administering drugs used to treat gout.

6. **Answer: b**
RATIONALE: The nurse should closely monitor the patient for adverse reactions as an ongoing assessment for patients receiving bisphosphonates for musculoskeletal disorders. Obtaining the patient's history of disorders, appraising the patient's physical condition and limitations, and assessing for pain in the upper and lower back or hip are preadministration assessments for patients receiving drugs for musculoskeletal disorders.

7. **Answer: a, b, e**
RATIONALE: Reporting adverse reactions (especially vision changes), being alert to reactions such as skin rash, fever, cough, or easy bruising, and being attentive to the patient's complaints such as tinnitus or hearing loss are the nursing interventions involved when a patient is administered hydroxychloroquine for a musculoskeletal disorder. A nurse encourages liberal fluid intake and measures intake and output when using uric acid inhibitors. A nurse need not ask the patient to compensate for missed dosages.

8. **Answer: a**
RATIONALE: The use of sulfinpyrazone is contraindicated in patients with peptic ulcer disease. The use of colchicine and not sulfinpyrazone is contraindicated in patients with renal, hepatic, and cardiac diseases.

9. **Answer: a**
RATIONALE: When a patient with rheumatic arthritis is administered the uric acid inhibitor sulfinpyrazone along with oral anticoagulants, the interaction between the two can lead to an increased risk of bleeding in the patient. Interaction of tolbutamide with uric acid inhibitor sulfinpyrazone can lead to an increased risk of hypoglycemia. Increased effect of verapamil is caused by the interaction between verapamil and sulfinpyrazone. Decreased effectiveness of probenecid results when the uric acid inhibitor probenecid is administered along with salicylates.

10. **Answer: a**
RATIONALE: The nurse should examine the appearance of the skin over joints in patients with gout. The nurse should examine affected joint mobility in patients with arthritis. The nurse should examine patients with osteoporosis for pain in the upper and lower back or hip and evidence of hearing loss for rheumatoid arthritis.

11. **Answer: a**
RATIONALE: Bisphosphonates are the class of medications used in the treatment of osteoporosis.

12. **Answer: c**
RATIONALE: Baclofen (Lioresal) is an example of a skeletal muscle relaxant.

13. **Answer: a**
RATIONALE: Zoledronic acid (Zometa) is an example of a bisphosphonate.

14. **Answer: d**
RATIONALE: Hydroxychloroquine (Plaquenil) is an example of a bisphosphonate disease-modifying antirheumatic drug (DMARD).

15. **Answer: b**
RATIONALE: Drowsiness is the most common adverse reaction to skeletal muscle relaxants like carisoprodol (Soma) that the nurse should discuss with the patient.

CHAPTER 32

SECTION I: ASSESSING YOUR UNDERSTANDING

Activity A MATCHING

1. **1.** c   **2.** b   **3.** d   **4.** a
2. **1.** b   **2.** d   **3.** c   **4.** a

Activity B FILL IN THE BLANKS

1. Expectorant
2. Opioid
3. Dextromethorphan
4. Atelectasis
5. Lozenge
6. Respiratory

Activity C SHORT ANSWERS

1. The nurse should perform the following preadministration assessments:
   - Document the type of cough (productive, nonproductive).
   - Describe the color and amount of sputum present.
   - Assess and record vital signs.
2. The nurse's role after the patient has been administered antitussives includes:
   - Monitor for a therapeutic effect.
   - Auscultate the lung sounds.
   - Take vital signs periodically.
   - Record the type of cough in the chart.
   - Record coughing frequency in the chart.
   - Note and record whether the cough interrupts sleep or causes pain in the chest or other parts of the body.

Activity D DOSAGE CALCULATION

1. 4 capsules
2. 6 tablets
3. 4 gelcaps
4. 6 tablets

SECTION II: APPLYING YOUR KNOWLEDGE

Activity E CASE STUDY

1. The triage nurse needs to ask Mr. Smith the following questions about his cough:
   - Is the cough productive or nonproductive?
   - Is sputum present?
   - What color and how much sputum is present?
   - What actions or home remedies has he used to treat his cough?
   - How long has he been coughing?
   - Are there any other symptoms present with his cough?
2. Based on the symptoms and duration of Mr. Smith's symptoms, the nurse should advise Mr. Smith to be seen by the doctor.

SECTION III: PRACTICING FOR NCLEX

Activity F NCLEX-STYLE

1. **Answer: b, c, e**
   RATIONALE: When caring for a patient that has been prescribed an expectorant for the treatment of a cough, the nurse should assess the respiratory status of the patient, document the lung sounds of the patient, and document the consistency of sputum. The nurse need not ask the patient about throat infection nor examine the patient's pulse rate every 30 minutes.

2. **Answer: b, c, e**
   RATIONALE: In the teaching plan for a patient undergoing antitussive drug therapy, the nurse should include instructions to avoid irritants such as cigarette smoke, avoid drinking fluids for 30 minutes after taking the drug, and avoid chewing or breaking open the oral capsules. The patient undergoing antitussive drug therapy need not take the medicine 1 hour before meals or take the medicine with milk to enhance absorption.

3. **Answer: b**
   RATIONALE: The nurse should monitor the patient for sedation as a reaction associated with the antitussive administration. The nurse need not monitor the patient for diarrhea, somnolence, and dehydration, as these are not reactions associated with antitussive administration.

4. **Answer: d**
   RATIONALE: The nurse should know that antitussives are contraindicated in the patient with hypersensitivity to the drug. Antitussives are not contraindicated in patients with cardiac problems, asthma, or liver dysfunction.

5. **Answer: a**
   RATIONALE: The nurse should be aware of hypokalemia as a possible effect of the interaction of potassium-containing medication with iodine products. Hypoglycemia, hypertension, and hemorrhage are not the effects of the interaction of potassium-containing medication with iodine products.

6. Answer: b
RATIONALE: The nurse should encourage fluid intake of up to 2000 mL per day, if this amount is not contraindicated by the patient's condition or disease process, to promote effective airway clearance. The nurse need not suggest avoiding the consumption of milk products, monitor fluid intake of the patient every 8 hours, or encourage taking mucolytics after each coughing episode.

7. Answer: b
RATIONALE: The nurse should instruct the patient to dilute the medicine before use. The nurse need not instruct the patient to take the medicine on an empty stomach, take the drug with warm milk, or warm the medicine before use.

8. Answer: a
RATIONALE: The nurse should instruct the patient to consult the PHCP if the cough lasts more than 10 days. The nurse need not instruct the patient to consult the PHCP if the patient's cough is accompanied by dizziness, the frequency of coughing is every 20 minutes, or the cough is accompanied by vomiting.

9. Answer: b
RATIONALE: The nurse should ensure that suction equipment is at the patient's bedside to be immediately available for the aspiration of secretions. The nurse need not ensure that the patient is not receiving any other drug therapy, the patient gets continuous oxygen supply, or the patient keeps drinking warm water.

10. Answer: a
RATIONALE: The nurse should monitor for hypotension in the patient. The nurse need not monitor the patient for dyspepsia, bronchitis, or opisthotonos as risks associated with the interaction of dextromethorphan with monoamine oxidase inhibitors.

11. Answer: a
RATIONALE: Dornase alfa (Pulmozyme) is a mucolytic use in the treatment of cystic fibrosis.

12. Answer: a
RATIONALE: Concurrent use of iodine products can increase the hypothyroid effects of antithyroid drugs.

13. Answer: a, c
RATIONALE: The adverse effects of benzonatate include sedation, headache, dizziness, constipation, nausea, GI upset, pruritus, and nasal congestion. It is recommended that patients with cough drink plenty of fluids (1500 to 2000 mL daily) unless fluids are contraindicated due to another disease state. Benzonatate should not be crushed or chewed, as a local anesthetic effect could result in choking. Consumption of alcohol while taking benzonatate can increase CNS depression and increased sedation. The maximum daily dose of benzonatate is 600 mg daily.

14. Answer: a, b, c, d, e
RATIONALE: Type of cough, presence of sputum, color and amount of sputum, home remedies used to treat the cough, and vital signs are all important to obtain from the patient and document for the provider to insure optimal and appropriate treatment of the client's cough.

15. Answer: a
RATIONALE: Thinning respiratory secretions is the mechanism of action for expectorants. Breaking down thick mucus in the lower lungs is the mechanism of action of mucolytics. Depressing the cough center in the brain is the mechanism of action for centrally acting antitussives. Anesthetizing stretch receptors in the respiratory passages is the mechanism of action for peripherally acting antitussives.

CHAPTER 33

SECTION I: ASSESSING YOUR UNDERSTANDING

Activity A MATCHING

1. 1. c 2. e 3. b 4. a 5. d
2. 1. d 2. e 3. a 4. b 5. c

Activity B FILL IN THE BLANKS

1. Mast
2. Decongestant
3. Vasoconstriction
4. Histamine
5. Sedating

Activity C SHORT ANSWERS

1. The nurse should include the following points in the teaching plan for a patient who is prescribed antihistamines to combat the symptoms of angioneurotic edema:
   - If there is drowsiness, do not drive or perform hazardous tasks. The drowsiness may diminish with continued use.
   - While taking the drug, avoid the use of alcohol and other drugs which can cause drowsiness.
   - Take frequent sips of water, suck on hard candy, or chew gum (preferably sugarless) to relieve mouth and throat dryness that may be caused by antihistamine use.
   - If there is gastric upset, take the drug with food. If the upset is not relieved, talk to the primary health care provider.
   - Avoid taking fexofenadine within 2 hours of taking an antacid.
   - Do not crush or chew the sustained-release preparations.
2. The decongestant used for sinusitis may be a topical or oral medication. The nurse should assure the patient that topical decongestants have minimal systemic effects on most individuals. Occasional side effects seen with topical decongestants include nasal burning or stinging, or dryness of the nasal mucosa. Topical decongestant liquid that is used frequently or swallowed may produce side effects similarto those seen with oral decongestants —i.e., tachycardia and other cardiac arrhythmias, nervousness, restlessness, insomnia, blurred vision, nausea, and vomiting.

Activity D DOSAGE CALCULATION

1. 2 teaspoonsful
2. 3 tablets
3. 4 tablets
4. 2.5 teaspoonsful
5. 4 tablets
6. 2 tablets

SECTION II: APPLYING YOUR KNOWLEDGE
Activity E CASE STUDY

1. Even though most medications to treat nasal congestion are available over the counter without a prescription, Mrs. Jones has hypertension, and decongestants should not be used by those with hypertension unless approved by the client's physician.

2. The triage nurse needs to ask Mrs. Jones the following questions about her cough.
   - What is the level/duration of Mrs. Jones' congestion?
   - What actions or home remedies has she used to treat her nasal congestion? (name of each product and frequency of use)
   - Are there any other symptoms present with her cough?
   What are Mrs. Jones' blood pressure and pulse rate?

SECTION III: PRACTICING FOR NCLEX
Activity F NCLEX-STYLE

1. **Answer: a, b, d**
   RATIONALE: The nurse should inform the patient taking prescribed antihistamines about the possible side effects, such as thickening of the bronchial mucosa, disturbed coordination and anaphylactic shock, or urticaria. Though antihistamines are used to treat allergies, they themselves can at times cause allergic reactions including anaphylactic shock and urticaria. Increased frequency of micturition and excessive sweating and salivation are not seen with antihistamines, which cause dryness of the oral mucosa.

2. **Answer: c**
   RATIONALE: The nurse should administer the antihistamine with precaution if there is angle-closure glaucoma. Acute conjunctivitis and allergic rhinitis are indications for the use of antihistamines. Precaution is also needed when the drug is given in hypertension and not in hypotension.

3. **Answer: a, c, d**
   RATIONALE: When caring for an elderly patient on decongestant therapy, the nurse should monitor for symptoms of overdosage such as hallucination, convulsion, and CNS depression. Dyspnea and fatigue are not commonly seen with the use of decongestants.

4. **Answer: d**
   RATIONALE: The nurse should tell the patient to administer the inhaler by warming it in his/her hand before use. The nasal spray should be administered by sitting upright and sniffing hard. The tip of the container should not touch the nasal mucosa. The nasal drop should be administered by reclining on the bed with the head hanging.

5. Answer: c

RATIONALE: The nurse should assess the blood pressure before administering promethazine in a patient who is also under an opioid analgesic. The bone density, urine output, and skin turgidity need not be assessed.

6. Answer: b

RATIONALE: The nurse should choose the deep intramuscular route for administering antihistamines, as certain antihistamines may irritate the skin and the subcutaneous tissue. Intravenous, intradermal, and subcutaneous routes are therefore not preferred.

7. Answer: c, a, e, b, d, f

RATIONALE: In response to injury, histamine is first released. It produces dilatation of the arterioles, which results in localized redness and an increased capillary permeability. This leads to escape of fluids from the blood vessels, producing localized swelling.

8. Answer: c

RATIONALE: The nurse should inform the patient that magnesium-based antacids can reduce the effects of antihistamines by reducing their absorption. Beta-blocking agents and opioid analgesics enhance the effects of antihistamines. Monoamine oxidase inhibitors do not reduce the effects of antihistamines.

9. Answer: a, b, e

RATIONALE: The nurse should administer decongestants cautiously in patients with hypertension, hyperthyroidism, and glaucoma. No extra caution is required when the drug is used in conjunctivitis or nephropathy.

10. Answer: b, d, e

RATIONALE: The nurse should instruct the patient taking antihistamines to avoid the use of alcohol and other sedatives as they can increase the CNS-depressant action of antihistamines. The drug should be taken with food to avoid gastric upset. Frequent sips of water or sucking on hard candy can help relieve the dryness of mouth, nose, and throat seen with the use of these drugs. Antihistamines should not be taken within 2 hours of taking an antacid. Aluminum- and magnesium-based antacids decrease the absorption of the medication. Sustained-release tablets should never be crushed or chewed before use; they should be taken whole.

11. Answer: c

RATIONALE: Diphenhydramine is a first-generation antihistamine. First-generation antihistamines elicit their antihistamine effects by nonselectively binding to central and peripheral H_1 receptors. The other answers listed are second-generation antihistamines.

12. Answer: b

RATIONALE: Desloratadine is a second-generation antihistamine. Second-generation antihistamines elicit their effects by selectively binding to peripheral H_1 receptors. The other answers listed are first-generation antihistamines.

13. Answer: a

RATIONALE: Antihistamines are administered intramuscularly because they irritate subcutaneous tissue.

14. Answer: a, b, c

RATIONALE: Antihistamines can be used to treat a variety of conditions including allergic rhinitis, treatment of Parkinsonism, and relief of nausea. Antihistamines can cause dry mouth and sedation.

15. Answer: d

RATIONALE: Vasoconstriction of small blood vessels of the nasal membrane is the mechanism of action for decongestants. First-generation antihistamines act to nonselectively bind to peripheral H_1 receptors; the mechanism of action for second-generation antihistamines is to selectively bind to peripheral H_1 receptors; and peripherally acting antitussives anesthetize stretch receptors in the respiratory passages.

CHAPTER 34

SECTION I: ASSESSING YOUR UNDERSTANDING

Activity A MATCHING

1. **1.** d **2.** c **3.** e **4.** a **5.** b
2. **1.** b **2.** e **3.** a **4.** c **5.** d

Activity B FILL IN THE BLANKS

1. Dilatation
2. Mucus
3. Wheezing
4. Calcium
5. Agonist

Activity C SHORT ANSWERS

1. The nurse should inform the patient about the following possible adverse effects of theophylline:
   - Restlessness
   - Nervousness
   - Tachycardia
   - Tremors
   - Headache
   - Palpitations
   - Increased respiration
   - Nausea
   - Vomiting
   - Fever
   - Hyperglycemia
   - Electrocardiographic changes

   The nurse should include the following points in the patient teaching plan:
   - Take the drug exactly as ordered.
   - Do not increase the dose or frequency on your own. Consult the health care provider if symptoms become worse.
   - Follow your primary health care provider's instructions concerning the monitoring of theophylline serum levels.
   - If gastric upset occurs, take the drug with food or milk.
   - Do not chew or crush sustained-release tablets.
   - Drink plenty of water each day to decrease the thickness of secretions.
   - Do not use any over thecounter drugs unless approved by your health care provider.
   - Avoid smoking while on the drug.
   - Avoid cola, coffee, chocolate, and charcoal-prepared foods
   - Do not change to any other brand without consulting your physician.

2. The nurse needs to carefully observe a patient with chronic bronchitis before administrating bronchodilator therapy. All preadministration assessments made must be carefully documented. The preadministration assessments include the following:
   - Assess the vital signs including blood pressure, pulse, and respiratory rate. If the respiratory rate is less than 12 breaths/min or above 24 breaths/min, it is considered abnormal.
   - Assess the lung fields and properly document the sounds heard.
   - Note any difficulty in breathing, coughing, wheezing, "noisy" respirations, or use of the accessory muscles when breathing.
   - If there is expectoration, record a description of the sputum.
   - Note and record the patient's general physical condition.
   - Record any signs of hypoxia-like mental confusion, restlessness, anxiety, and cyanosis.
   - The health care provider may order arterial blood gas analysis or pulmonary function tests.
   - Ask the patient questions concerning allergies, the frequency and severity of attacks, factors that cause or relieve the attacks, and any antiasthma drugs used currently or taken previously.

Activity D DOSAGE CALCULATION

1. 2 teaspoonsful
2. 0.25 mL
3. 0.5 mL of the diluted solution
4. 0.25 mL
5. 300 mg
6. 0.1 mL

SECTION II: APPLYING YOUR KNOWLEDGE

Activity E CASE STUDY

1. Step 3 persistent asthma patient should be treated daily with a low-dose inhaled corticosteroid plus a long-acting β_2 agonist (LABA) or medium-dose inhaled corticosteroid. He should also have a short-acting, inhaled β_2-agonist (SABA) for rescue.

2. Environmental controls used to help control asthma include not smoking, not allowing smoking in the home, being aware of and avoiding asthma triggers (pollen, sulfites, etc.), washing bedding once a week in hot water, and wearing a scarf over the mouth and nose if cold air bothers the patient.

SECTION III: PRACTICING FOR NCLEX

Activity F NCLEX-STYLE

1. **Answer: c**
   RATIONALE: Terbutaline is a safer drug to administer to a pregnant patient with acute respiratory distress. Terbutaline comes under FDA Pregnancy Category B and can be used with caution. All other sympathomimetic bronchodilators, including albuterol, epinephrine, and salmeterol, are under Pregnancy Category C. These drugs can be used only if the expected benefits clearly outweigh the potential risks to the fetus.

2. **Answer: d**
   RATIONALE: The nurse should inform the patient that beta-blockers could increase the effects of aminophylline. Ketoconazole, rifampin, and loop diuretics decrease the effects of theophyllines, including aminophylline.

3. **Answer: a**
   RATIONALE: The nurse should assess the electrocardiographic changes to check for the occurrence of adverse effects with aminophylline. Aminophylline belongs to the group theophylline, which causes electrocardiographic changes as side effects. Changes in blood hemoglobin, fluid intake and output, or the consistency of stool are not adverse effects associated with aminophylline.

4. **Answer: b**
   RATIONALE: The nurse may observe increased sweating or diaphoresis in a patient with asthma. Increased micturition, decreased pulse rate, or decreased blood pressure is not seen in patients with asthma. During an asthmatic attack there may be an increased pulse rate.

5. **Answer: b**
   RATIONALE: When zafirlukast is given to a patient on aspirin, there may be an increase in the plasma levels of zafirlukast. The absorption of zafirlulast is not decreased in a patient taking aspirin along with zafirlulast. There is no decrease in the plasma levels or increase in the thrombolytic effects of aspirin due to such an interaction.

6. **Answer: c, d, b, e, a**
   RATIONALE: In asthma, the mast cells release histamine. This causes increased mucus formation and edema of the airway leading to bronchospasm and inflammation. This leads to narrowing of the airway along with clogging due to excessive mucus. When the airways are narrowed, there is decreased airflow to the lungs.

7. **Answers: a, b, d**
   RATIONALE: Corticosteroids, leukotriene formation inhibitors, and mast cell stabilizers may be used as adjunct therapy along with bronchodilators in asthmatic patients. They relieve the inflammation associated with asthma. Uricosuric agents and leukotriene receptor antagonists are not used as adjunct therapy to treat asthma. Uricosuric agents are used in the treatment of gout. Leukotriene receptor agonists may be used as adjunct therapy to treat asthma.

8. **Answers: b, c, e**
   RATIONALE: Flunisolide, beclomethasone, and triamcinolone are inhalational corticosteroid agents used in the treatment of asthma. Cromolyn and ipratropium are not used in the treatment of asthma. Cromolyn is a mast cell stabilizer. Ipratropium is an anticholinergic drug.

9. **Answers: b, d, e**
   RATIONALE: When a patient on antiasthmatic drugs experiences nausea, the nurse should instruct the patient to eat small frequent meals, limit fluids with meals, and rinse the mouth properly after food. These interventions will help alleviate the symptoms of nausea. Keeping the head end of the bed elevated helps in preventing the symptoms of heartburn and not nausea. Sucking on sugarless candy may help alleviate the unpleasant taste sensation experienced with certain antiasthmatic drugs, and may not alleviate the symptoms of nausea.

10. **Answer: a**
    RATIONALE: The nurse should instruct the patient to take montelukast orally only once in the evening. This drug should be taken even when there are no symptoms. The health care provider should be contacted if asthma is not well controlled, even with therapy. The patient should not take the drug more than once daily.

11. **Answer: c**
    RATIONALE: Albuterol is a SABA. Formoterol, Salmeterol, and Arformoterol are long-acting β_2-agonists (LABA)

12. **Answer: a**
    RATIONALE: Long-acting β_2-agonists have been shown in studies to increase the risk of asthma-related death.

13. **Answer: a, b, e**
    RATIONALE: Worsening of cough, tachypnea, dyspnea, and generalized wheezing and chest tightness usually precede an asthma exacerbation.

14. **Answer: a**
    RATIONALE: Nicotine decreases theophylline levels. If a client is no longer using nicotine, his/her theophylline levels will increase warranting a decrease in theophylline dose.

15. **Answer: b**
    RATIONALE: Stimulation of the central nervous system is the mechanism of action for xanthine derivatives. Stimulation of beta-adrenergic receptors is the mechanism of action for β_2-agonists. Reduction of airway hyper-responsiveness is the mechanism of action for inhaled corticosteroids. Stabilization of mast cell membranes is the mechanism of action for mast cell stabilizers.

CHAPTER 35

SECTION I: ASSESSING YOUR UNDERSTANDING

Activity A MATCHING

| 1. | 1. d | 2. a | 3. b | 4. c |
| 2. | 1. c | 2. a | 3. d | 4. b |

Activity B FILL IN THE BLANKS

1. Hyperlipidemia
2. Lipid
3. Liver
4. Catalyst
5. Rhabdomyolysis

Activity C SHORT ANSWERS

1. The nurse should perform the following assessments before administration of an anti-hyperlipidemic drug:
   - Documentation of serum cholesterol levels and liver functions tests
   - Note of dietary history, focusing on the types of foods normally included in the diet
   - Recording of vital signs and weight
   - Inspection of skin and eyelids for evidence of xanthomas
2. The nurse's role after an antihyperlipidemic drug is administered includes:
   - Frequent monitoring of blood cholesterol and triglyceride levels
   - Checking of vital signs and assessing bowel functioning
   Notifying the PHCP of change in serum transaminase levels

Activity D DOSAGE CALCULATIONS

1. 4 packets
2. 5 tablets
3. 2 tablets
4. 3 tablets
5. 4 tablets

SECTION II: APPLYING YOUR KNOWLEDGE

Activity E CASE STUDY

1. Pravastatin is an HMG-CoA reductase inhibitor or statin. The patient should be told to take the pravastatin 1 tablet daily at bedtime and not to stop taking the medication even if she begins to feel better. Mrs. Smith should be advised to contact her physician as soon as possible if muscle pain, tenderness, or weakness occurs. She should also be made aware of potential adverse reactions including headache, nausea, vomiting, and diarrhea.
2. Mrs. Smith should be encouraged to stop smoking, decrease intake of saturated fat and cholesterol, increase intake of fiber, increase physical activity with the physician's permission, and maintain a healthy weight.

SECTION III: PRACTICING FOR NCLEX

Activity F NCLEX-STYLE

1. **Answer: a**
   RATIONALE: The nurse should instruct the patient to take the drug 2 hours before cholestyramine, a bile acid sequestrant. The nurse need not instruct the patient to ensure a time gap of 1 hour when taking these drugs, take both the drugs 30 minutes before the meals, or take a bile acid sequestrant with warm water, as these are not the appropriate instructions.

2. **Answer: c**
   RATIONALE: The atorvastatin drug is contraindicated in patients with serious liver disorders. The atorvastatin drug should be used cautiously in patients with visual disturbances. Bile acid sequestrants are contraindicated in patients with complete biliary obstruction. The fibric acid derivatives are contraindicated in patients with renal dysfunction.

3. **Answer: d**
   RATIONALE: The nurse should monitor for arthralgia in the patient. Vertigo, headache, and cholelithiasis are the adverse reactions to gemfibrozil drug administration.

4. **Answer: c**
   RATIONALE: The nurse should observe enhanced effects of the anticoagulant in the patient as the effect of the interaction of clofibrate with anticoagulants. Increased hypoglycemic effect is an effect of the interaction of sulfonylureas with fibric acid derivatives (particularly with

gemfibrozil). Increased risk of severe myopathy is an effect of the interaction of HMG-CoA reductase inhibitors with macrolides, erythromycin, clarithromycin, amiodarone, niacin, and verapamil. Increased risk of hypertension is not an effect of the interaction of clofibrate with anticoagulants.

5. **Answer: b, c, e**
RATIONALE: The nurse should use HMG-CoA reductase inhibitors with caution in patients with a history of acute infection, visual disturbances, endocrine disorders, alcoholism, hypotension, trauma, and myopathy. The fibric acid derivatives should be used cautiously in patients with peptic ulcer disease. Niacin is used cautiously in patients with unstable angina.

6. **Answer: a**
RATIONALE: The nurse should monitor the patient who is receiving garlic therapy with warfarin for bleeding. The nurse need not monitor the patient for irritation, as it is an adverse reaction to garlic and is not caused due to the interaction of warfarin with garlic. The nurse need not monitor the patient receiving garlic therapy for peptic ulcers and skin rashes.

7. **Answer: a, b, c**
RATIONALE: The nurse should monitor for difficulty in passing stools, hard dry stools, and complaints of constipation when caring for an elderly patient on bile acid sequestrants. The nurse need not monitor the patient for mouth dryness or urinary hesitancy, as these are adverse reactions to antispasmodic drugs.

8. **Answer: a**
RATIONALE: In case of a paradoxical elevation of blood lipid levelsin the patient receiving an antihyperlipidemic drug, the nurse should notify the PHCP for a different antihyperlipidemic drug. The nurse need not collect the blood samples for further examination, administer the next dose of the drug with milk, or record the fluid intake and output every hour, as these interventions will not help improve the patient's condition.

9. **Answer: b**
RATIONALE: The nurse should inform the patient that dyspnea is a toxic reaction to flax consumption. Abdominal pain, cramps, and dyspepsia are the adverse reactions to atorvastatin and are not toxic reactions associated with the consumption of flax powder.

10. **Answer: a, b, d**
RATIONALE: The nurse should instruct the patient to increase fluid intake, eat foods high in dietary fiber, and exercise daily to help prevent constipation. The nurse should instruct the patient to take oral vitamin K supplements to prevent the deficiency of vitamin K. The nurse need not instruct the patient to take the drug 1 hour after meals, as this will not help prevent constipation.

11. **Answer: a, b**
RATIONALE: Modifiable risks factors for hyperlipidemia are weight, diet, and physical inactivity. Nonmodifiable risk factors for hyperlipidemia are age, gender, and family history.

12. **Answer: d**
RATIONALE: Increased levels of LDL in combination with other risk factors can lead to the development of atherosclerotic heart disease.

13. **Answer: c**
RATIONALE: The benefits of garlic include lowering serum cholesterol and triglyceride levels.

14. **Answer: a, b, c**
RATIONALE: HMG-CoA reductase inhibitors, fibric acid derivatives, and bile acid resins are classes of medications used to treat hyperlipidemia. Calcium-channel blockers and angiotensin II receptor blockers are used to treat hypertension.

15. **Answer: b**
RATIONALE: Bile acid resins can decrease the gastrointestinal absorption of several medications.

CHAPTER 36

SECTION I: ASSESSING YOUR UNDERSTANDING

Activity A MATCHING

1. 1. c 2. a 3. e 4. b 5. d
2. 1. b 2. d 3. e 4. a 5. c

Activity B FILL IN THE BLANKS

1. Vasoconstrictor
2. Diuretic
3. Hypertensive
4. Sodium
5. Hyponatremia

Activity C SHORT ANSWERS

1. When caring for a patient on captopril therapy, the nurse should perform the following assessments:
   - Monitor the blood pressure in the same arm in the same position every time. The blood pressure should be recorded every 15 to 30 minutes after the first dose of captopril is administered for at least 2 hours. This to monitor for hypotension, which occurs with ACEIs. Notify the health care provider if there is an increase or decrease in blood pressure.
   - Weigh the patient regularly during the initial period of the therapy. A weight gain of 2 lb or more per day should be reported.
   - Assess for edema of the extremities and also in the sacral area. If edema is present, the nurse should notify the health care provider.
2. When caring for a patient taking antihypertensive drug therapy, the nurse should include the following points in the patient teaching plan:
   - Take the drug regularly and do not discontinue or stop the drug on the patient's own. The health care provider should be notified before doing so.
   - Have regular blood pressure checkups and record the readings.
   - Avoid over thecounter drugs unless advised by the health care provider.
   - Avoid the consumption of alcohol, unless approved by the practitioner.
   - Educate the patient about precautions to be taken to prevent dizziness or lightheadedness.
   - If drowsiness occurs. avoid performing hazardous tasks or tasks involving the need for alertness.
   - Educate the patient about the adverse effects occurring with the therapy.
   - Inform the patient to contact the health care provider if adverse effects occur.
   - Implement diet recommendations given.

Activity D DOSAGE CALCULATIONS

1. 8 tablets
2. 2 ampoules
3. 2 tablets
4. 3 tablets
5. 4 tablets
6. Half a tablet

SECTION II: APPLYING YOUR KNOWLEDGE
Activity E CASE STUDY

1. Mr. Dunn's hypertension would be classified as Stage 2 because his systolic blood pressure is greater than or equal to 160. He will most likely require a 2-drug combination for control of his hypertension.
2. Mr. Dunn should be encouraged to follow the DASH diet, decrease salt intake, increase physical activity with the physician's permission, decrease stress, maintain a healthy weight, and take his medication every day, even if he begins to feel better.

SECTION III: PRACTICING FOR NCLEX
Activity F NCLEX-STYLE

1. **Answer: a**
   RATIONALE: Systolic pressure between 120 and 139 mm Hg is indicative of prehypertension. Prehypertension poses a risk for the development of hypertension. Individuals with such blood pressure changes should practice certain lifestyle changes.

2. **Answer: b**
   RATIONALE: Captopril is an angiotensin-converting enzyme inhibitor (ACEI), which is contraindicated in patients with renal impairment. Hydralazine and minoxidil are vasodilating drugs used for hypertension management, and are administered to patients with renal impairment after dose adjustments. Doxazosin is an alpha-adrenergic blocker used for the treatment of hypertension, and may be administered with caution to patients with renal impairment.

3. **Answer: d**
   RATIONALE: Nitroprusside is the drug which is to be administered in hypertensive emergencies. In hypertensive emergencies, nitroprusside, which is a potent vasodilator, should be given IV to bring down the blood pressure rapidly. If the blood pressure is not lowered it results in damage to the kidneys, eyes, and heart. Amlodipine, acebutolol, and diltiazem are not the preferred drugs in case of hypertensive emergencies.

4. **Answer: c**
   RATIONALE: An increased risk of hypoglycemia occurs with the simultaneous use of insulin and ACEI drugs like enalapril. Use of potassium-sparing diuretics along with ACEI drugs

increases the risk of electrolyte imbalance. Concomitant allopurinol usage increases the risk of hypersensitivity reactions. Increased risk of hypotensive effects occurs with the concomitant use of diuretics. Increased risk of hypersensitivity, hypotensive effect, and electrolyte imbalance do not occur when both drugs are used.

5. **Answers: c, d, e**
   RATIONALE: Headache is a common adverse effect of antiadrenergic drugs. The nurse should instruct the patient to apply a cool cloth over the forehead, to engage in progressive body relaxation, and to take an analgesic drug. Elevating the legs above the head in a supine position increases the blood gushing to the head and worsens the headache. Stopping prazosin will not relieve the headache.

6. **Answers: s, d, e**
   RATIONALE: The nurse should report changes such as swelling of the face, difficulty in breathing, and angina or severe indigestion to the practitioner in patients receiving minoxidil. Minoxidil is a vasodilating drug used in the treatment of hypertension. Minoxidil causes a rapid rise in the heart rate. A rise in the heart rate of 20 beats per minute or more should be reported. Weight gain of 5 lb, and not 1 lb, or more should be reported.

7. **Answer: s**
   RATIONALE: The nurse should ensure that captopril is taken 1 hour before or 2 hours after food; this is to enhance the absorption of captopril. Captopril should not be given along with food. This will retard absorption. Rubbing the patient's back prior to administration and engaging the patient in exercise will not affect absorption. Hence, the nurse need not be involved in such activities.

8. **Answers: a, d, e**
   RATIONALE: Orthostatic hypotension is common during the initial therapy with antihypertensives such as terazosin. The nurse should instruct the patient to rise slowly from a sitting or lying position, to rest on the bed for 1 or 2 minutes before rising, and to stand still for a few minutes after rising for patients experiencing orthostatic hypotension. Increasing the fluid intake or applying a cool cloth on the forehead will not relieve dizziness.

9. **Answers: b, c, d**
   RATIONALE: Heart disease, blindness, and stroke will occur as a consequence of hypertension.

Hypertension causes the heart to work harder and leads to the production of atherosclerosis. Obesity and adrenal tumor are risk factors for the development of hypertension, and are not the consequences of hypertension.

10. **Answers: a, b, e**
    RATIONALE: The nurse should inform the patient that hypotension, sedation, and arrhythmia are the adverse effects seen with hawthorn use. Hawthorn is a natural agent used in the treatment of cardiovascular problems. Neutropenia and pruritus are the adverse effects of ACEI drugs, and not of hawthorn use.

11. **Answer: a**
    RATIONALE: Prehypertension is defined as a systolic pressure between 120 and 130 mm Hg or a diastolic pressure between 80 and 89 mm Hg.

12. **Answer: c**
    RATIONALE: Angiotensin-converting enzyme inhibitors (ACEIs) act primarily to suppress the rennin-angiotensin-aldosterone system and lisinopril is an ACEI. Verapamil and diltiazem are calcium-channel blockers and furosemide is a diuretic.

13. **Answer: a, b, c, d**
    RATIONALE: Hypertension increases a person's risk for heart failure, stroke, blindness, kidney disease, and heart disease.

14. **Answer: c**
    RATIONALE: Once primary hypertension develops, management of the disorder becomes a lifetime task.

15. **Answer: a**
    RATIONALE: Bile acid resins can decrease the gastrointestinal absorption of several medications.

CHAPTER 37

SECTION I: ASSESSING YOUR UNDERSTANDING

Activity A MATCHING

1. 1. b   2. d   3. a   4. c
   5. f   6. g   7. e
2. 1. b   2. c   3. a

Activity B FILL IN THE BLANKS

1. Coronary
2. Calcium
3. Smooth
4. Dermatitis
5. Claudication

Activity C SHORT ANSWERS

1. The nurse should educate patients having anginal attacks about certain aspects of the disease and also about the use of antianginal drugs. The teaching plan should include the following:
   - Take the drug regularly, as recommended by the health care provider.
   - Notify the health care provider if the pain worsens or if the pain is not relieved by the medication.
   - Take the oral medications on an empty stomach, unless advised by the health care provider.
   - Avoid the consumption of alcohol, unless directed otherwise by the health care provider.
   - Keep an additional supply of the drug for events such as vacations and bad weather conditions.
   - Maintain a record of acute anginal attacks. This should include date, time of attack, and dose used to relieve pain.
2. The nurse should make certain assessments in a patient receiving vasodilator therapy. These include the following:
   - Assess the involved extremity daily for color and temperature changes.
   - Record the patient's comments regarding pain improvement or relief following therapy.
   - Monitor the pulse and blood pressure once or twice a day. This is to detect any decrease in blood pressure, which occurs with the use of these drugs.
   - When cilostazol is used for treating intermittent claudication, assess an improvement in the walking distance.

Activity D DOSAGE CALCULATIONS

1. 2 tablets
2. 2 tablets
3. 2 tablets
4. 2.5 mL
5. 2 tablets
6. 7 tablets

SECTION II: APPLYING YOUR KNOWLEDGE
Activity E CASE STUDY

1. Nitrates are used for the treatment of angina.
2. Mr. Rollins should be instructed to place 1 tablet under his tongue at the onset of chest pain. He should not swallow the tablet. The dose may be repeated every 5 minutes until chest pain is relieved or until he has administered 3 doses in a period of 15 minutes. If the pain is not relieved after the third dose he should call the nurse, who will notify the physician and instruct him on the steps that need to be taken. Finally, he should make sure the tablets are stored in the original container away from heat and moisture, and should obtain new tablets every 6 months even if he hasn't used all the old ones.

SECTION III: PRACTICING FOR NCLEX
Activity F NCLEX-STYLE

1. **Answer: a**
   RATIONALE: The nurse should administer 3 doses of sublingual nitroglycerin in a 15-minute period. If the pain worsens or if there is no improvement in the pain, the health care provider should be notified. In such cases, a change of dosage or alternate drug therapy may be required.

2. **Answer: d**
   RATIONALE: Cilostazol should be taken 30 minutes before food or 2 hours after food. This is to ensure optimal absorption of the drug. Cilostazol should not be administered with grape juice, as it increases the blood concentration of cilostazol. Antianginal drugs and not cilostazol need to be given in the supine position to prevent postural hypotension.

3. **Answer: b**
   RATIONALE: The nurse should identify that L-arginine brings about its action by increasing the nitric oxide concentration. L-arginine is an herb used in the treatment of heart failure, hypertension, and peripheral vascular diseases. Abnormalities of the vascular endothelium cause the degradation of nitric oxide. L-arginine is used in vascular conditions, as it increases nitric oxide levels. Calcium-channel blockers, and not L-arginine, are involved in blocking calcium channels. L-arginine is not involved in promoting sodium retention or in blocking alpha adrenergic receptors.

4. **Answer: c**
   RATIONALE: Isoxsuprine is a vasodilator used in the treatment of peripheral vascular diseases (PVD). This drug should not be given in the immediate postpartum period as it brings about uterine relaxation. Nitroglycerin and isosorbide dinitrate are nitrates used in the treatment of angina. These drugs are used cautiously in pregnancy and lactation. Nifedipine is a calcium-channel blocking drug, which is used cautiously in pregnancy and lactation. Nitroglycerin, isosorbide dinitrate, and nifedipine are not used in the treatment of PVD.

5. **Answer: b**
   RATIONALE: Papaverine can be given in the management of peripheral vascular diseases (PVD). Papaverine is a vasodilating drug which acts on the smooth muscle layer of the blood vessel. Nitroglycerin, isosorbide mononitrate, and amyl nitrite are vasodilating drugs used in the management of angina, and not for peripheral vascular diseases.

6. **Answers: b, c, e**
   RATIONALE: The effects of the calcium-channel blockers on the heart include retarding the conduction velocity, dilating the coronary arteries, and depressing myocardial contractility. Calcium-channel blockers act by blocking the calcium channel present in the cardiac and vascular smooth muscle layer. By depressing the myocardial contractility, these drugs do not increase, but rather decrease, the heart rate. Some of the calcium-channel blockers are used in atrial fibrillation, which is the rapid contractions occurring in the atrial muscle. Calcium-channel blockers do not cause rapid atrial contractions.

7. **Answers: c, d, e**
   RATIONALE: The nurse should monitor for asthenia, arrhythmia and flushing in patients receiving diltiazem. Diltiazem is a calcium-channel blocker used in the treatment of angina. The adverse effects occurring with diltiazem therapy include dizziness, peripheral edema, headache, nausea, and constipation. It also causes hypotension and bradycardia. Hypertension and tachycardia do not occur with diltiazem use.

8. **Answers: b, c, e**
   RATIONALE: Increase in painless walking distance, decreased pain and cramping in the legs, and reduced scaling of the affected area indicate improvement with cilostazol therapy. During therapy with cilostazol the nurse should assess for decreased pain and cramping, improvement of skin color and temperature, and increase in painless walking distance. There will be increased warmth in the extremities and not coldness on improvement following therapy. There will also be an increase, and not decrease, in the amplitude of the peripheral pulses.

9. **Answers: b, c, e**
   RATIONALE: The nurse should assess for adverse effects such as sedation, flushing, and headache in patients taking isoxsuprine. Isoxsuprine is a vasodilating drug used in the treatment of peripheral vascular disease. Hypotension and tachycardia are the other adverse effects seen with the use of peripheral vasodilators. Hypertension and bradycardia are the adverse effects associated with peripheral vasodilators.

10. **Answer: b, d, c, a**
    RATIONALE: The nurse should instruct the patient taking translingual nitrates as follows: To read the instructions supplied with the product properly before using nitrates. The nurse should instruct the patient to use the drug prophylactically 5 to 10 minutes before engaging in strenuous activities. The patient should be instructed to spray 1 to 2 metered doses of nitrate under or onto the tongue when chest pain occurs. The patient should be instructed to report to the health care provider if the pain does not subside after taking 3 metered doses in a 15-minute period.

11. **Answer: a, b, e**
    RATIONALE: Nitrates relax the smooth muscle of blood vessels, increase the lumen of the artery or arteriole, and increase the amount of blood flowing through the vessel.

12. **Answer: a, b, c**
    RATIONALE: Nitrates are available in the following dosage forms: sublingual, translingual spray, transdermal, and parenteral.

13. **Answer: a, b, e**
    RATIONALE: Calcium-channel blockers slow the conduction velocity of the cardiac impulse, depress myocardial contractility, and dilate coronary arteries and arterioles.

14. **Answer: a, b, d**

    RATIONALE: Adverse reactions associated with antianginal medications include headache, dizziness, weakness, restlessness, hypotension, flushing, and rash.

15. **Answer: a**

    RATIONALE: Nitrates are contraindicated in clients with known hypersensitivity, severe anemia, closed-glaucoma, head trauma, cerebral hemorrhage, and constrictive pericarditis.

CHAPTER 38

SECTION I: ASSESSING YOUR UNDERSTANDING

Activity A MATCHING

1. 1. d   2. c   3. a   4. b
2. 1. b   2. d   3. a   4. c

Activity B FILL IN THE BLANKS

1. Prothrombin
2. Thrombus
3. Arterial
4. Thrombolytics
5. Enzyme
6. Heparin

Activity C SHORT ANSWERS

1. The following factors should be considered by the nurse to determine the success of the treatment plan:
   - The therapeutic drug effect is achieved.
   - Adverse reactions are identified, reported to the primary health care provider, and managed successfully using appropriate nursing interventions.
   - The patient demonstrates an understanding of the drug regimen.
   - The patient verbalizes the importance of complying with the prescribed therapeutic regimen.
   - The patient lists or describes early signs of bleeding.
2. The nurse should offer the following instructions to the patient:
   - Follow the dosage schedule prescribed by the primary health care provider, and report any signs of active bleeding immediately.
   - Use a soft toothbrush, and consult a dentist regarding routine oral hygiene, including the use of dental floss.

- Use an electric razor when possible to avoid small skin cuts.
- Take the drug at the same time each day.
- Avoid changing brands of anticoagulants without consulting a physician or pharmacist.
- Contact the PHCP in case of bleeding and bruising on any part of the body.
- Limit foods high in vitamin K.
- Avoid alcohol unless use has been approved by the PHCP .

Activity D DOSAGE CALCULATIONS

1. 5 tablets
2. 3 tablets
3. 4 tablets
4. 4 tablets
5. 6 tablets

SECTION II: APPLYING YOUR KNOWLEDGE

Activity E CASE STUDY

1. Initially a PT/INR will need to be drawn every 1 to 3 days. Once PT/INR are stable, they will need to be drawn at least every 4 weeks.
2. Signs of warfarin overdosage include melena (blood in the stool), petechiae (pinpoint-size red hemorrhagic spots on the skin), bleeding from gums after teeth brushing, oozing from superficial injuries, or excessive menstrual bleeding.

SECTION III: PRACTICING FOR NCLEX

Activity F NCLEX-STYLE

1. **Answers: a, c, d**

   RATIONALE: The nurse should monitor the patient receiving alteplase for gingival bleeding, epistaxis, and ecchymosis. Thrombolytic drugs such as alteplase will dissolve all clots encountered, both occlusive and those repairing vessel leaks; hence, bleeding is a great concern when using these agents. Erythema is an adverse reaction to phytonadione, sodium, and heparin administration. Anemia is the adverse effect of reteplase and tenecteplase administration.

2. **Answer: c**

   RATIONALE: The nurse should observe an increased risk of bleeding as the effect of the interaction of abciximab with aspirin in the patient. Decreased effectiveness of aspirin, increased effectiveness of abciximab, and decreased absorption of abciximab are not the effects of interaction between abciximab and aspirin.

3. **Answers: b, d, e**
RATIONALE: Anticoagulants are contraindicated in patients with tuberculosis, leukemia, and hemorrhagic disease. Thrombolytics should be used with caution in patients with diabetic retinopathy and GI bleeding.

4. **Answer: d**
RATIONALE: The nurse should continually assess the patient for any signs of bleeding after the anifsindione drug is administered. Blood for a complete blood count is usually drawn before the administration of the thrombolytic agents. The international normalized ratio (INR) is determined before an anticoagulant or thrombolytic therapy begins. Blood for a baseline PT/INR test is drawn before the first dose of warfarin is given.

5. **Answer: a**
RATIONALE: The nurse should instruct the patient to use a soft toothbrush, and to consult a dentist regarding routine oral hygiene, including the use of dental floss. The nurse need not include instructions such as taking foods high in vitamin K, taking medication with food, and taking the drug at a different time each day in the teaching plan for the patient. Instead, the nurse should instruct the patient to limit foods high in vitamin K, and to take the drug at the same time each day.

6. **Answer: c**
RATIONALE: The nurse should inspect for bright red to black stools which are an indication of GI bleeding. The nurse need not inspect the urine for red-orange color. Oral anticoagulants may impart a red-orange color to alkaline urine, making it difficult to detect hematuria;, in such conditions a urinanalysis would be necessary to detect hematuria. The nurse need not monitor the patient's fluid intake and output. If bleeding occurs, the nurse should stop the drug and monitor the vital signs every hour or more frequently for at least 48 hours after the drug is discontinued, instead of monitoring them every 4 hours.

7. **Answer: a**
RATIONALE: The nurse should monitor for internal and external bleeding in the patient after the administration of heparin. The nurse need not monitor for difficulty in breathing, excessive perspiration, and skin rash in the patient.

Difficulty in breathing and skin rash are the signs of an allergic (hypersensitivity) reaction when thrombolytic drugs are administered.

8. **Answer: d**
RATIONALE: The nurse should avoid the intramuscular (IM) administration of heparin to avoid the possibility of the development of local irritation, pain, or hematoma. The application of firm pressure after injection helps to prevent hematoma formation. The nurse need not avoid administration sites such as buttocks and lateral thighs, as these are also areas of heparin administration by the SC route. When heparin is given by the SC route, the nurse should avoid areas within 2 inches of the umbilicus because of the increased vascularity of that area.

9. **Answer: c**
RATIONALE: The nurse should observe the patient for new evidence of bleeding if administration of the drug is necessary. The nurse need not measure the patient's body temperature every hour, monitor the patient's pulse rate every 2 hours, or administer the drug to the patient via the IV route. The nurse should monitor the patient's blood pressure and pulse rate every 15 to 30 minutes for 2 hours or more after administration of the heparin antagonist. Protamine sulfate, which is used to treat overdosage of LMWHs, is given slowly via the IV route during a period of 10 minutes.

10. **Answer: a, b, e**
RATIONALE: The nurse should observe for symptoms such as abdominal pain, coffee-ground emesis, black tarry stools, hematuria, joint pain, and spitting or coughing up blood in the patient. Petechiae is a symptom of warfarin overdosage. Chest pain is an adverse effect of clopidogrel.

11. **Answer: c**
RATIONALE: Phytonadione (vitamin K) is indicated for the treatment of warfarin overdose.

12. **Answer: a**
RATIONALE: St. John's wort in combination with warfarin can result in an increased risk of bleeding.

13. **Answer: d**
RATIONALE: Clopidogrel (Plavix) 300 mg should only be administered as a single loading dose.

14. Answer: a, b, d

RATIONALE: The use of thrombolytic drugs is contraindicated in a client with known hypersensitivity to the medication, active bleeding, and a history of stroke, aneurysm, and recent intracranial surgery.

15. Answer: a

RATIONALE: Enoxaparin (Lovenox) is administered via subcutaneous injection.

CHAPTER 39

SECTION I: ASSESSING YOUR UNDERSTANDING

Activity A MATCHING

1. **1.** c   **2.** a   **3.** d   **4.** b
2. **1.** d   **2.** f   **3.** a   **4.** c
   5. b   **6.** e

Activity B FILL IN THE BLANKS

1. Intravenous
2. Left
3. Neonatal
4. Bradycardia
5. Digitalized

Activity C SHORT ANSWERS

1. Before starting digoxin, the nurse should make the following physical assessments:
   - Record the patient's blood pressure, apical-radial pulse rate, and respiratory rate.
   - Measure the patient's weight.
   - Check for distension of the jugular veins.
   - Examine for edema in the extremities.
   - Look for cyanosis, dyspnea, and mental changes.
   - Auscultate the lungs for any unusual sounds during inspiration or expiration.
   - Inspect any sputum expelled and note its appearance.
2. The nurse should include the following points in the teaching plan for patients taking digitalis:
   - Take the drug at the same time every day.
   - Record the patient's pulse before taking the drug. Withhold the drug and notify the primary health care provider if the pulse is less than 60 or more than 100 beats per minute.
   - Do not stop or discontinue the drug or take an extra dose without consulting the primary health care provider.

- Report to the health care center if signs of digitalis toxicity such as nausea, vomiting, diarrhea, unusual fatigue, weakness, and vision changes occur.
- Carry or wear a medical alert band.
- Do not take over the counter drugs unless the health care provider approves them.
- Keep the drug in its original container.

Activity D DOSAGE CALCULATIONS

1. 2 tablets
2. 5 ampoules
3. 10 vials
4. 5 mL
5. 8 vials
6. 3 ampoules

SECTION II: APPLYING YOUR KNOWLEDGE

Activity E CASE STUDY

1. The nurse should prepare 1.5 milliliters for slow IV infusion.

$$0.75 mg \times 1.0 mL/0.5 mg = 1.5 mL$$

2. Prior to administering the IV digoxin the nurse should complete a physical assessment of the patient which includes blood pressure, apical-radial pulse, respiratory rate, auscultation of the lungs, examining extremities for edema, checking for jugular vein distention, measurement of weight, inspection of sputum if present, and evidence of other problems (mental status changes, cyanosis, shortness of breath on exertion).

SECTION III: PRACTICING FOR NCLEX

Activity F NCLEX-STYLE

1. **Answer: a**

RATIONALE: These signs and symptoms indicate that the patient is experiencing heart failure. The symptoms of heart failure are cough, dyspnea, weakness, anorexia, and unusual fatigue. The signs of heart failure include pitting edema and distended jugular veins. There is also reduced ejection fraction. These signs and symptoms are not seen in glomerulonephritis, pulmonary disease, or hypothyroidism.

2. **Answer: b**

RATIONALE: The nurse should monitor for signs of digoxin toxicity. The effect of benzodiazepine-digoxin interaction results in increased plasma digoxin levels. Increasing the dosage of digoxin or benzodiazepine will result in digoxin toxicity. Signs of reduced effectiveness of digoxin are seen with thyroid hormone administration and not with benzodiazepines.

3. **Answer: c**
RATIONALE: Digitalis can be used in atrial fibrillation. Digitalis is contraindicated in ventricular tachycardia, atrioventricular block, and ventricular failure.

4. **Answer: d**
RATIONALE: The nurse should withhold the drug and notify the practitioner. A pulse rate of less than 60 beats per minute indicates digoxin toxicity. The nurse should withhold the drug and notify the practitioner. Increasing the infusion rate will augment the toxicity. Gastrointestinal suctioning causes hypokalemia, which sensitizes the heart to digoxin toxicity. Milrinone lactate is given in unresponsive cases of heart failure, not in toxic states.

5. **Answer: b**
RATIONALE: The nurse should administer approximately half the total dose as the first dose. During rapid digitalization several doses are administered over a period of time. The first dose is approximately half the total dose. Additional doses are administered at intervals of 6 to 8 hours.

6. **Answer: a, d, e**
RATIONALE: The signs of digoxin toxicity that the nurse should assess for are anorexia, blurred vision, and vomiting. Headache and weakness are the adverse effects of digoxin, even at normal dosage, and do not signify digoxin toxicity.

7. **Answer: b, c, d**
RATIONALE: The nurse should report electrolyte changes such as hypokalemia, hypomagnesemia, and hypocalcemia to the practitioner. These changes increase the sensitivity of the heart muscle to the effects of digitalis. This in turn increases the risk for developing digitalis toxicity. Hyponatremia and hypophosphatemia do not increase the risk of developingdigitalis toxicity.

8. **Answer: b, d, e**
RATIONALE: The appropriate intervention is to ensure that the patient consumes small frequent meals, restricts fluid intake at meals, and rinses mouth after meals. These are techniques that help control nausea and vomiting.

Fluid intake at meals will increase the feeling of nausea. Fluid intake should be avoided 1 hour before meals. Doubling the drug dosage will worsen the condition.

9. **Answer: c, d, e**
RATIONALE: The adverse effects of digitalis administration that the nurse should assess for are drowsiness, vomiting, and arrhythmias. Hepatotoxicity is the adverse effect of inamrinone administration, and not of digitalis administration. Angina is the adverse effect of milrinone administration, and not of digitalis administration.

10. **Answer: b, c, d, a, e**
RATIONALE: The nurse should teach the steps involved in the calculation of the pulse. Place the nondominant arm on the table or arm of the chair. Place index and third fingers of the other hand on the wrist bone. Feel for a beating or pulsing sensation, which is the pulse. Record the number of times the pulse beats in a minute. If the pulse beats more than 100 beats per minute, notify the practitioner.

11. **Answer: a, d**
RATIONALE: Cardiotonic drugs are used to treat heart failure if other treatments fail to improve patient status, and to treat atrial fibrillation.

12. **Answer: a**
RATIONALE: Milrinone (Primacor) is only to be given intravenously.

13. **Answer: A, B, E**
RATIONALE: The symptoms of right ventricular dysfunction include peripheral edema, neck vein distention, hepatic engorgement, weight gain, nausea, weakness, anorexia, and nocturia.

14. **Answer: a, b, d**
RATIONALE: ACEIs, beta-blockers, and loop diuretics are currently first-line treatments for heart failure.

15. **Answer: a**
RATIONALE: Positive inotropes increase cardiac output.

CHAPTER 40

SECTION I: ASSESSING YOUR UNDERSTANDING

Activity A MATCHING

1. 1. d   2. a   3. e   4. b   5. c
2. 1. c   2. a   3. d   4. e   5. b

Activity B FILL IN THE BLANKS

1. Threshold
2. Sympathetic
3. Proarrhythmic
4. Sodium
5. Hypertension

Activity C SHORT ANSWERS

1. When a patient is prescribed an antiarrhythmic agent, the nurse should inform him about the following possible adverse effects that are common to most antiarrhythmic agents:
   - Central Nervous System (lightheadedness, weakness, somnolence)
   - Cardiovascular (hypotension, arrhythmia, bradycardia)
   - Other (urinary retention, local inflammation)
   All of the antiarrhythmic drugs need to be used cautiously in cases of:
   - Renal disease
   - Hepatic disease
   - Electrolyte imbalance
   - Congestive heart failure (CHF)
   - Pregnancy
   - Lactation
   - Administration to children
   The drug disopyramide is used cautiously in those with myasthenia gravis, urinary retention, glaucoma, and prostate enlargement.
2. Before administrating an antiarrhythmic agent, the nurse should perform the following assessments:
   - Assess and record blood pressure, apical and radical pulses, and respiratory rate for comparison during therapy.
   - Assess and record the patient's general condition including skin color, orientation, level of consciousness, and general status.
   - Record any symptoms described by the patient.
   - Review and report any abnormalities in any laboratory and diagnostic tests, renal and hepatic function tests, complete blood count, and serum enzymes and electrolyte analyses, as directed by the health care provider.
   - The patient may be put on a cardiac monitor before initiating therapy.
   - An ECG may be ordered by the primary health care provider to provide baseline data for comparison during therapy.

Activity D DOSAGE CALCULATIONS

1. 1.5 tablets per dose
2. 2 tablets per dose
3. 5.5 mL
4. 80 mg in each dose
5. 3500 mg
6. 195 mg per dose

SECTION II: APPLYING YOUR KNOWLEDGE

Activity E CASE STUDY

1. The nurse should give Mrs. Simpson 340 mg in one dose.

   176 lb × 1 kg/2.2 lb = 80 kg

   80 kg × 50 mg/1 kg = 4000 mg/day

   4000 mg/8 = 500 mg per dose

2. Mrs. Simpson would need 2 capsules per dose.
   500 mg/250 mg = 2

SECTION III: PRACTICING FOR NCLEX

Activity F NCLEX-STYLE

1. **Answer: b**
   RATIONALE: Disopyramide is an example of a class IA antiarrhythmic drug. Disopyramide decreases the depolarization of myocardial fibers during the diastolic phase of the cardiac cycle, prolongs the refractory period, and increases the action potential duration of normal cardiac cells. Lidocaine belongs to class IB drugs, propafenone to class IC drugs, and amiodarone to class III antiarrhythmic drugs.

2. **Answer: d**
   RATIONALE: Flecainide depresses the sodium channels in the heart. It is an antihypertensive belonging to the class IC drugs. It depresses fast sodium channels, decreases the height and rate of rise of action potentials, and slows conduction of all areas of the heart. It does not depress the calcium, chloride, and oxygen channels of the heart.

3. **Answer: c**
RATIONALE: Lightheadedness is a possible adverse effect seen with antiarrhythmic drug therapy. Other adverse effects include hypotension, somnolence, and urinary retention. Hypertension, insomnia, and frequent urination are not seen as adverse effects of antiarrhythmic drugs.

4. **Answer: c**
RATIONALE: Amiodarone belongs to FDA Pregnancy Category D. Drugs in this category have demonstrated a risk to the fetus in adequate well-controlled or observational studies in pregnant women. However, the drug may be given in a life-threatening situation if safer drugs cannot be used or are ineffective. The Category B drugs show a risk to the fetus in animal studies. Either there are no controlled human studies, or well-controlled human studies fail to show any risk to the fetus. These drugs may be used cautiously in pregnancy. The Category C drugs may be used in pregnancy only if the possible benefits clearly outweigh the potential hazards to the fetus. In Category X drugs the risks clearly outweigh the benefits. Therefore these drugs are clearly contraindicated in pregnancy.

5. **Answer: d**
RATIONALE: The nurse should notify the primary health care provider immediately when the pulse rate is below 60 beats per minute or above 120 beats per minute. Pulse rates of 82 beats per minute, 92 beats per minute and 102 beats per minute fall within the controllable range seen in patients with tachycardia.

6. **Answer: c**
RATIONALE: The nurse should instruct the patient to eat small frequent meals instead of larger ones. This will help alleviate nausea, which is a common adverse effect seen with the use of antiarrhythmic drugs. The nurse should instruct the patient to avoid lying flat for at least 2 hours after meals in order to prevent nausea. The drug should be administered with meals to avoid gastric upset. Drinking lots of fluid after the drug may lead to vomiting, if there is nausea.

7. **Answer: d**
RATIONALE: When taken concurrently with disopyramide, rifampicin can decrease the serum levels of disopyramide. When taken concurrently with disopyramide, erythromycin and quinidine increase the levels of disopyramide in the serum. Thioridazine increases the risk of life-threatening arrhythmias and does not decrease the serum levels of disopyramide, if taken concurrently.

8. **Answer: c**
RATIONALE: The nurse should report a lidocaine blood level of 6.0 mcg/mL to the health care provider. A blood level higher than that is associated with an increased risk of central nervous system and cardiovascular depression. Blood lidocaine levels of 1.5 mcg/mL, 3.0 mcg/mL, and 4.5 mcg/mL are not a cause of alert and need not be reported immediately to the health care provider.

9. **Answer: a, d, e**
RATIONALE: Weakness, arrhythmias, and lightheadedness are possible adverse effects of antiarrhythmic drugs. Another possible adverse effect is hypotension, and not hypertension. Somnolence, and not insomnia, may occur as another adverse effect associated with antiarrhythmic drugs.

10. **Answer: b**
RATIONALE: Shortness of breath may be seen as a sign of heart failure in elderly patients on antiarrhythmic drug therapy. Other signs include an increase in weight and a decrease in urine output. There is no decrease in weight or increase in urine volume due to heart failure. Chills and fever may be seen with antiarrhythmic drug therapy, but are not due to heart failure; rather, they may be due to agranulocytosis seen as an adverse reaction to antiarrhythmic drugs.

11. **Answer: c**
RATIONALE: Atrial flutter is described as rapid contraction of the atria (up to 300 bpm) at a rate too rapid for the ventricles to pump efficiently.

12. **Answer: a**
RATIONALE: Urinary retention may occur during therapy with disopyramide because of the drug's anticholinergic properties.

13. **Answer: a, b, d**
RATIONALE: All antiarrhythmics can cause new arrhythmias or worsen existing arrhythmias.

14. **Answer: a, e**
RATIONALE: Acebutolol and propranolol are class II antiarrhythmics.

15. **Answer: c**
RATIONALE: Flecainide is a class IC antiarrhythmic.

CHAPTER 41

SECTION I: ASSESSING YOUR UNDERSTANDING

Activity A MATCHING

1. **1.** c   **2.** e   **3.** a   **4.** b   **5.** d
2. **1.** b   **2.** c   **3.** a   **4.** e   **5.** d

Activity B FILL IN THE BLANKS

1. Gastrointestinal
2. Esophagus
3. Vomiting
4. Dronabinol
5. Duodenal

Activity C SHORT ANSWERS

1. The nurse should perform the following preadmission assessments:
   - Question the patient regarding the type and intensity of symptoms.
   - Document the number of vomiting experiences and approximate amount of fluid lost.
   - Record vital signs and assess signs of fluid and electrolyte imbalances,
   - Explain the rationale for preventing an episode of a condition.
2. The nurse's role after the administration of the drug includes:
   - Monitoring the patient frequently for continued complaints of pain, sour taste, or spitting of blood or coffee-ground–colored emesis.
   - Suction equipment should be kept available in case the need for insertion of a nasogastric tube or suctioning is warranted to prevent aspiration of the emesis.
   - Observing the patient for signs and symptoms of electrolyte imbalance if vomiting is severe.
   - Monitoring the blood pressure, pulse, and respiratory rate every 2 to 4 hours.
   - Carefully measuring intake and output until vomiting ceases.
   - Documenting on the chart each case of vomiting.
   - Notifying the PHCP if there is blood in the emesis or if vomiting suddenly becomes more severe.
   - In those with prolonged and repeated episodes of vomiting, measuring the patient's weight daily to weekly.
   - Assessing the patient at frequent intervals for the drug's effectiveness.
   - Notifying the primary health care provider if the drug fails to relieve or diminish symptoms.

Activity D DOSAGE CALCULATIONS

1. 6 capsules
2. 2 capsules
3. 4 tablets
4. 4 tablets
5. 6 tablets

SECTION II: APPLYING YOUR KNOWLEDGE

Activity E CASE STUDY

1. The following drugs may be utilized in the prevention of motion sickness: promethazine (Phenergan), buclizine (Bucladin-S), cyclizine (Marezine), dimenhydrinate (Dramamine), diphenhydramine (Benadryl), meclizine (Antivert), and scopolamine (Transderm-Scop).
2. The nurse should advise Ms. Myers about the following when using the scopolamine patch:
   - One patch is applied behind the ear approximately 4 hours before the antiemetic effect is needed.
   - Discard any disk that becomes detached and replace it with a fresh disk applied behind the opposite ear.
   - Wash hand thoroughly after patch application and removal to avoid drug coming in contact with the eyes.
   - The disk will last about 3 days, at which time Ms. Meyers may remove the disk and apply another, if needed.
   - Only use one disk at a time.
   - Stress the importance of observing caution when driving or performing hazardous tasks while using the medication.

SECTION III: PRACTICING FOR NCLEX

Activity F NCLEX-STYLE

1. **Answer: c**
   RATIONALE: The nurse should monitor the patient for euphoria, which is an adverse reaction to dronabinol. Sedation and hypoxia are adverse reactions to ondansetron HCl. Asthenia is an adverse reaction to granisetron hydrochloride.

2. **Answer: a**

RATIONALE: The nurse should observe an increased risk of respiratory depression in the patient as the interaction between antacids and opioid analgesics. There will be a decrease in white blood cell count when the antacid is administered with carmustine. There will be an increased risk of bleeding when antacids are administered with oral anticoagulants. There is an increased risk of dehydration if the patient has vomiting and diarrhea.

3. **Answers: a, b, d**

RATIONALE: The nurse should administer promethazine with caution to patients with hypertension, sleep apnea, or epilepsy. Trimethobenzamide is used cautiously in children with a viral illness. Cholinergic blocking antiemetics are used cautiously in patients with glaucoma.

4. **Answer: b**

RATIONALE: The nurse should monitor the patient for coffee-ground–colored emesis after the administration of aluminum hydroxide gel. The nurse need not monitor for complaints of headache, signs of electrolyte imbalances, or the amount of fluid lost. The nurse assesses for signs of electrolyte imbalances before starting antiemetic therapy for a patient. The nurse should document the approximate amount of fluid lost as part of the preadministration assessment for a patient receiving a drug for nausea and vomiting.

5. **Answer: d**

RATIONALE: The nurse should instruct the patient to avoid driving or performing other hazardous tasks when taking the drug, because drowsiness may occur with use. The nurse need not instruct the patient to increase frequency of dose if symptoms worsen, avoid direct exposure to sunlight, or take other drugs 1 hour before taking the antacid. The nurse should instruct the patient not to increase the frequency of use or the dose if symptoms become worse; instead, patient should see the primary health care provider as soon as possible. Since the antacids impair the absorption of some drugs, the other drugs should not be taken within 2 hours before or after taking the antacid.

6. **Answer: a, c, e**

RATIONALE: Before an emetic is given to the patient, the nurse should obtain information such as substances that have been ingested, the time the substances were ingested, and symptoms noted before seeking medical treatment. Cause for ingesting the poison and the patient's mental status before taking the poison are not related to the administration of the emetic.

7. **Answer: b, c, e**

RATIONALE: The nurse should monitor the patient for symptoms of dehydration such as decreased urinary output, concentrated urine, dry mucous membranes, poor skin turgor, restlessness, irritability, and confusion. Increased respiratory rate is a symptom of dehydration. White streaks in stools are a normal observation when the patient is administered antacids.

8. **Answer: a**

RATIONALE: The nurse should monitor the patient for rate of infusion at frequent intervals during administration through IV because too rapid an infusion may induce cardiac arrhythmias. Recording body temperature every hour, observing for irritation due to drug administration, or checking blood pressure every 2 hours are not relevant interventions in this case.

9. **Answer: d**

RATIONALE: The nurse should record the fluid intake and output of the patient who experiences diarrhea after taking the antacid drug as a measure to monitor dehydration. The nurse removes items with strong odor from the room if the patient has symptoms of nausea and vomiting. Changing to a different antacid usually alleviates the problem. Recording the patient's temperature every hour will not help when caring for a patient with diarrhea.

10. **Answer: c**

RATIONALE: The nurse should remove items with a strong smell and odor to prevent vomiting and to enhance the patient's appetite. Suggesting that the patient consume milk products or perform physical exercises will not help the patient improve his appetite. The nurse should give frequent oral rinses to the patient to remove the disagreeable taste that accompanies vomiting.

11. **Answer: c**

RATIONALE: Magaldrate (Riopan) is a combination product that contains magnesium and aluminate. Magaldrate (Riopan) treats heartburn by neutralizing stomach acidity, by combining with hydrochloric acid (HCl) and increasing the pH of the stomach acid.

12. Answer: a
RATIONALE: The nurse should warn a patient taking magnesium- and sodium-containing antacids concerning the risk of diarrhea associated with taking products containing either medication.

13. Answer: d
RATIONALE: The nurse should warn a patient taking aluminum- and calcium-containing antacids concerning the risk of constipation associated with taking products containing either medication.

14. Answer: a
RATIONALE: Sodium bicarbonate is the antacid that is contraindicated in patients with cardiovascular problems such as hypertension and congestive heart failure, and those on sodium-restricted diets, as sodium bicarbonate can alter the body's sodium-water balance and cause fluid retention.

15. Answer: b
RATIONALE: Administering an antacid to a patient taking digoxin will decrease the absorption of digoxin and result in a decreased digoxin effect.

CHAPTER 42

SECTION I: ASSESSING YOUR UNDERSTANDING

Activity A MATCHING

1. 1. c   **2.** a   **3.** d   **4.** b
2. 1. d   **2.** b   **3.** a   **4.** c

Activity B FILL IN THE BLANKS

1. Diarrhea
2. Chamomile
3. Laxative
4. Pruritus
5. Aminosalicylates

Activity C SHORT ANSWERS

1. The nurse should perform the following preadministration assessment:
   - Question the patient regarding the type and intensity of symptoms such as pain, discomfort, diarrhea, or constipation.
   - Listen to the bowel sounds and palpate the abdomen.
   - Monitor the patient for signs of guarding or discomfort.
2. The nurse's role after the administration of the drug to the patient includes:
   - Assessing the patient for relief of symptoms such as diarrhea, pain, or constipation.
   - Notifying the primary health care provider if the drug fails to relieve symptoms.
   - Monitoring vital signs on a daily basis or more frequently.
   - Observing the patient for adverse drug reactions.
   - Evaluating the effectiveness of drug therapy.
   - Evaluating the patient's response to therapy.

Activity D DOSAGE CALCULATIONS

1. 168 capsules
2. 2 tablets
3. 2 capsules
4. 24 tablets
5. 2 tablets

SECTION II: APPLYING YOUR KNOWLEDGE
Activity E CASE STUDY

1. Mr. Jackson's amitriptyline and ferrous sulfate may be contributing to his constipation. The following is a list of medication that may cause constipation in patients: anticholinergics, antihistamines, phenothiazines, tricyclic antidepressants, opioids, non–potassium-sparing diuretics, iron preparations, barium, clonidine, and antacids containing calcium or aluminum.
2. The nurse could recommend the following non-pharmacological treatments to Mr. Jackson to help with his constipation: increase his daily fluid and fiber intake and if possible increase his physical activity.

SECTION III: PRACTICING FOR NCLEX
Activity F NCLEX-STYLE

1. Answer: c
RATIONALE: The nurse should monitor for increased blood glucose level in the patient as a result of the interaction between mesalamine and hypoglycemic drugs. When the patient is administered warfarin with mesalaminem, there will be increased risk of bleeding. Neither the decreased absorption of hypoglycemic drugs nor the reduced effect of mesalamine will result due to the interaction of mesalamine and hypoglycemic drugs.

2. **Answer: b**
RATIONALE: The nurse should monitor for constipation, dry skin and mucous membranes, nausea, and lightheadedness on administering loperamide to a patient with acute diarrhea. Cramping is an adverse reaction to olsalazine. Administration of infliximab could cause sore throat as an adverse reaction. Anorexia is an adverse reaction to sulfasalazine.

3. **Answer: a**
RATIONALE: The nurse should administer bismuth subsalicylate with caution to patients with severe hepatic impairment. Aminosalicylates are contraindicated in patients with intestinal obstruction. Laxatives are contraindicated in patients with signs of acute appendicitis and rectal bleeding.

4. **Answer: b**
RATIONALE: The nurse should instruct the patient to chew the drug thoroughly because complete particle dispersion enhances antiflatulent action. The nurse need not instruct the patient to take the drug early in the morning. Instead, the nurse should instruct the patient to take the drug after each meal and at bedtime. The nurse gives bulk-producing or stool-softening laxatives with a full glass of juice. The administration of a bulk-producing laxative is followed by an additional full glass of water.

5. **Answer: a**
RATIONALE: The nurse should encourage the patient with chronic diarrhea to drink extra fluids. The nurse need not instruct the patient to avoid the use of commercial electrolytes or encourage the patient to take food high in fiber. When diarrhea is severe, the nurse should use commercial electrolytes. The nurse should encourage patients with constipation to take food high in fiber and to exercise often.

6. **Answer: b, c, e**
RATIONALE: The nurse should instruct an outpatient undergoing antidiarrheal therapy to observe caution when driving, as the drug may cause drowsiness, and avoid the use of alcohol and other nonprescription drugs unless their use has been approved by the primary health care provider. The nurse instructs the patient who is prescribed laxatives to eat foods high in roughage and to get sufficient exercise.

7. **Answer: d**
RATIONALE: The nurse should instruct the patient to take mineral oil in the evening on an empty stomach for optimal response to therapy. The nurse should not instruct the patient to take it half an hour after a meal, before breakfast, or at bedtime after dinner, as these methods will not promote an optimal response to therapy.

8. **Answer: c**
RATIONALE: The nurse should instruct the patient to eat foods high in bulk or roughage, drink plenty of fluids, and exercise to avoid constipation. The nurse need not instruct the patient to take commercial electrolytes, take the drug with food, or avoid milk products, as these interventions are not appropriate and will not help in preventing constipation.

9. **Answer: b**
RATIONALE: The nurse should monitor for serious electrolyte imbalances in the patient, an effect of the prolonged use of laxatives. Obstruction of the small intestine occurs when bulk-forming laxatives are administered without adequate fluid intake or in patients with intestinal stenosis. Renal impairment and fecal impaction do not result from the prolonged use of laxatives.

10. **Answer: c**
RATIONALE: Antidiarrheals are contraindicated in patients with obstructive jaundice, pseudomembranous colitis, and abdominal pain of unknown origin. Constipation, nausea, and abdominal distention are adverse reactions associated with the administration of antidiarrheals.

11. **Answer: c**
RATIONALE: Patients with a sulfonamide allergy should avoid the use of aminosalicylate such as mesalamine (Asacol) to treat an ulcerative colitis flare.

12. **Answer: a**
RATIONALE: Chamomile is an herbal product that has been used to treat digestive upset and stomach ulcers.

13. **Answer: c**
RATIONALE: Diphenoxylate (Lomotil) is chemically related to opioid drugs, and treats diarrhea by decreasing intestinal peristalsis.

14. **Answer: c**

RATIONALE: The nurse should counsel a patient to discontinue use of over-the-counter antidiarrheals and seek treatment from a physician if diarrhea persists for more than 2 days.

15. **Answer: b**

RATIONALE: The nurse could recommend simethicone (Mylicon) to a patient to treat flatulence.

CHAPTER 43

SECTION I: ASSESSING YOUR UNDERSTANDING

Activity A MATCHING

1. **1.** b   **2.** c   **3.** a
2. **1.** c   **2.** d   **3.** a   **4.** b

Activity B FILL IN THE BLANKS

1. Insulin
2. Polyuria
3. Glycogen
4. Hypokalemia
5. Hyperglycemia
6. Hemoglobin
7. Ketoacidosis

Activity C SHORT ANSWERS

1. The nurse should consider the following factors when evaluating the success of the treatment plan:
   - The therapeutic drug effect is achieved, and normal or near-normal blood glucose levels are maintained.
   - Hypoglycemic reactions are identified, reported to the primary health care provider, and managed successfully.
   - Anxiety is reduced.
   - The patient begins to demonstrate the ability to cope with the disorder and its required treatment.
   - The patient demonstrates a positive outlook and adjustment to the diagnosis.
   - The patient verbalizes a willingness to comply with the prescribed treatment regimen.
   - The patient demonstrates an understanding of the drug regimen.
   - The patient demonstrates an understanding of the information presented in teaching sessions.

   - The patient is able to use the glucometer correctly to monitor blood glucose levels or test urine for glucose and ketones.
2. The nurse should provide the following instructions to the patient and his/her family:
   - Take the drug exactly as directed on the container.
   - Follow the diet and drug regimen prescribed by the primary health care provider exactly.
   - Never stop taking the drug or increase or decrease the dose unless told to do so by the PHCP.
   - Take the drug at the same time or times each day.
   - Avoid alcohol, dieting, commercial weight-loss products, and strenuous exercise programs.
   - Maintain good foot and skin care and routine eye and dental examinations for early detection.
   - Notify the primary health care provider if any of the following occur: episodes of hypoglycemia, apparent symptoms of hyperglycemia, elevated blood glucose levels, positive results of urine tests for glucose or ketone bodies, or pregnancy.
   - An antidiabetic drug is not oral insulin and cannot be substituted for insulin.
   - Test blood for glucose and urine for ketones as directed by the primary health care provider.
   - Wear identification, such as a MedicAlert bracelet, to inform medical personnel and others of diabetes and the drug or drugs currently being used to treat the disease.

Activity D DOSAGE CALCULATION

1. 4 tablets
2. 5 tablets
3. 6 tablets
4. 3 tablets
5. 6 tablets

SECTION II: APPLYING YOUR KNOWLEDGE

Activity E CASE STUDY

1. The nurse should give Mrs. Arthur the following instructions on the injecting of insulin and rotation of injection sites:
   - Insulin injections can be given in the following: upper arms, outer aspect, stomach (except for a 2-inch margin around the umbilicus), back, right, and left sides just below the waist, or upper thighs, both front and side.

- Swab the injection site and vial top with an alcohol pad.
- Draw up the correct dose.
- Inject the needle into the skin at a 45° angle.
- Site rotation instruction should include the following: note the site of the last injection, place the side of the thumb at the old site and measure across its width (about 1 inch). Select a site on the other side of the thumb for the next injection, repeating the procedure for each subsequent injection and using the same area for a total of about 10 to 15 injections before moving to another area.

2. The nurse should tell Mrs. Arthur the following about hypoglycemia: Onset is sudden, characterized by blood glucose less than 60 mg/dL; signs include fatigue, weakness, nervousness, agitation, confusion, headache, diplopia, convulsions, dizziness, unconsciousness, rapid and shallow breathing, hunger, nausea, pale, moist, cool sweaty skin, and numbness or tingling of the lips or tongue.

SECTION III: PRACTICING FOR NCLEX
Activity F NCLEX-STYLE

1. **Answer: b**
   RATIONALE: The nurse should monitor for myalgia, headache pain, aggravated diabetes, infections, and fatigue in the patient receiving pioglitazone HCl drug therapy. The nurse need not monitor for congestive heart failure, sodium retention, and glycosuria in the patient receiving pioglitazone HCl drug therapy, as these are the adverse reactions observed in patients receiving diazoxide drug therapy.

2. **Answer: a**
   RATIONALE: Chlorpropamide sulfonylureas is contraindicated in patients with coronary artery disease and liver or renal dysfunction. α-glucosidase inhibitors are contraindicated in patients with colonic ulceration, chronic intestinal diseases, and inflammatory bowel disease.

3. **Answer: c**
   RATIONALE: The nurse informs the patient that the need for insulin is greatest during the third trimester of pregnancy. Insulin requirements usually decrease in the first trimester, increase during the second and third trimester, and decrease rapidly after delivery.

Insulin is not required before conception, as gestational diabetes occurs during pregnancy.

4. **Answer: b**
   RATIONALE: The nurse should administer regular insulin to the patient 30 to 60 minutes before a meal to achieve optimal results. Insulin aspart is administered within 5 to 10 minutes of a meal. Insulin lispro is administered 15 minutes before a meal, and insulin glargine is administered once at bedtime via the SC route.

5. **Answer: c**
   RATIONALE: The nurse should administer dextrose rather than sugar to the patient if the administration of miglitol results in hypoglycemia. The nurse should discuss the disease and methods of controlling the disease with the patient after he/she is diagnosed as diabetic. The nurse should not administer acetohexamide with insulin to the patient, as it may enhance the hypoglycemic effect. The capillary blood specimens of the patient are obtained by the nurse when the patient has deficient fluid volume.

6. **Answer: b**
   RATIONALE: When preparing an insulin mixture, the nurse should draw up insulin lispro first in the syringe and then draw the long-acting insulin. The nurse should confirm if the ratio of insulin NPH to regular to be administered is 70/30 or 50/50. When the patient is to receive regular insulin and NPH insulin, or regular and Lente insulin, the nurse must clarify with the primary health care provider whether two separate injections are to be given or if the insulins may be mixed in the same syringe. The premixed solutions may not be effective in patients who have difficulty controlling their diabetes, and hence the nurse need not keep the mixture for 1 hour.

7. **Answer: c**
   RATIONALE: The nurse should instruct the patient to keep a source of glucose ready for signs of low blood glucose for the patient receiving α-glucosidase inhibitors. The nurse should instruct patients prescribed meglitinides therapy to avoid drug administration in case of a skipped meal. The nurse should instruct the patient prescribed metformin therapy to report to the PHCP respiratory distress or muscular aches. The nurse should instruct the patient to take the drug at the same time or times each day.

8. **Answer: d**

   RATIONALE: The insulin pump method is used for the patient who has undergone renal transplantation and pregnant women with diabetes with early long-term complications, since it attempts to mimic the body's normal pancreatic function. Needle and syringe method using microfine needles, jet injection system method, and syringes with prefilled cartridges are used in general for most diabetic patients.

9. **Answer: a**

   RATIONALE: Before insulin administration the nurse should make sure that air bubbles are eliminated from the syringe barrel and the hub of the needle. The nurse should not shake the vial vigorously just before withdrawal; instead, the vial should be tilted end-to-end very gently. The nurse need not ensure that the vial has been standing for an hour. If the vial has been standing for an hour the insulin will be in suspension and the nurse should tilt the vial gently and rotate it in the palm of the hands. The nurse should not use a syringe labeled with a higher concentration; instead, the nurse should always use a syringe marked with the required concentration.

10. **Answer: b**

    RATIONALE: The nurse should instruct the patient to change the needle every 1 to 3 days when administering insulin with an insulin pump. The blood glucose levels should be monitored 4 to 8 times per day. The amount of insulin to be injected is not the same every time; instead, it should be adjusted according to blood glucose levels. A mixture of isophane and regular insulin should not be used for the patient; only regular insulin should be administered through the insulin pump.

11. **Answer: d**

    RATIONALE: Glycosylated hemoglobin measures glucose control over the past 2 or 3 months.

12. **Answer: a**

    RATIONALE: Insulin is produced by the pancreas.

13. **Answer: a**

    RATIONALE: Insulin lispro (Humalog) is an example of rapid-acting insulin.

14. **Answer: b**

    RATIONALE: Insulin glargine (Lantus) is an example of long-acting insulin.

15. **Answer: a**

    RATIONALE: Insulin aspart (Apidra) is given immediately before a meal or within 5 to 10 minutes of beginning a meal.

CHAPTER 44

SECTION I: ASSESSING YOUR UNDERSTANDING

Activity A MATCHING

1. **1.** b **2.** a **3.** d **4.** c
2. **1.** c **2.** d **3.** b **4.** a

Activity B FILL IN THE BLANKS

1. Corticosteroids
2. Prolactin
3. Gonadotropins
4. Rhinyle
5. Menotropin

Activity C SHORT ANSWERS

1. The nurse plays the following role in promoting an optimal response to the growth hormone therapy:
   - The nurse should administer the growth hormone subcutaneously.
   - The nurse should not shake the vial containing the hormone.
   - The nurse should swirl the vial containing the hormone.
   - The nurse should not administer the solution if it is cloudy.
   - The nurse should divide the weekly dosage and give it in 3 to 7 doses throughout the week.
   - The nurse should give the drug at bedtime to closely adhere to the body's natural release of the hormone.
   - The nurse should conduct periodic testing of the growth hormone levels, glucose tolerance, and thyroid functioning during the treatment.

2. The nurse's role in educating the patient and the family includes the following:
   - The nurse discusses in detail the therapeutic regimen for increasing the growth of the child.
   - The nurse instructs the parents on the proper injection technique if the drug is to be given at bedtime and not in the outpatient clinic.

- The nurse encourages parents and child to keep all clinic or office visits.
- The nurse explains that the child may experience sudden growth and increase in appetite.
- The nurse instructs the parents to report lack of growth, symptoms of diabetes such as increased hunger, increased thirst, or frequent voiding, or symptoms of hypothyroidism such as fatigue, dry skin, and intolerance to cold.

Activity D DOSAGE CALCULATION

1. 8 tablets
2. 12 tablets
3. 10 tablets
4. 6 tablets
5. 4 tablets

SECTION II: APPLYING YOUR KNOWLEDGE
Activity E CASE STUDY

1. The nurse should instruct Mr. Smallwood to hold the bottle upright, place the tip of the bottle just inside one of his nares with his head in a vertical position. and to squeeze one spray into his nose.
2. The nurse should warn Mr. Smallwood that the adverse effects of desmopressin (DDAVP) include headache, nausea, nasal congestion, abdominal cramps, and water intoxication.

SECTION III: PRACTICING FOR NCLEX
Activity F NCLEX-STYLE

1. **Answer: a, c, e**
   RATIONALE: The nurse should cautiously administer corticotropin to patients with diabetes, diverticulosis, renal insufficiencies, myasthenia gravis, tuberculosis, hypothyroidism, cirrhosis, nonspecific ulcerative colitis, heart failure, seizures, or febrile infections. Sinus bradycardia and arthralgia are not related to the adverse reactions to corticotropin. Sinus bradycardia is an adverse reaction to octreotide acetate. Arthralgia is an adverse reaction to somatropin.

2. **Answer: d**
   RATIONALE: The nurse should mention the decreased antidiuretic effect to the patient as the effect of the interaction between vasopressin and oral anticoagulants. Increased risks of hypokalemia, increased need for antidiabetic medication or decreased muscle

function are not the effects of interaction between vasopressin and oral anticoagulants. When the patient is administered a diuretic or amphotericin with ACTH, there is an increased risk of hypokalemia. Increased need for antidiabetic medication occurs when the patient is administered insulin or an oral antidiabetic with ACTH. When the patient is administered cholinergic blockers with ACTH, there is decreased muscle function.

3. **Answer: b, c, d.**
   RATIONALE: The nurse should monitor for adverse reactions such as acneiform eruptions, increased sweating, and perineal itching in patients receiving dexamethasone for mycosis fungoides. Nasal congestion and abdominal cramps are not the adverse reactions associated with the use of dexamethasone for mycosis fungoides. Nasal congestion and abdominal cramps are adverse reactions to desmopressin acetate.

4. **Answer: b**
   RATIONALE: The nurse should monitor for a rise in blood glucose level in a patient receiving adrenocorticotropic hormones for nonsuppurative thyroiditis. The nurse need not record the patient's abdominal girth, measure specific gravity of the urine, or monitor the bone age in a patient receiving adrenocorticotropic hormones. The nurse records the patient's abdominal girth before administering vasopressin to relieve abdominal distension. Specific gravity of the urine is measured when the patient needs to self-administer vasopressin by the parenteral route. Bone age is monitored periodically as an ongoing assessment of a patient receiving growth hormones.

5. **Answer: a**
   RATIONALE: The nurse should give the drug with food or a full glass of water to minimize gastric irritation. The nurse need not give an enema, supply large amounts of drinking water, or auscultate the abdomen to minimize gastric irritation. An enema may be given when vasopressin is administered before abdominal roentgenography. Patients with diabetes insipidus are continually thirsty and need to be supplied with large amounts of drinking water. The nurse auscultates the abdomen before administering vasopressin to relieve abdominal distention.

6. Answer: c

RATIONALE: The nurse should monitor for hypertension in the patient receiving fludro-cortisone acetate for primary adrenocortical deficiency. The nurse need not monitor for joint pain, hyperthyroidism, or insulin resistance in the patient receiving fludrocortisone acetate. Joint pain, hyperthyroidism, and insulin resistance are adverse reactions to the growth hormone.

7. Answer: a

RATIONALE: The nurse should discontinue the drug therapy if the infertile patient receiving ganirelix acetate complains of visual disturbances. The nurse need not administer the drug with food, assess the skin integrity, or perform a complete blood count in the patient receiving ganirelix. Oral corticosteroids are given with food to minimize gastric irritation. Assessing skin integrity and performing a complete blood count (CBC) test are preadministration assessments for a patient receiving corticotropin.

8. Answer: c

RATIONALE: The nursing diagnosis checklist for a patient receiving glucocorticoids for systemic lupus erythematosus should include: disturbed body image related to adverse reactions; risk for infection related to immune suppression or impaired wound healing; risk for injury related to muscle atrophy, osteoporosis, or spontaneous fractures; acute pain related to epigastric distress of gastric ulcer formation; excess fluid volume related to adverse reactions such as sodium and water retention; disturbed thought processes related to adverse reactions such as depression, psychosis, and other changes in mental status. The nursing diagnosis checklist for a patient receiving glucocorticoids need not include pain related to abdominal distention, deficient fluid volume related to inability to replenish fluid intake, or risk for infection related to masking of signs of infection. The diagnosis checklist for a patient receiving vasopressin includes pain related to abdominal distention and deficient fluid volume related to inability to replenish fluid intake when the patient is administered vasopressin. The nurse should include risk for infection related to masking of signs of infection in the diagnosis checklist when the patient is administered ACTH.

9. Answer: a

RATIONALE: When the drug is administered before abdominal roentgenography, the nurse administers 2 injections of 10 units each. The first dose is given 2 hours before an x-ray examination, and the nurse should give an enema before administering the first dose of vasopressin to the patient undergoing abdominal roentgenography. The nurse need not check stools, monitor for rash, urticaria, and hypotension, or ensure that the daily oral doses are given before 9 AM for a patient receiving vasopressin and undergoing abdominal roentgenography. The nurse should check stools for evidence of bleeding or monitor the patient for rash, urticaria, and hypotension when the patient is administered ACTH. Daily oral doses are generally given before 9 AM to minimize adrenal suppression in patients administered glucocorticoids or mineralocorticoids.

10. Answer: b, d, e

RATIONALE: The nurse is likely to observe buffalo hump, moon face, oily skin and acne, osteoporosis, purple striae on the abdomen and hips, altered skin pigmentation, and weight gain in the patient undergoing an overdose of prednisone. The nurse need not observe for swelling and muscle pain as the adverse reactions to overdose of prednisone. Swelling and muscle pain are adverse reactions to somatropin.

11. Answer: a

RATIONALE: Vasopressin is a hormone secreted by the posterior pituitary gland.

12. Answer: c

RATIONALE: Diabetes insipidus is treated with replacement of vasopressin.

13. Answer: a

RATIONALE: Vasopressin is the hormone responsible for the regulation of reabsorption of water by the kidneys.

14. Answer: b

RATIONALE: Somatotropin is the hormone responsible for the growth of the body during childhood, especially the growth of muscles and bones.

15. Answer: a

RATIONALE: Clomiphene (Clomid) is the medication that binds to estrogen receptors, decreasing the amount of available estrogen receptors and causing the anterior pituitary to increase secretion of FSH and LH.

CHAPTER 45

SECTION I: ASSESSING YOUR UNDERSTANDING

Activity A MATCHING

1. **1.** b   **2.** c   **3.** a
2. **1.** c   **2.** a   **3.** d   **4.** b

Activity B FILL IN THE BLANKS

1. Hyperthyroidism
2. Hypothyroid
3. Iodine
4. Euthyroid
5. Antithyroid

Activity C SHORT ANSWERS

1. The nurse should provide the following information to the patient and family, emphasizing the importance of taking the thyroid hormone replacement therapy:
   - Replacement therapy is for life, with the exception of transient hypothyroidism seen in those with thyroiditis.
   - Do not increase, decrease, or skip a dose unless advised to do so by the primary health care provider.
   - Notify the primary health care provider if any of the following occur: headache, nervousness, palpitations, diarrhea, excessive sweating, heat intolerance, chest pain, increased pulse rate, or any unusual physical changes or events.
   - Weigh yourself weekly and report any significant weight gain or loss to the primary health care provider.
2. The nurse should consider the following factors to determine the success of the therapy:
   - The therapeutic effect is achieved.
   - Adverse reactions are identified and reported to the primary health care provider.
   - The patient verbalizes the importance of complying with the prescribed treatment regimen.
   - The patient verbalizes an understanding of the treatment modalities and importance of continued follow-up care.
   - The patient and family demonstrate an understanding of the drug regimen.

Activity D DOSAGE CALCULATION

1. 3 tablets
2. 6 tablets
3. 3 tablets
4. 2 tablets
5. 12.5 mcg

SECTION II: APPLYING YOUR KNOWLEDGE

Activity E CASE STUDY

1. The nurse should instruct Ms. Higgs to take the levothyroxine (Synthroid) in the morning before breakfast to ensure better drug absorption.
2. Early effects of levothyroxine (Synthroid) treatment can occur in as few as 48 hours; however, the full effects of thyroid hormone replacement may not be apparent for several weeks.

SECTION III: PRACTICING FOR NCLEX

Activity F NCLEX-STYLE

1. **Answer: b**
   RATIONALE: The nurse should notify the primary health care provider if agranulocytosis, an adverse reaction to the methimazole drug, occurs. The nurse need not report tachycardia, weight loss, and fatigue as adverse reactions to the methimazole drug, as these are the common adverse reactions to levothyroxine sodium (T_4), liothyronine sodium (T_3), and sodium iodine (^{131}I), liotrix (T_3, T_4), and thyroid USP desiccated.

2. **Answer: a**
   RATIONALE: The nurse should observe decreased effectiveness of the cardiac drug when the thyroid hormones are administered with digoxin to the patient. The nurse need not observe increased risk of prolonged bleeding, decreased effectiveness of the thyroid drug, and increased potential for bleeding in the patient as the effect of interaction between the thyroid hormones and digoxin. There is an increased risk of prolonged bleeding when the patient is administered thyroid hormones with oral anticoagulants. When the patient is administered thyroid hormones with antidepressants, there is an increased and not decreased effectiveness of the thyroid drug. When the patient is administered antithyroid drugs with propylthiouracil, there is an increased potential for bleeding.

3. **Answer: c**
RATIONALE: The nurse should monitor mild diuresis as a sign of therapeutic response after the thyroid hormone is administered to the patient. The nurse need not monitor agranulocytosis, headache, and loss of hair as the sign of therapeutic response after the thyroid hormone is administered to the patient. Agranulocytosis, headache, and loss of hair are the adverse reactions to antithyroid preparations.

4. **Answers: b, c, e**
RATIONALE: The nurse should document cold intolerance, confusion, and unsteady gait as the symptoms of hypothyroidism during the preadministration assessment. The nurse need not document weight loss and sweating as the symptoms of hypothyroidism. Weight loss and sweating are the adverse reactions to the levothyroxine sodium (T_4) drug.

5. **Answers: a, c, e**
RATIONALE: The nurse should instruct the patient to take the drug at regular intervals, record weight twice a week, and avoid taking the drug in larger doses. The nurse need not instruct the patient undergoing propylthiouracil drug therapy to take the drug before breakfast, or to notify the primary health care provider if a palpitation occurs. The nurse should instruct the patient taking thyroid hormones to take the drug before breakfast and notify the primary health care provider if headache, nervousness, palpitations, diarrhea, excessive sweating, heat intolerance, chest pain, increased pulse rate, or any unusual physical change or event occurs.

6. **Answer: b**
RATIONALE: The nurse should notify the primary health care provider of the development of chest pain in the patient so that the dosage of the thyroid hormone can be reduced. The nurse need not notify the development of high fever, sweating, and headache to the primary health care provider to reduce the dosage of the thyroid hormone. High fever is a sign of thyroid storm, which occurs in patients whose hyperthyroidism is inadequately treated. Sweating is the adverse reaction to levothyroxine sodium (T_4). Headache is the adverse reaction to levothyroxine sodium (T_4) and methimazole.

7. **Answer: d**
RATIONALE: The nurse should monitor the patient for altered mental status, high fever, and extreme tachycardia as the signs of thyroid storm during the ongoing assessment. The nurse need not monitor the patient for anxiety, increased pulse rate, and nervousness as the signs of thyroid storm during the ongoing assessment. Anxiety and nervousness are the signs of hyperthyroidism. Increased pulse rate is the sign of a therapeutic response.

8. **Answer: a**
RATIONALE: When the patient is prescribed an iodine procedure, it is essential that the nurse take a careful allergy history, particularly to iodine or seafood. The nurse need not monitor the signs of agranulocytosis, assess the patient for mouth infection, or monitor the patient's stool color in the patient who has been prescribed an iodine procedure.

9. **Answer: b**
RATIONALE: Thyroid hormones are contraindicated in patients with known hypersensitivity to the drug, an uncorrected adrenal cortical insufficiency, or thyrotoxicosis. The drug is not contraindicated in patients with agranulocytosis, granulocytopenia, and hypoprothrombinemia. Agranulocytosis, granulocytopenia, and hypoprothrombinemia are some of the severe systemic reactions to antithyroid drugs.

10. **Answer: a, c, d**
RATIONALE: The nurse should report signs of hyperthyroidism such as moist skin, moderate hypertension, and increased appetite to the primary health care provider before the next dose is due, because it may be necessary to decrease the daily dosage. Easy bruising, sore throat, fatigue, fever, and bleeding are the signs and symptoms indicating an adverse reaction related to a decrease in blood cells.

11. **Answer: a**
RATIONALE: Iodine is the essential element for the manufacturing of thyroxine and triiodothyronine.

12. **Answer: c**
RATIONALE: Levothyroxine (Synthroid) is the drug of choice for hypothyroidism because it is relatively inexpensive, requires once-a-day dosing, and has a more uniform potency than do other thyroid hormone replacement drugs.

13. Answer: a

   RATIONALE: The nurse should advise patients to take levothyroxine (Synthroid) in the morning on an empty stomach.

14 Answer: a

   RATIONALE: A nurse should be cautious not to administer levothyroxine (Synthroid) to a patient who has recently had myocardial infarction.

15. Answer: a

   RATIONALE: Levothyroxine (Synthroid) is in pregnancy category A, and it is safe to use during pregnancy.

CHAPTER 46

SECTION I: ASSESSING YOUR UNDERSTANDING

Activity A MATCHING

1. 1. c   **2.** a   **3.** e   **4.** b   **5.** d
2. 1. e   **2.** c   **3.** d   **4.** a   **5.** b

Activity B FILL IN THE BLANKS

1. Menarche
2. Endogenous
3. Catabolism
4. Prostate
5. Androgens

Activity C SHORT ANSWERS

1. Treatment with androgens may lead to an increase in fluid volume. When a nurse is monitoring patients on androgen therapy, the following assessments should be made:
   - The nurse should observe the patient for any signs of edema as a result of sodium and water retention making the patient edematous. She should also make a note of any puffiness of the eyelids. If the patient is ambulatory, there may be dependent swelling of the hands or feet. If the patient is nonambulatory, the nurse may need to look for swelling of the sacral area.
   - The patient's weight should be noted prior to androgen therapy, to be used as a guide. As part of the ongoing assessment, the nurse needs to compare the patient's weight with the preadministration weight on a daily basis.

The nurse needs to monitor daily fluid intake and output to calculate the fluid balance. The nurse should be aware that older adults with heart and kidney diseases pose a greater risk, as they are at an increased risk of developing sodium and water retention.

2. The nurse should include the following points in the teaching plan when educating a patient about oral contraceptives:
   - Read the package insert carefully. Discuss any questions with the health care provider.
   - Take the first dose as directed by the instructions or by the primary health care provider.
   - The drug should be taken at intervals not exceeding once every 24 hours. It is best taken with the evening meal or at bedtime. The dose schedule has to be followed for proper efficacy of the drug. Failure to comply may lead to pregnancy.
   - Until the first week of the next cycle, an additional birth control method should be used.
   - If one day's dose is missed, the missed dose should be taken as soon as remembered, or 2 tablets taken the next day.
   - If 2 days are missed, then 2 tablets need to taken for the next 2 days and then the normal dosing schedule should be continued. Another form of birth control must be used until the cycle is completed and a new cycle has begun.
   - If 3 days in a row or more are missed, the drug should be discontinued. Another form of birth control may be used until a new cycle can begin. Before restarting the regimen, absence of pregnancy, due to a break in the regimen, needs to be confirmed.
   - If the patient is not sure what to do about a missed dose, the primary health care provider needs to be contacted.
   - Both active and passive smoking should be avoided while taking oral contraceptives.
   - Any adverse reactions such as fluid retention or edema to the extremities; weight gain; pain, swelling, or tenderness in the legs; blurred vision; chest pain; yellowed skin or eyes; dark urine; or abnormal vaginal bleeding should be reported.
   - Periodic examinations by the primary health care provider and laboratory tests are needed during the therapy.

Activity D DOSAGE CALCULATION

1. 4 tablets
2. 3 tablets
3. 2 tablets
4. 1.5 tablets
5. 2 capsules
6. 7.5 tablets in a day

SECTION II: APPLYING YOUR KNOWLEDGE
Activity E CASE STUDY

1. High-dose levonorgetrel (Plan B) should be given within 72 hours after unprotected intercourse or contraceptive failure.
2. Levonorgestrel (Plan B) should be taken the following way: 1st dose within 72 hours of event and a second dose 12 hours later. If vomiting occurs within 1 hour after taking either dose, the physician should be notified.

SECTION III: PRACTICING FOR NCLEX
Activity F NCLEX-STYLE

1. **Answer: b**
   RATIONALE: The nurse should consider that the androgen therapy might have been prescribed for testosterone deficiency. The male hormone testosterone and its derivatives are collectively called *androgens*. Thus, androgen therapy may be prescribed for testosterone deficiency. Adrenal cortical cancer is treated with adrenal steroid inhibitors such as mitotane, and not by androgen therapy. Symptoms of benign prostatic hypertrophy are treated by androgen hormone inhibitors, and not by androgen therapy. Male pattern baldness occurs due to androgens, and androgen hormone inhibitors are used for its prevention.

2. **Answer: d**
   RATIONALE: Anabolic steroids may be used to promote weight gain following profound weight loss due to surgery, trauma, or infections. Anabolic steroids are not intended for increase in muscle mass and strength in young, healthy individuals. Such abuse can cause serious adverse effects and is considered illegal. Androgens, progestins, and conjugated estrogens are not prescribed for the promotion of weight gain following profound weight loss, though some of these drugs may cause some weight gain as a side effect.

3. **Answer: a**
   RATIONALE: Increased antidiuretic effects may be seen when androgens or androgen hormone inhibitors are used concomitantly in a patient on oral anticoagulant therapy. Decreased anticoagulant effects are seen when female hormones, and not male hormones, are used with oral anticoagulant therapy. Increased risk of hypoglycemia may be seen when male hormone therapy is used in patients taking sulfonylureas, and not oral anticoagulants. There is an increased risk of paranoia when imipramine, and not oral anticoagulants, are given with male hormones or male-hormone inhibitors.

4. **Answer: b**
   RATIONALE: Gynecomastia or enlargement of the breast is a complication of androgen therapy seen among male patients. Testicular atrophy, and not enlargement of testes, may be seen as another side effect of androgen therapy. Virilization is the appearance of male secondary sexual characteristics in females and is seen as a side effect of androgen therapy in females, and not males. Water retention, and not frequent urination, is seen in patients on androgen therapy.

5. **Answer: c**
   RATIONALE: In menopausal women with an intact uterus, progestins are given along with estrogen to reduce the risk of an endometrial carcinoma. GI irritation may be caused by estrogen. However, taking the medication with food can reduce this. Progestins do not reduce GI irritation caused by estrogen. The associated atrophic vaginitis is treated with estrogen therapy, and not progestin therapy. Risk of osteoporosis is also reduced by taking estrogens, and not by taking progestins.

6. **Answer: c**
   RATIONALE: Impaired vision may occur as an adverse effect of the herb black cohosh. It may cause high, and not low, blood pressure. It does not cause ringing in the ears, but rather is used to treat this symptom seen during menopause. The herb causes weight gain, and not weight loss.

7. **Answer: b**
   RATIONALE: The nurse should keep in mind that Depo-Provera is to be shaken vigorously before administration to ensure a uniform suspension. The drug is not implanted in the subdermal tissue, but rather given as a deep intramuscular injection. The initial dosage is

given within the first 5 days of menstruation or within 5 days postpartum. It is not given on the 10th day of the menstruation cycle. Depo-Provera is given IM every 3 months, and does not provide contraceptive protection for as long as 5 years.

8. **Answers: a, b, d**
   RATIONALE: The risk of iron-deficiency anemia, ovarian cancer, and osteoporosis is decreased with the use of oral contraceptives. The risks of cervical erosion and vaginal candidiasis are increased, and not reduced, with the use of oral contraceptives.

9. **Answer: d**
   RATIONALE: If a woman has missed 1 day's dose of an oral contraceptive, she should be advised to take the missed dose as soon as remembered or to take 2 tablets the next day. Discontinue the drug and using another form of birth control until the next cycle is needed when the doses for 3 days in a row or more have been missed, not when only one day's dose is missed. Remembering to take 1 tablet the next day and forgetting about the missed dose does not help, as it may reduce the contraceptive effectiveness and lead to pregnancy.

10. **Answer: d**
    RATIONALE: The nurse should explain that the female hormone estropipate is a synthetic estrogen. Estropipate is not produced endogenously and must be obtained from outside as a drug. Estradiol, estrone, and estriol are estrogens that are produced endogenously in the body. These are not synthetic hormones. Estradiol is available as a drug, but it is also produced endogenously and need not be obtained only as a drug.

11. **Answer: a**
    RATIONALE: Dutasteride (Avodart) is an example of an androgen hormone inhibitor used to treat patients with benign prostatic hypertrophy.

12. **Answer: a**
    RATIONALE: Fluoxymesterone is an androgen that can be used to treat hypogonadism.

13. **Answer: b**
    RATIONALE: Oxymetholone is an anabolic steroid that can be used to treat anemia.

14. **Answer: a**
    RATIONALE: Nandrolone is an example of an anabolic steroid.

15. **Answer: a**
    RATIONALE: Testosterone is not able to be given intravenously.

CHAPTER 47

SECTION I: ASSESSING YOUR UNDERSTANDING

Activity A MATCHING

1. 1. c   2. b   3. a   4. e   5. d
2. 1. b   2. c   3. a   4. e   5. d

Activity B FILL IN THE BLANKS

1. Contractions
2. Posterior
3. Eclampsia
4. Ergotism
5. Antidiuretic

Activity C SHORT ANSWERS

1. The nurse should immediately discontinue the oxytocin infusion if any of these changes are noted:
   - A significant change in the FHR or rhythm
   - A marked change in the frequency, rate, or rhythm of uterine contractions
   - A marked increase or decrease in the patient's blood pressure or pulse or any significant change in the patient's general condition
2. During the ongoing assessment of a patient receiving a tocolytic drug, the role of a nurse includes:
   - Recording blood pressure, pulse, and respiratory rate
   - Monitoring FHR
   - Checking the IV infusion rate
   - Examining the area around the IV needle insertion site for signs of infiltration
   - Monitoring uterine contractions (frequency, intensity, length)
   - Measuring maternal intake and output

Activity D DOSAGE CALCULATION

1. 4 ampoules
2. 4 mL
3. 2 tablets
4. 10 mL
5. 0.25 mL
6. 0.5 mL

SECTION II: APPLYING YOUR KNOWLEDGE
Activity E CASE STUDY

1. The nurse should obtain the following information during the preadministration assessment of Mrs. Stevens: obstetric history (parity, gravidity, previous obstetric problems, type of labor, still births, abortions, live-birth infant abnormalities), and a general health history. Immediately before starting the IV infusion of oxytocin (Pitocin), the nurse assesses the fetal heart rate and the patient's blood pressure, pulse, and respiratory rate.
2. The adverse effects of oxytocin (Pitocin) include: fetal bradycardia, uterine rupture, uterine hypertonicity, nausea, vomiting, cardiac arrhythmias, anaphylactic reactions, and water intoxication.

SECTION III: PRACTICING FOR NCLEX
Activity F NCLEX-STYLE

1. **Answer: a**
   RATIONALE: When administering oxytocin intranasally to facilitate the letdown of milk, the nurse should place the patient in an upright position, and with the squeeze bottle held upright, should administer the prescribed number of sprays to one or both nostrils. The supine and lateral positions are not favorable in breastfeeding the infant or collecting milk. The standing position will be inconvenient to the patient and is not the appropriate position when administrating oxytocin intranasally to the patient.

2. **Answers: a, d, e**
   RATIONALE: The patient receiving oxytocin to induce labor may have concern over the use of the drug. In order to reduce anxiety, the nurse should explain the purpose of the IV infusion and the expected results to the patient. Not explaining the expected results or outcome will increase the patient's anxiety. The nurse should spend time with the patient and offer encouragement and reassurance. Without prior instructions from the primary health care provider, the nurse should not administer any drug as it might lead to drug interaction and complications.

3. **Answer: c**
   RATIONALE: In some patients who are calcium deficient, the uterus may not respond well to ergonovine. The nurse should immediately report a lack of response to ergonovine.

Administering calcium by IV injection usually restores response to the drug. Magnesium sulfate is a tocolytic drug and cannot be used in this condition. Increasing the dosage of the drug might lead to complications such as ergotism. Terbutaline is a tocolytic used to prevent preterm labor and is not used in this situation.

4. **Answer: d**
   RATIONALE: Magnesium sulfate is contraindicated in eclampsia. The other contraindications include hypersensitivity to the drug, heart block, myocardial damage, and severe preeclampsia within 2 hours of delivery. Oxytocin is contraindicated in conditions such as cephalopelvic disproportion and total placenta previa. Ergonovine is contraindicated in hypertension and not magnesium sulfate.

5. **Answer: c**
   RATIONALE: The nurse should place a cardiac monitor on the patient during the administration of magnesium sulfate, as a dosage change might be required. The blood pressure and the pulse range should be monitored to determine when the IV infusion has to be stopped. Urinary output should be monitored only if the patient develops vomiting. Vaginal bleeding is an adverse effect of indomethacin and not magnesium sulfate; hence, monitoring for vaginal bleeding is not required. Monitoring of urine output, pedal edema, and vaginal bleeding is not required during the administration of magnesium sulfate.

6. **Answer: d**
   RATIONALE: Ergonovine is contraindicated in hypertension, before delivery of the placenta, and in hypersensitivity of the drug. In renal disease, lactation, and heart disease the drug should be used cautiously, and is not strictly contraindicated.

7. **Answer: a, c, d**
   RATIONALE: When administering methylergonovine for controlling postpartum bleeding, the nurse should monitor the vital signs every 4 hours, and should note the character and amount of vaginal bleeding. The nurse should immediately notify the primary health care provider when abdominal cramping is moderate to severe. The termination of the drug is decided by the primary health care provider depending on the condition and not by the nurse. The nurse need not put the patient in the lateral position after administering the drug.

8. *Answer: a*

RATIONALE: When oxytocin is administered IV, there is a danger of excessive fluid volume (water intoxication) because oxytocin has an antidiuretic effect. Therefore, it is necessary for hourly measurements of fluid intake and output. Ergonovine, methylergonovine, and magnesium sulfate are not associated with water intoxication.

9. Answer: a, c, e

RATIONALE: Symptoms of ergotism include coolness, numbness, and tingling of extremities, dyspnea, nausea, confusion, tachycardia or bradycardia, chest pain, hallucinations, and convulsions. Water intoxication and diplopia are not the symptoms of ergotism. Water intoxication may be seen in patients receiving oxytocin, and diplopia is an adverse reaction associated with magnesium sulfate.

10. Answer: a

RATIONALE: Magnesium sulfate is used to manage preterm labor in pregnancies of greater than 27 weeks' gestation. It is a calcium antagonist and works to decrease the force of uterine contractions. Indomethacin is an NSAID that blocks the production of prostaglandins, which contribute to uterine contractions. Magnesium sulfate does not block the production of prostaglandin. Magnesium sulfate, not being an oxytocic drug, does not stimulate the uterus. Oxytocin, and not magnesium sulfate, has an antidiuretic action.

11. Answer: a

RATIONALE: Oxytocin (Pitocin) is used antepartum to induce uterine contractions.

12. Answer: b

RATIONALE: Oxytocin is an endogenous hormone produced by the posterior pituitary gland.

13. Answer: a

RATIONALE: The nurse should administer oxytocin (Pitocin) intranasally to a patient to stimulate the mild ejection reflex.

14. Answer: a

RATIONALE: A nurse should monitor a patient receiving oxytocin (Pitocin) for the following adverse effects: fetal bradycardia, uterine rupture, uterine hypertonicity, nausea, vomiting, cardiac arrhythmias, and anaphylactic reactions.

15. Answer: c

RATIONALE: Water intoxication is an adverse effect caused by all uterine stimulants because of their antidiuretic effect.

CHAPTER 48

SECTION I: ASSESSING YOUR UNDERSTANDING

Activity A MATCHING

1. 1. e   2. a   3. b   4. c   5. d
2. 1. c   2. a   3. d   4. b

Activity B FILL IN THE BLANKS

1. Edema
2. Carbonic
3. Potassium
4. Paresthesias
5. Dermatologic

Activity C SHORT ANSWERS

1. The nurse should perform the following preadministration assessments before the administration of a diuretic drug to a patient:
   - The nurse should take the vital signs and weigh the patient.
   - Current laboratory test results, especially the levels of serum electrolytes, should be carefully reviewed.
   - Patients with renal dysfunction should also have blood urea nitrogen (BUN) and creatinine clearance levels monitored.
   - If the patient has peripheral edema, the nurse should inspect the involved areas and record in the patient's chart the degree and extent of edema.
   - If the patient is receiving a carbonic anhydrase inhibitor for increased IOP, the nurse should obtain the patient's description of pain and vital signs.
   - The preadministration physical assessment of the patient receiving a diuretic for epilepsy includes vital signs and weight. The nurse should review the patient's chart for a description of the seizures and their frequency.
   - If the patient is to receive an osmotic diuretic, the focus of the assessment is on the patient's disease or disorder and the symptoms being treated. For example, if the patient has a low urinary output and the

osmotic diuretic is given to increase urinary output, then the nurse should review the intake and output ratio and symptoms the patient is experiencing. In addition, the nurse should also weigh the patient and take the vital signs as part of the physical assessment before drug therapy starts.

2. The nurse should perform the following assessments after the administration of a diuretic drug:
   - During initial therapy, the nurse should observe the patient for the effects of drug therapy. The type of assessment will depend on such factors as the reason for administration of the diuretic, type of diuretic administered, route of administration, and condition of the patient.
   - The nurse should measure and record fluid intake and output, and report to the primary health care provider any marked decrease in the output.
   - During ongoing therapy, the nurse should weigh the patient at the same time daily, making certain that the patient is wearing the same amount or type of clothing.
   - Depending on the specific diuretic, frequent serum electrolyte, uric acid, and liver and kidney function tests should be performed during the first few months of therapy, and periodically thereafter.

Activity D DOSAGE CALCULATION

1. 3 tablets
2. 4 tablets
3. 3 tablets
4. 20 mL solution
5. 2.5 tablets

SECTION II: APPLYING YOUR KNOWLEDGE
Activity E CASE STUDY

1. The nurse will need to administer 3.4 mL to Mr. Morton every 6 hours.

   150 lb × 1 kg/2.2 lb = 68.2 kg

   68.2 kg × 1 mg/kg = 68.2 mg

   68.2 mg × 1 mL/20 mg = 3.4 mL

2. The adverse effects of furosemide (Lasix) include: electrolyte and hematologic imbalances, anorexia, nausea, vomiting, dizziness, rash, photosensitivity, orthostatic hypotension, hypokalemia, and glycosuria.

SECTION III: PRACTICING FOR NCLEX
Activity F NCLEX-STYLE

1. **Answer: a, c, d**
   RATIONALE: The nurse should take a daily measurement and record the patient's weight to monitor fluid loss. The nurse should measure fluid intake and output every 8 hours and assess respiratory rate every 4 hours to assess that the patient is achieving optimal response to therapy. The nurse need not check the pupil of the eye every 2 hours for dilation, or check patient's response to light; these interventions are done for patients with acute closed-angle glaucoma.

2. **Answer: b**
   RATIONALE: When caring for a patient receiving diuretics and experiencing GI upset, the nurse should instruct the patient to take the drug with food or milk. The nurse need not instruct the patient to take the drug on an empty stomach, or avoid intake of fibrous food, as these are not appropriate interventions to reduce the symptoms or discomforts due to GI upset. The nurse should not instruct the patient to reduce fluid intake to prevent discomfort associated with GI upset. Patients may exhibit anxiety with the frequent need to urinate as a result of the diuretic therapy, but the nurse should not reduce their fluid intake, explaining that the need to urinate frequently decreases after a few weeks of therapy.

3. **Answer: c**
   RATIONALE: The nurse should closely observe the patient receiving the spironolactone drug for signs of hyperkalemia, which is a serious and potentially fatal electrolyte imbalance. This medication is a potassium-sparing medication. The nurse should closely observe the patient for paresthesias and anorexia after administering acetazolamide. The patient needs to be observed for vertigo after administering bendroflumethiazide.

4. **Answer: b**
   RATIONALE: The nurse should monitor the patient for an increased risk of hyperglycemia as an effect of interaction between the chlorothiazide and anitdiabetic drug. The patient will not develop hypersensitivity to the drug as a result of the interaction between chlorothiazide and the antidiabetic drug. The nurse should monitor for an increased risk of ototoxicity when loop diuretics are adminis-

tered with cisplatin or aminoglycosides to a patient. Increased risk of ototoxicity is not known to occur due to the interaction between chlorothiazide and the antidiabetic drug. An increase in the effect of chlorothiazide is also not known to occur due to the interaction of chlorothiazide and the antidiabetic drug.

5. **Answer: a, b, d**
   RATIONALE: The nurse should inform the patient that herbal diuretics should not be taken unless approved by the PHCP. The nurse should inform the patient that most plant and herbal extracts available as OTC diuretics are nontoxic and that most herbal diuretics are either ineffective or no more effective than caffeine. The nurse should not encourage the patient to consume diuretic teas like juniper berries because they are contraindicated. Juniper berries have been associated with renal damage, and horsetail contains severely toxic compounds. Teas with ephedrine should be avoided, especially by individuals with hypertension.

6. **Answer: a**
   RATIONALE: The nurse should know that endocrine disturbances, heart failure, and kidney and liver diseases cause excess fluid retention in the body. Hematological changes, gastric distress, and hyperkalemia are the adverse reactions to bendroflumethiazide and are not known to cause excess fluid retention in the body. Hyperkalemia is also most likely to occur in patients with diabetes.

7. **Answer: b, d, e**
   RATIONALE: The nurse should monitor for levels of serum electrolytes, blood urea nitrogen (BUN), and creatinine clearance levels before administering metolazone to a patient with renal dysfunction. Patients with edema caused by heart failure are weighed daily to monitor fluid loss. Serum potassium levels are monitored for patients at risk for hypokalemia.

8. **Answer: b**
   RATIONALE: The nurse should know that the patient is experiencing an electrolyte imbalance. Warning signs of a fluid and electrolyte imbalance include dry mouth, thirst, weakness, lethargy, drowsiness, restlessness, muscle pains or cramps, confusion, gastrointestinal disturbances, hypotension, oliguria, tachycardia, and seizures. Hyperkalemia, hypercal

cemia, and hyponatremia are characterized by high levels of potassium and calcium and low levels of sodium ions circulating in the blood respectively. Symptoms of hyperkalemia include paresthesia (numbness, tingling, or prickling sensation), muscular weakness, fatigue, flaccid paralysis of the extremities, bradycardia, shock, and electrocardiographic (ECG) abnormalities. Hypercalcemia and hyponatremia are not characterized by muscle pain, cramps, oliguria, hypotension, and GI disturbances.

9. **Answer: c**
   RATIONALE: If the serum potassium levels in the patient exceed 5.3 mEq/mL, the nurse should discontinue the drug and notify the physician immediately, since this could be a sign of hypokalemia. The drug is not to be discontinued if the patient experiences gout attacks, or if the urine tests positive for glucose, or excess fluid has been removed from the patient's body. Thiazide diuretic drug therapy may cause gout attacks in patients, during which they could experience joint pain. Patients who have diabetes mellitus and take loop or thiazide diuretics may test positive for the presence of glucose in their urine, in which case the PHCP has to be contacted immediately. The patient needs to continue diuretic drug therapy to prevent further accumulation of fluid, as the excess fluid has been removed from the body due to the drug therapy.

10. **Answer: a**
    RATIONALE: Furosemide (Lasix) is an example of a loop diuretic.

11. **Answer: b**
    RATIONALE: Acetazolamide (Diamox) is a carbonic anhydrase inhibitor that exerts its effect by inhibiting the enzyme carbonic anhydrase.

12. **Answer: a**
    RATIONALE: Mannitol (Osmitrol) is an osmotic diuretic that exerts its diuretic effects by increasing the density of the filtrate in the glomerulus.

13. **Answer: a**
    RATIONALE: Spironolactone (Aldactone) is a potassium-sparing diuretic that exerts its diuretic effect by antagonizing the action of aldosterone.

14. Answer: d

RATIONALE: Triamterene (Dyrenium) is a potassium-sparing diuretic that exerts its effect by depressing the reabsorption of sodium in the kidney tubules, thereby increasing sodium and water excretion.

15. Answer: a

RATIONALE: Hydrochlorothiazide (Microzide) is a thiazide diuretic that exerts its diuretic effect by inhibiting the reabsorption of sodium and chloride ions in the ascending portion of the loop of Henle and the early distal tubule of the nephron.

CHAPTER 49

SECTION I: ASSESSING YOUR UNDERSTANDING

Activity A MATCHING

1. 1. b   **2.** a   **3.** d   **4.** c
2. 1. c   **2.** a   **3.** d   **4.** b

Activity B FILL IN THE BLANKS

1. Cystitis
2. Antispasmodic
3. Neurogenic
4. Nocturia
5. Urge

Activity C SHORT ANSWERS

1. The nurse should consider the following factors to determine the success of the treatment plan:
   - Achievement of the therapeutic effect
   - Identification, reporting, and successful management of adverse reactions through appropriate nursing interventions
   - Demonstration of the understanding of the drug regimen by the patient and family
   - Verbalization of the importance of complying with the prescribed therapeutic regimen by the patient
2. The nurse should include the following teaching points in the teaching plan:
   - Take the drug with food or meals (nitrofurantoin must be taken with food or milk). If GI upset occurs despite taking the drug with food, contact the primary health care provider.
   - Take the drug at the prescribed intervals and complete the full course of therapy. Do

not discontinue taking the drug even though the symptoms have disappeared, unless directed to do so by the primary health care provider.
   - If drowsiness or dizziness occurs, avoid driving and performing tasks that require alertness.
   - During therapy with this drug, avoid alcoholic beverages, and do not take any nonprescription drug unless its use has been approved by the primary health care provider.
   - Notify the primary health care provider immediately if symptoms do not improve after 3 or 4 days.
   - Take nitrofurantoin with food or milk to improve absorption. Continue therapy for at least 1 week or for 3 days after the urine shows no signs of infection. Notify the primary health care provider immediately if any of the following occur: fever, chills, cough, shortness of breath, chest pain, or difficulty breathing. Do not take the next dose of the drug until the primary health care provider has been contacted. The urine may appear brown during therapy with this drug; this is not abnormal.

Activity D DOSAGE CALCULATIONS

1. 3 tablets
2. 10 tablets
3. 8 tablets
4. 8 capsules

SECTION II: APPLYING YOUR KNOWLEDGE
Activity E CASE STUDY

1. Prior to leaving the office the nurse should discuss the following adverse reactions to nitrofurantoin (Macrobid) with Ms. Anthony: nausea, anorexia, peripheral neuropathy, headache, and bacterial superinfection.
2. The nurse should recommend the following nonpharmacological measures to Ms. Anthony: Increase fluid intake to at least 2000 mL/day to aid in physical removal of bacteria; urge her to drink fluids every hour; offer suggestions for fluids to drink based on her likes and dislikes; demonstrate the procedure for measuring intake and output using household measures; inform her about urine appearance when intake is increased; and describe drug-induced urine color changes that can stain undergarments.

SECTION III: PRACTICING FOR NCLEX
Activity F NCLEX-STYLE

1. Answer: a
RATIONALE: When caring for a patient experiencing dry mouth, the nurse should instruct the patient to suck on sugarless lozenges. Sucking on hard candy can also bring relief to patients with dry mouth, and so the nurse need not instruct the patient to refrain from consuming them. The nurse need not instruct the patient to increase the intake of fibrous foods because doing so will not bring relief from dry mouth. The nurse should instruct the patient to take the nitrofurantoin with food or milk to improve absorption of the drug. Taking the drug with milk in case of a dry mouth will not lessen the discomforts or the symptoms of the patient's condition.

2. Answer: b
RATIONALE: The nurse should monitor for dry eyes in the patient on solifenacin drug therapy. Dry eyes, blurred vision, and dry mouth are common adverse reactions to antispasmodic drugs. Headache, pruritus, and rash are the adverse reactions to the phenazopyridine drug and are not known to occur with the administration of solifenacin.

3. Answer: a
RATIONALE: The nurse should monitor the patient for an increased risk of bleeding when sulfamethoxazole is administered with oral anticoagulants. Delay in gastric emptying is observed in the patient when anticholinergics are administered with nitrofurantoin. Decreased effect of the sulfamethoxazole is not known to occur as a result of the interaction of sulfamethoxazole with oral anticoagulants. Urinary tract excretion of the anti-infective (particularly fosfomycin) and lowered plasma concentrations occur when metoclopramide is administered with fosfomycin.

4. Answer: c
RATIONALE: The nurse should know that antispasmodics are contraindicated in patients with myasthenia gravis. Antispasmodics are not contraindicated in patients with hepatic impairment, with cerebral arteriosclerosis, or in patients with convulsive disorders. Anti-infectives should be used cautiously in those with renal or hepatic impairment. Nalidixic acid (NegGram), an anti-infective, is contraindicated in patients who have convulsive disorders. Nitrofurantoin, an anti-infective, and nalidixic acid are used cautiously in patients with cerebral arteriosclerosis.

5. Answer: c
RATIONALE: The nurse should administer the urinary tract anti-infective with prune juice to decrease the pain experienced by the patient on voiding. The nurse can also administer cranberry juice to the patient. Even other fluids, preferably water, are encouraged during drug administration, though the nurse need not administer the drug strictly with warm water. The nurse should not administer the drug after meals or strictly with milk to prevent pain experienced by the patient on voiding. Nitrofurantoin is generally administered with milk to prevent the irritation it causes in the stomach.

6. Answer: c
RATIONALE: The nurse should avoid administration of phenazopyridine for more than 2 days when the patient is also receiving an antibacterial drug for the UTI. When used for more than 2 days, the drug may mask the symptoms of a more serious disorder. The nurse should encourage the patient to drink at least 2000 mL of fluid daily and administer the urinary tract anti-infectives with cranberry or prune juice to dilute urine and decrease pain on voiding. The nurse need not administer phenazopyridine 2 hours before giving the antibacterial drug, as this is not the appropriate intervention to be followed.

7. Answer: a
RATIONALE: The nurse should instruct the patient to increase the intake of fluids to alleviate the effect of constipation due to flavoxate. The nurse need not increase the patient's intake of citrus fruits, decrease the patient's consumption of milk products, or administer the drug with warm water, as these interventions will not help alleviate the effect of constipation.

8. Answer: b
RATIONALE: The nurse should administer the drug with milk to prevent irritation in the stomach of the patient receiving a nitrofurantoin urinary tract anti-infective. The nurse need not administer the drug with apple juice, at bedtime, or 1 hour before meals as these interventions will not prevent irritation in the stomach of the patient receiving nitrofurantoin.

9. Answer: b, c, d

RATIONALE: During preadministration assessment, the nurse should question the patient regarding symptoms of infection before instituting therapy, take and record the patient's vital signs, and record the color and appearance of the urine. The nurse also assesses for and documents pain, urinary frequency, bladder distension, or other symptoms associated with the urinary system. The nurse constantly monitors the patient's body temperature as part of the ongoing assessment. Any significant rise in body temperature is reported to the primary health care provider because methods of reducing the fever may need to be altered, or culture and sensitivity tests may need to be repeated. Though urine culture and sensitivity tests are performed to determine bacterial sensitivity to the drugs before drug administration, periodic urinalysis and culture-sensitivity tests are performed only during ongoing assessments to monitor the effects of drug therapy.

10. Answer: c

RATIONALE: The nurse should use anti-infective drugs cautiously in patients with renal impairment. Antispasmodics drugs are used cautiously in patients with GI infections, urinary retention, and hypertension.

11. Answer: a

RATIONALE: Phenazopyridine (Pyridium) is a dye that exerts a topical analgesic effect on the lining of the urinary tract.

12. Answer: c

RATIONALE: The use of nitrofurantoin (Macrobid) has been known to cause acute and chronic reactions in the respiratory system.

13. Answer: a

RATIONALE: The nurse should advise patients taking phenazopyridine (Pyridium) that their urine may become discolored and may appear a dark-orange to brown color.

14. Answer: a

RATIONALE: The use of nalidixic (NegGram) is contraindicated in patients with convulsion disorders.

15. Answer: b

RATIONALE: Patients who are allergic to tartrazine should not be administered methenamine (Hiprex) because it contains tartrazine dye and an allergic reaction may result.

CHAPTER 50

SECTION I: ASSESSING YOUR UNDERSTANDING

Activity A MATCHING

1. 1. c   2. a   3. d   4. b   5 e
2. 1. e   2. a   3. d   4. e   5. c

Activity B FILL IN THE BLANKS

1. Reye
2. Artificially
3. Booster
4. Immunity
5. Cell

Activity C SHORT ANSWERS

1. The nurse should document the following information in the patient's chart or form provided by the institution:
   - Date of vaccination
   - Route and site of administration, vaccine type, and its manufacturer
   - Expiration date and drug lot number
   - Name, address, and title of individual administering the vaccine
2. When educating the parents of a child receiving a vaccination, the nurse should include the following information:
   - Risks of contracting vaccine-preventable diseases and benefits of immunization
   - Importance of bringing immunization records during all visits
   - Date for next vaccination
   - Common adverse reactions (e.g., fever or soreness at the injection site) and methods to combat these reactions (e.g., acetaminophen, warm compresses)
   - Importance of reporting any adverse reactions after vaccine is administered

Activity D DOSAGE CALCULATIONS

1. 7.5 mL
2. 6 patients
3. 3 mL
4. 0.35 mL
5. 8 patients
6. 0.5 mL

SECTION II: APPLYING YOUR KNOWLEDGE
Activity E CASE STUDY

1. Immunization is a form of artificial active immunity.

2. Once the nurse administers Susan's vaccine, the nurse needs to document the following information in her chart: date of vaccination, route and site, vaccine type, manufacturer, lot number, expiration date, and name, address, and title of individual administering the vaccine.

SECTION III: PRACTICING FOR NCLEX
Activity F NCLEX-STYLE

1. **Answer: a, b, c**
   RATIONALE: The benefits of lentinan, a derivative of the shiitake mushroom, include boosting the body's immune system, lowering the cholesterol level, and prolonging the survival time of patients with cancer by increasing immunity. The benefit of this herb in lowering cholesterol levels is achieved by increasing the rate at which cholesterol is excreted from the body. Mild side effects such as skin rashes and gastrointestinal upset have been reported. Lentinan does not help in lowering blood pressure or reducing the risks of heart diseases.

2. **Answer: a**
   RATIONALE: The recommended dosage of shiitake mushrooms is 1 to 5 capsules per day. It is used to maintain general health and also to lower cholesterol levels. The other recommended dosages include 3 to 4 fresh shiitake mushrooms, and 1 dropper 2 to 3 times a day. Increasing dosage (such as 10 mushrooms and 1 dropper 8 times daily) might lead to severe adverse effects, such as skin rashes and gastrointestinal upset. Drinking 12 cups of shiitake juice is not prescribed.

3. **Answer: c**
   RATIONALE: Lymphocytes play a major role in providing cellular and humoral immunity. Immunity refers to the ability of the body to identify and resist potentially harmful microorganisms. This ability enables the body to inhibit tissue and organ damage. T lymphocytes play a major role in maintaining cellular immunity, and B lymphocytes in maintaining humoral immunity. Neutrophils, basophils and eosinophils do not play any major role in humoral immunity.

4. **Answer: a, b, d**
   RATIONALE: The uses of vaccines and toxoids include routine immunization of infants and children, immunization of adults against tetanus, adults at high risk for certain diseases

(e.g., pneumococcal and influenza vaccines), and children or adults at risk for exposure to a particular disease (e.g., hepatitis A for those going to endemic areas). The rubella vaccine is never given in pregnant women as it might lead to infection. It is given for immunization of nonpregnant women of childbearing age. Vaccines and toxoids are contraindicated in leukemia.

5. **Answer: d**
   RATIONALE: Antivenins should be administered within 4 hours of exposure to yield the most effective response. Antivenins are used for passive, transient protection from the toxic effects of bites by spiders (black widow and similar spiders) and snakes (rattlesnakes, copperhead, cottonmouth, and coral). The nurse should know that the most effective response is obtained when the drug is administered within 4 hours after exposure. If the drug is administered beyond 4 hours, it might lessen the therapeutic value and its action against the venom.

6. **Answer: c**
   RATIONALE: The nurse should alert the patient about herpes zoster, which is a complication of chickenpox. Chickenpox can cause herpes zoster (shingles), which is a painful condition, later in life. When salicylates are administered to patients with chickenpox, they may develop Reye's syndrome. Hepatitis, Reye's syndrome, and acute renal failure are not the late complications of chickenpox.

7. **Answer: a, b, d**
   RATIONALE: The diseases preventable by vaccination before traveling to endemic areas include cholera, diphtheria, typhoid, and yellow fever. Other diseases that can be prevented by vaccination before traveling to endemic areas include Japanese encephalitis, Lyme disease, and smallpox. Tetanus and rubella vaccines are given as routine vaccinations to prevent tetanus and rubella, and are not required prior to traveling to endemic areas.

8. **Answer: a, d**
   RATIONALE: To reduce the pain, general interventions such as increasing fluid intake, allowing for adequate rest, and keeping the atmosphere quiet and nonstimulating may be beneficial. The primary health care provider may prescribe acetaminophen every 4 hours

to relieve pain. Local irritation at the injection site may be treated with warm or cool compresses. Warm or cool compresses do not help in relieving pain at the injection site. Decreasing fluids in the diet and massaging the injected site do not help in relieving pain at the injection site.

9. **Answer: a**
   RATIONALE: In lactation, vaccines are to be used with caution. The other conditions include minor illness, allergies, and pregnancy. The contraindication for the use of vaccines includes acute febrile illnesses, leukemia, lymphoma, immunosuppressive illness, drug therapy, and nonlocalized cancer.

10. **Answer: a, b, c**
    RATIONALE: After administering an immunologic agent, patients are usually advised to stay in the clinic for observation for about 30 minutes to assess for signs of hypersensitivity, if any. The signs of hypersensitivity that a nurse should assess for include pruritus, dyspnea, and laryngeal edema. The other signs of hypersensitivity include angioneurotic edema, hives, and severe dyspnea. Renal failure and convulsions are not the signs associated with hypersensitivity.

11. **Answer: c**
    RATIONALE: Cell-mediated immunity depends on the actions of T lymphocytes.

12. **Answer: d**
    RATIONALE: T lymphocytes are responsible for a delayed type immune response seen in cell-mediated immunity.

13. **Answer: a**
    RATIONALE: Immunizations are a form of what type of artificial active immunity?

14. **Answer: c**
    RATIONALE: The administration of immune globulins or antivenins is a form of passive immunity.

15. **Answer: a**
    RATIONALE: The nurse must administer toxoids and vaccines to a patient prior to exposure to the disease-causing organism in order for the patient to be protected against the disease.

CHAPTER 51

SECTION I: ASSESSING YOUR UNDERSTANDING

Activity A MATCHING

1. **1.** b **2.** e **3.** a **4.** c **5.** d
2. **1.** c **2.** a **3.** e **4.** b **5.** d

Activity B FILL IN THE BLANKS

1. Malignant
2. Myelosuppression
3. Neutropenia
4. Erythemia
5. Chemotherapy

Activity C SHORT ANSWERS

1. Nursing care for a patient receiving antineoplastic drugs depends on:
   - Drug or combination of drugs given
   - Drug dosage
   - Route of administration
   - Patient's physical response to therapy
   - Response of tumor to chemotherapy
   - Type and severity of adverse reactions
2. The nurse should observe the following guidelines when caring for a patient receiving chemotherapeutic drugs:
   - Follow policies established by the health care provider.
   - Increase frequency of assessments if the patient's condition changes.
   - Incorporate health care setting guidelines into the individualized nursing care plan.
   - Review the drugs being given before their administration.
   - Ensure the drugs are prescribed by a provider trained specifically in the care of oncology patients.
   - Consult appropriate references to obtain information on the drug—preparation, administration, average dose ranges, and adverse reactions.

Activity D DOSAGE CALCULATIONS

1. 2 vials
2. 5 vials
3. 3 vials
4. 2 capsules
5. 2 vials
6. 4 tablets

SECTION II: APPLYING YOUR KNOWLEDGE
Activity E CASE STUDY

1. Vincristine (Oncovin) is a plant alkaloid which interferes with amino acid production in the S phase and formation of microtubules in the M phase.
2. Following the administration of vincristine (Oncovin) to Mrs. Lopez, the nurse bases the ongoing assessment on the following factors: her general health, individual response to the drug, adverse reactions that may occur, guidelines established by the oncology physician or clinic, and results of periodic laboratory test and radiographic scans.

SECTION III: PRACTICING FOR NCLEX
Activity F NCLEX-STYLE

1. **Answer: a, d, e**
   RATIONALE: Chemotherapy is administered in a series of cycles to allow for the recovery of the normal cells, to destroy more of the malignant cells, and to affect cells that rapidly divide and reproduce. Chemotherapy is administered at the time the cell population is dividing as part of a strategy to optimize cell death. Green tea releases antioxidants, polyphenols, and flavonoids into the system.

2. **Answer: a, b, d**
   RATIONALE: The nurse informs the patient with hypertension to drink green tea with caution as it causes nervousness, insomnia, and GI upset. Green tea does not cause mouth ulcers or stomatitis. Mouth ulcers or stomatitis may be caused by injury, deficiency in vitamin B_{12}, folic acid or iron, or viral infections.

3. **Answer: d**
   RATIONALE: The nurse should explain that a cell-cycle–specific drug targets the cells in one of the phases of cell division. Cell-cycle–nonspecific drugs target the cells at any phase of the cycle or cells in various stages of cell division. Cell-cycle–specific drugs do not affect only malignant cells; they affect all cells that rapidly divide and reproduce, and in the process affect normal cells that line the oral cavity and gastrointestinal (GI) tract, and cells of the gonads, bone marrow, hair follicles, and lymph tissue.

4. **Answer: b**
   RATIONALE: The nurse should explain that an antimetabolite incorporates itself into the cel-lular components during the S phase of cell division, thus interfering with the synthesis of RNA and DNA. Alkylating agents change the cell to a more alkaline environment, which in turn damages the cell. Plant alkaloids interfere with amino acid production in the S phase, of cell division, and formation of the micro-tubules in the M phase.

5. **Answer: a, c, d**
   RATIONALE: When preparing a nursing care plan for ongoing assessment of the patient, the nurse should consider the guidelines established by the health care facility, the patient's general condition, and individual response to the drug. The patient's appetite is of concern to the nurse after the administration of the drug, as a decreased appetite could result in imbalanced nutrition. Adequacy of health insurance coverage is of importance to the nurse as part of the preadministration assessment procedure for the patient.

6. **Answer: a**
   RATIONALE: When administering a subcutaneous injection, the nurse should use no more than 1 mL of the drug. An angiocath is used for intravenous administration. The Z-track method of administration is recommended for all IM injection administrations. The injection for subcutaneous administration should contain no more than 1 mL of the drug; 3 mL is the maximum to administer for IM injections.

7. **Answer: c**
   RATIONALE: The nurse should provide the patient frequent small meals, which are better tolerated than three large meals. The nurse should not provide the patient with fatty or greasy foods, which may not be tolerated by the patient. The nurse should not provide the patient unsalted food ; instead, cold, dry, and salty foods are better tolerated by these patients.

8. **Answer: b**
   RATIONALE: The nurse must apply pressure to the injection site for at least 3 to 5 minutes to avoid the formation of a hematoma. The nurse must not use the same site for withdrawals and injections, and instead should rotate the site of injections. The nurse must suggest that the patient avoid the use of electric razors and nail trimmers to prevent the occurrence of any injury leading to bleeding.

9. **Answer: d**

   RATIONALE: The nurse should offer consistent and empathetic care to the patient and the family, as treatment is spread over time and provides the nurse with several opportunities to help relieve their anxiety. The health care team, and not the nurse alone, assists in making critical decisions regarding treatment, emphasizes safety requirements for chemotherapy, and plans and institutes therapy to control the disease.

10. **Answer: b**

    RATIONALE: The nurse should inform the patient to take the drug as directed on the prescription container. The nurse should instruct the patient to take the exact amount of the drug at the same time every day. The nurse should instruct the patient to inform the dentist or any other physician of the antineoplastic drug therapy being followed. The nurse should instruct the patient not to decrease the dose according to the decrease in symptoms of the illness, and instead continue the dose as prescribed by the physician.

11. **Answer: c**

    RATIONALE: The part of cell growth that entails RNA and protein synthesis preparing for division is known as G_2 phase

12. **Answer: a**

    RATIONALE: The normal cells that line the oral cavity and GI tract, and cells of the gonads, bone marrow, hair follicles, and lymph tissues are rapidly-dividing cells that are subject to the affects of antineoplastic drugs and are the cause of the drugs' adverse effects.

13. **Answer: d**

    RATIONALE: Green tea, loaded with antioxidants. is the herbal product that has the benefits of overall well-being, cancer prevention, dental health, and maintenance of heart and liver health.

14. **Answer: b**

    RATIONALE: The vinca alkaloids, like vinblastine (Velban), are the class of antineoplastic drugs that interfere with amino acid production in the S phase and the formation of microtubules in the M phase.

15. **Answer: a**

    RATIONALE: Podophyllotoxins are the class of antineoplastic drugs that stop cells in the S and G_2 phase, thereby causing cell division to cease.

CHAPTER 52

SECTION I: ASSESSING YOUR UNDERSTANDING

Activity A MATCHING

1. 1. d   2. c   3. b   4. a
2. 1. d   2. c   3. b   4. a

Activity B FILL IN THE BLANKS

1. Erythropoiesis
2. Anemia
3. Leucovorin
4. Megaloblastic
5. Macrocytic

Activity C SHORT ANSWERS

1. Before administering the first dose of ferrous gluconate, the nurse should perform the following assessments in the patient:
   - Obtain a general health history and ask about the symptoms of anemia.
   - Take vital signs to provide a baseline during therapy.
   - Other physical assessments may include patient's general appearance and, in the severely anemic, evaluation of the patient's ability to carry out the activities of daily living.
   - If iron dextran is to be given, an allergy history is necessary because this drug is given with caution to those with significant allergies or asthma.
   - Record the patient's weight and hemoglobin level to calculate dosage.
2. The nurse should monitor the following adverse reactions in a patient who is administered sodium ferric gluconate complex for the treatment of iron-deficiency anemia:
   - Flushing
   - Hypotension
   - Syncope
   - Tachycardia
   - Dizziness
   - Pruritus
   - Dyspnea
   - Conjunctivitis
   - Hyperkalemia

Activity D DOSAGE CALCULATIONS

1. 1.5 mL
2. 1 mL
3. 14 tablets
4. 2 mL

SECTION II: APPLYING YOUR KNOWLEDGE
Activity E CASE STUDY

1. The common adverse reactions seen with the use of filgrastim (Neupogen) are bone pain, nausea, vomiting, diarrhea, and alopecia.
2. Filgrastim (Neupogen) should be used cautiously in patients with hypthroidism and is contraindicated in patients with known hypersensitivity to the drug or any of its components.

SECTION III: PRACTICING FOR NCLEX
Activity F NCLEX-STYLE

1. **Answer: b**
   RATIONALE: The nurse should monitor the patient administered a Folvite injection for allergic hypersensitivity. The nurse need not monitor the patient for anorexia, arthralgia, or adrenal hyperplasia. Arthralgia is an adverse reaction associated with the use of epoetin alfa. Adrenal hyperplasia is caused due to an unusual increase in the production of androgens by the adrenal glands. Anorexia nervosa is an eating disorder characterized by voluntary starvation and exercise stress.

2. **Answer: a**
   RATIONALE: Epoetin alfa is contraindicated in patients with hypersensitivity to human albumin. Epoetin alfa is not contraindicated in patients with allergy to cyanocobalamin, patients undergoing treatment for pernicious anemia, or patients with hemolytic anemia. Vitamin B_{12} is contraindicated in patients who are allergic to cyanocobalamin. Folic acid and leucovorin are contraindicated in patients undergoing treatment for pernicious anemia. Iron supplements are contraindicated in patients with hemolytic anemia.

3. **Answer: a, c, e**
   RATIONALE: The nurse should know that patients who consume alcohol, neomycin, or colchicine show a reduced absorption of vitamin B_{12} when they are administered vitamin B_{12} to counter its deficiency. Caffeine and nicotine are not known to reduce the absorption of vitamin B_{12} in patients taking vitamin B_{12} supplements for its deficiency.

4. **Answer: a**
   RATIONALE: The nurse should obtain the patient's weight and hemoglobin level to calculate the dosage of iron dextran to be administered to the patient. The patient's heart rate, blood pressure, and body temperature are not required for calculating the dosage of iron dextran. Heart rate, blood pressure, and body temperature are the patient's vital signs and have to be taken by the nurse when conducting preadministration and ongoing assessments.

5. **Answer: c**
   RATIONALE: When a patient is administered iron supplements along with methyldopa, the patient should be monitored for the decreased effect of Parkinson's medication. The interaction of iron supplements with methyldopa is not known to lead to a decrease in blood pressure or an increase in heart rate. The increased absorption of iron is observed in patients taking iron supplements with ascorbic acid or vitamin C.

6. **Answer: a, b, c**
   RATIONALE: In order to fulfill the nutritional deficiency of vitamin B_{12} through a balanced diet, the nurse should ask the patient to consume a diet consisting of seafood, meat, eggs, and dairy products, as these are rich sources of vitamin B_{12}. The nurse need not instruct the patient to consume leafy vegetables, breads, and cereals to increase the intake of vitamin B_{12}, as leafy vegetables are rich in iron and fiber and breads and cereals are rich in carbohydrates and proteins, but not in vitamin B_{12}.

7. **Answer: b**
   RATIONALE: In the teaching plan, the nurse should instruct the patient receiving ferrous fumarate to take the drug with water on an empty stomach or with food or meals if the patient experiences gastrointestinal upset. The nurse should ask the patient not to take antacids in case of acidity, as antacids may interfere with the absorption of iron. The nurse should not ask the patient to drink the liquid iron preparation directly from a glass, as doing so can stain the patient's teeth. Instead, the patient should use a straw while drinking. The patient should avoid multivitamin preparations unless advised otherwise by the PHCP in case the patient is taking folic acid. The patient need not avoid taking multivitamin preparations when taking ferrous fumarate.

8. **Answer: a, b, e**

   RATIONALE: The nurse should monitor adverse reactions such as urticaria, dyspnea, and rashes in patients receiving parenteral administration of iron for the treatment of anemia. Insomnia and diabetes are not known to occur due to the parenteral administration of iron.

9. **Answer: a**

   RATIONALE: When conducting the ongoing assessment for a patient receiving oral iron supplements, the nurse should inform the patient that the color of his or her stools will be black. Administering oral supplements does not result in high palpitations, weight gain, or the development of rashes.

10. **Answer: a**

    RATIONALE: The nurse should instruct patients receiving iron supplements to avoid milk, which interferes with iron absorption. The nurse need not ask the patients to avoid poultry, meat, and fish, as these products do not interfere with iron absorption.

11. **Answer: c**

    RATIONALE: Red blood cells, also known as erythrocytes, supply cells with oxygen from the lungs.

12. **Answer: a**

    RATIONALE: Megakaryocytes divide into platelets that control the bleeding from microscopic or major tears in our tissues.

13. **Answer: d**

    RATIONALE: Infection is likely to occur when a patient is neutropenic.

14. **Answer: c**

    RATIONALE: Anemia can cause decreased platelet production.

15. **Answer: a**

    RATIONALE: Hematopoiesis is the process by which the body is stimulated to make more of a specific type of blood cells.

CHAPTER 53

SECTION I: ASSESSING YOUR UNDERSTANDING

Activity A MATCHING

1. **1.** b   **2.** d   **3.** a   **4.** c
2. **1.** d   **2.** a   **3.** b   **4.** c

Activity B FILL IN THE BLANKS

1. Superinfection
2. Immunocompromised
3. Hypersensitivity
4. Antiseptic
5. Germicide
6. Antipsoriatics

Activity C SHORT ANSWERS

1. The preadministration assessment involves a visual inspection and palpation of the involved area(s). The nurse should carefully record the areas of involvement, including size, color, and appearance. A specific description is important so that changes can be readily identified indicating worsening or improvement of the lesions. The nurse should note the presence of scales, crusting, drainage, or any complaint of itching. Some agencies may provide a figure on which the lesions can be drawn, indicating the shape and distribution of the involved areas.

2. At the time of each application, the nurse inspects the affected area for changes (e.g., signs of improvement or worsening of the infection) and for adverse reactions such as redness or rash. The nurse contacts the primary health care provider and the drug is not applied if these or other changes are noted, or if the patient reports new problems such as itching, pain, or soreness at the site.

Activity D DOSAGE CALCULATIONS

1. 56
2. 42

SECTION II: APPLYING YOUR KNOWLEDGE
Activity E CASE STUDY

1. Common adverse reactions seen with the use of calcipotriene (Dovonex) are: burning, itching, skin irritation, erythema, dry skin, peeling, rash, worsening of psoriasis, dermatitis, and hyperpigmentation.

2. The nurse should instruct Mr. Vasquez to apply the calcipotriene (Dovonex) in the following way:
   - Gather all necessary supplies and wash hands before starting.
   - First wash the area to remove any debris and old drug.
   - Pat area dry with a clean cloth.

- Open container or tube and place the lid or cap upside down on the counter or surface.
- Use a tongue blade, gloved finger (either with a nonsterile gloved hand or finger cot), cotton swab, or gauze pad to remove the drug, then apply to the skin.
- Wipe drug onto the affected area using long, smooth strokes in the direction of hair growth.
- Apply thin layer of drug to the area; more is not better.
- Do not re-use applicator to remove additional drug from the container. Use a new applicator or clean gloved finger each time.
- Apply a clean, dry dressing (if appropriate) over the area.

SECTION III: PRACTICING FOR NCLEX
Activity F NCLEX-STYLE

1. Answer: a
RATIONALE: Masoprocol is a keratolytic, and keratolytics are contraindicated in patients with known hypersensitivity to the drugs; for use on moles, birthmarks, or warts with hair growing from them; on genital or facial warts; on warts on mucous membranes; or on infected skin. Masoprocol is not contraindicated as monotherapy for bacterial skin infections, for use on the face, groin, or axilla, or as sole therapy in plaque psoriasis. The topical corticosteroids are contraindicated in patients with known hypersensitivity to the drug or any of its components ; as monotherapy for bacterial skin infections; for use on the face, groin, or axilla (only the high-potency corticosteroids); or as sole therapy in plaque psoriasis and ophthalmic use.

2. Answer: b
RATIONALE: Alclometasone dipropionate is a topical corticosteroid, and topical corticosteroids are contraindicated in patients with known hypersensitivity to the drug or any component of the drug; as sole therapy in plaque psoriasis, as monotherapy for bacterial skin infections; for use on the face, groin, or axilla (only the high-potency corticosteroids); and ophthalmic use. Alclometasone dipropionate is not contraindicated for use on moles, birthmarks, or warts with hair growing from them; on genital or facial warts; on warts on mucous membranes; or on infected skin. Keratolytics are contraindicated in patients with known hypersensitivity to the drugs and for use on moles, birthmarks, or warts with hair growing from them; on genital or facial warts; on warts on mucous membranes; or on infected skin.

3. Answer: c
RATIONALE: Benzocaine is a topical anesthetic, and topical anesthetics are used cautiously in patients receiving class I antiarrhythmic drugs such as tocainide and mexiletine because the toxic effects are additive and potentially synergistic. Benzocaine need not be used cautiously during pregnancy and lactation. Benzocaine is not associated with immuno-compromised patients with herpes simplex virus infections, cutaneous candidiasis, or tinea pedis. The topical antibiotics are pregnancy Category C drugs and are used cautiously during pregnancy and lactation. Immuno-compromised patients with herpes simplex virus infections are treated with antiviral drugs. Patients having cutaneous candidiasis or tinea pedis are treated with antifungal drugs.

4. Answer: d
RATIONALE: Anthralin may cause skin irritation as well as temporary discoloration of the hair and fingernails. Hypothalamic-pituitary-adrenal axis suppression, Cushing's syndrome, hyperglycemia, and glycosuria are not the adverse reactions associated with anthralin. Hypothalamic-pituitary-adrenal axis suppression, Cushing's syndrome, hyperglycemia, and glycosuria are the systemic adverse reactions to topical corticosteroids.

5. Answer: a
RATIONALE: Alclometasone dipropionate is a topical corticosteroid and in the use of topical corticosteroids, systemic reactions may occur with hypothalamic-pituitary-adrenal axis suppression, Cushing's syndrome, hyperglycemia, and glycosuria. Numbness and dermatitis, mild and transient pains, and flu-like syndrome are not the adverse reactions associated with alclometasone dipropionate. Numbness and dermatitis and mild and transient pains are the adverse reactions to the application of collagenase. Flu-like syndrome is an adverse reaction to keratolytic drugs.

6. Answer: b
RATIONALE: Numbness and dermatitis and mild and transient pains are the adverse reactions to the application of collagenase. Flu-like syndrome, Cushing's syndrome, hyperglycemia,

and glycosuria are not the adverse reactions associated with the application of collagenase. Flu-like syndrome is an adverse reaction to keratolytic drugs. Cushing's syndrome, hyperglycemia, and glycosuria are the systemic adverse reactions to topical corticosteroids.

7. **Answer: c**
RATIONALE: Salicylic acid is a keratolytic, and flu-like syndrome is an adverse reaction to keratolytic drugs. Numbness and dermatitis, mild and transient pains, temporary discoloration of the hair, hyperglycemia, and glycosuria are not the adverse reactions to salicylic acid. Numbness and dermatitis, and mild and transient pains are the adverse reactions to the application of collagenase. Anthralin may cause skin irritation as well as temporary discoloration of the hair and fingernails. Hyperglycemia and glycosuria, hypothalamic-pituitary-adrenal axis suppression, and Cushing's syndrome are the systemic adverse reactions to topical corticosteroids.

8. **Answer: d**
RATIONALE: Accuzyme is a topical enzyme that is used to help remove necrotic tissue from chronic dermal ulcers. Accuzyme is not used for the treatment of psoriasis, eczema, or insect bites. Psoriasis, eczema, or insect bites are treated with topical corticosteroids.

9. **Answer: a**
RATIONALE: Topical corticosteroids exert localized anti-inflammatory activity. When applied to inflamed skin, they reduce itching, redness, and swelling. Topical corticosteroids do not act to reduce the number of bacteria on the skin surface, to prevent infection in cuts and wounds, or to cleanse the skin thoroughly. Topical antibiotics and germicides are used to reduce the number of bacteria on the skin surface, to prevent infection in cuts and wounds, and to cleanse the skin thoroughly.

10. **Answer: b**
RATIONALE: Topical antiseptics and germicides are used for washing the hands before and after caring for patients, as a surgical scrub, and as a preoperative skin cleanser. Topical antipsoriatics, topical enzymes, and topical antifungals are not used for washing hands before and after caring for patients. Topical antipsoriatics are drugs used to treat psoria-

sis. A topical enzyme is used to help remove necrotic tissue from chronic dermal ulcers and severely burned areas. Topical antifungals are used to inhibit the growth of fungi.

11. **Answer: a**
RATIONALE: Clindamycin (Clindagel), a topical antibiotic drug, might be used topically by a patient with acne vulgaris.

12. **Answer: c**
RATIONALE: Ciclopirox (Penlac) is a topical antifungal drug that might be used to treat onychomycosis (a nail fungus).

13. **Answer: d**
RATIONALE: Lemon balm is an herbal product with antiviral properties against HSV.

14. **Answer: a**
RATIONALE: Docosanol (Abreva) is available over the counter and can be recommended for patient HSV.

15. **Answer: b**
RATIONALE: Aloe vera is an herbal product that can be used topically to prevent infection and promote healing of minor burns and wounds.

CHAPTER 54

SECTION I: ASSESSING YOUR UNDERSTANDING

Activity A MATCHING

1. 1. b   2. d   3. a   4. c
2. 1. c   2. a   3. b

Activity B FILL IN THE BLANKS

1. Superinfection
2. Glaucoma
3. Miosis
4. Antibacterial
5. Natamycin
6. Cycloplegia

Activity C SHORT ANSWERS

1. The nurse may be responsible for examining the outer structures of the ear—namely, the earlobe and skin around the ear. The nurse should document a description of any drainage or impacted cerumen and check with the primary health care provider before administering an otic preparation to a patient with a perforated ear drum.

2. The nurse assesses the patient's response to therapy by confirming whether a decrease in pain or inflammation has occurred. The nurse should examine the outer ear and ear canal for any local redness or irritation that may indicate sensitivity to the drug.

Activity D DOSAGE CALCULATIONS

1. 16 drops
2. 24 drops

SECTION II: APPLYING YOUR KNOWLEDGE
Activity E CASE STUDY

1. The nurse should tell Mr. Owens that the drops may sting on instillation, especially the first few doses; do not use if the solution is brown or contains a precipitate; and do not use while wearing soft contact lenses.
2. The nurse should advise Mr. Owens to administer the brimonidine (Alphagan) drops in the following way:
   - Wash hands thoroughly before beginning.
   - Hold bottle (drops) or tube (ointment) in hand for a few minutes before applying.
   - Cleanse area around the eye of any secretions.
   - Squeeze bottle to fill the drop chamber.
   - Tilt head slightly back and toward the eye to be treated.
   - Pull affected lower lid down.
   - Position dropper, bottle, or tube over lower conjunctival sac.
   - Steady hand by resting fingers against cheek or resting base of hand on cheek; look up at ceiling.
   - Squeeze bottle; instill prescribed number of drops into middle of lower conjunctival sac.
   - Close eyes gently and release lower lid; do not squeeze eyes shut after instilling drug.
   - Place finger on inner canthus to avoid absorption through tear duct (when instilling drops and only if ordered).
   - Repeat procedure with other eye (if ordered).
   - If more than one type of ophthalmic preparation is being instilled, wait the recommended time before instilling the second drug (usually 5 minutes for drops and 10 to 15 minutes for ointment).
   - Replace cap of the eye preparation immediately after instilling; Do not touch the tip of the bottle or tube.

SECTION III: PRACTICING FOR NCLEX
Activity F NCLEX-STYLE

1. **Answer: a**
   RATIONALE: Prolonged use of otic preparations containing an antibiotic such as ofloxacin may result in a superinfection, due to an overgrowth of bacterial or fungal microorganisms not affected by the antibiotic being administered. Systemic effects of cholinesterase inhibitors, exacerbation of existing hypertension, and additive CNS depressant effects are not related to the use of otic antibiotics. Individuals working with organophosphate insecticides or pesticides are at risk for systemic effects of the cholinesterase inhibitors from absorption through the respiratory tract or the skin. Older adults are at risk for exacerbation of existing disorders such as hypertension if systemic absorption of sympathomimetic ophthalmic drugs occurs. When brimonidine is used with central nervous system depressants such as alcohol, barbiturates, opiates, sedatives, or anesthetics, there is a risk for an additive CNS depressant effect.

2. **Answer: b**
   RATIONALE: Ofloxacin is a pregnancy Category C drug and should be administered in pregnancy only if the potential benefit justifies the risk to the fetus. Brimonidine tartrate, being an alpha$_2$-adrenergic blocker, is contraindicated in patients taking monoamine oxidase inhibitors. Brimonidine may cause fatigue or drowsiness and therefore must be used cautiously for patients with activities requiring mental alertness. Dapiprazole may cause difficulty in dark adaptation and may reduce field of vision, and therefore must be used cautiously when driving at night or performing activities in dimly lit areas.

3. **Answer: c**
   RATIONALE: Before instilling floxacin otic, the nurse informs the patient that while the solution remains in the ear canal, a feeling of fullness may be felt in the ear and that hearing in the treated ear may be temporarily impaired. Fatigue and drowsiness and local effects such as headache and visual blurring may be experienced as systemic effects in treatment with brimonidine tartrate.

4. **Answer: d**
   RATIONALE: The nurse should hold the container in the hand for a few minutes to warm

it to body temperature. Cold and warm (above body temperature) preparations may cause dizziness or other sensations after being instilled in the ear. The number of drops needs to be confirmed as per the prescription when being instilled and while the applicator is inside the bottle. The nurse need not hold the container in the hand for a few minutes to confirm if it has been refrigerated. If the drops are in a suspension form, the nurse should shake the container well for 10 seconds before using.

5. Answer: a
RATIONALE: When instilling ear drops, the nurse has the patient lie on his or her side with the ear toward the ceiling. If the patient wishes to remain in an upright position, the head is tilted toward the untreated side with the ear toward the ceiling. To straighten the ear canal in adults and children ages 3 and older, the cartilaginous portion of the outer ear is gently pulled up and back. The dropper or applicator tip should never be inserted into the ear canal.

6. Answer: c
RATIONALE: The nurse should stop using Cerumenex if ear drainage, discharge, pain, or irritation occurs. Also Cerumenex should not be used for more than 4 days. If excessive cerumen remains, the primary health care provider should be consulted. Cold and warm (above body temperature) preparations may cause dizziness or other sensations after being instilled into the ear and this can be avoided by the nurse holding the container in the hand for a few minutes to warm it to body temperature.

7. Answer: b
RATIONALE: Being a sympathomimetic drug, dipivefrin hydrochloride may cause transient local reactions such as brow ache, headache, burning and stinging, eye pain, allergic lip reactions, and ocular irritation. Deposits may occur in the conjunctiva and cornea with prolonged use of adrenochrome (a red pigment contained in epinephrine). Ocular allergic reactions and foreign body sensation are the local effects of the administration of brimonidine tartrate.

8. Answer: d
RATIONALE: Dapiprazole hydrochloride, being an alpha-adrenergic blocker, may cause local effects such as ptosis (drooping of the upper eyelid), burning in the eye, eyelid edema, itching, corneal edema, brow ache, dryness of the eye, tearing, and blurred vision. Abnormal corneal staining and decreased night vision are the local adverse reactions associated with the β-adrenergic blocking drugs. Frequent urge to urinate is a systemic adverse reaction to direct-acting miotic drugs.

9. Answer: a
RATIONALE: Echothiophate iodide is a cholinesterase inhibitor ophthalmic preparation and therefore the ophthalmic adverse reactions could include eyelid muscle twitching, iris cysts, burning, lacrimation, eyelid muscle twitching, conjunctivitis, ciliary redness, brow ache, and headache. Abdominal cramps, cardiac irregularities, and urinary incontinence are systemic adverse reactions to cholinesterase inhibitors.

10. Answer: b
RATIONALE: Travoprost, being a prostaglandin agonist, is likely to cause local adverse reactions that include eyelid discomfort, blurred vision, burning and stinging, foreign body sensation, itching, increased pigmentation of the iris, dry eye, and excessive tearing. Unpleasant taste, asthma and cold/flu symptoms are the systemic adverse reactions associated with the mast cell inhibitors.

11. Answer: c
RATIONALE: Antipyrine is used as an analgesic in otic preparations.

12. Answer: a
RATIONALE: The nurse can recommend carbamide peroxide to aid in the removal of cerumen from the ear canal.

13. Answer: c
RATIONALE: If medication is needed in the other ear, it is best to wait at least 5 minutes after instillation of the first ear drops before administering drops to the other ear.

14. Answer: b
RATIONALE: Cerumenex should not be allowed to stay in the ear canal more than 30 minutes before irrigation.

15. Answer: a
RATIONALE: A patient should not use over the counter ear wax removal products for more than 4 days; if excessive cerumen remains, the patient should consult a physician.

CHAPTER 55

SECTION I: ASSESSING YOUR UNDERSTANDING

Activity A MATCHING

1. 1. c   **2.** a   **3.** d   **4.** b

Activity B FILL IN THE BLANKS

1. Electrolyte
2. Alkaline
3. Overload
4. Hyponatremia
5. Substrates

Activity C SHORT ANSWERS

1. The nurse should consider the following factors when evaluating the intravenous replacement solution therapy to determine its effectiveness:
   - The therapeutic effect of the drug is achieved.
   - The fluid volume deficit is corrected.
   - The nutrition deficit is corrected.
   - The patient and family demonstrate an understanding of the procedure.
2. The nurse should include the following points for the intake of potassium in a patient teaching plan:
   - Take the drug exactly as directed on the prescription container. Do not increase, decrease, or omit doses of the drug unless advised to do so by the primary health care provider.
   - Take the drug immediately after meals or with food and a full glass of water.
   - Avoid the use of nonprescription drugs and salt substitutes (many contain potassium) unless use of a specific drug or product has been approved by the primary health care provider.
   - Contact the primary health care provider if tingling of the hands or feet, a feeling of heaviness in the legs, vomiting, nausea, abdominal pain, or black stools should occur.
   - If the tablet has a coating (an enteric-coated tablet), swallow it whole. Do not chew or crush the tablet.
   - If effervescent tablets are prescribed, place the tablet in 4 to 8 oz of cold water or juice. Wait until the fizzing stops before drinking. Sip the liquid during a period of 5 to 10 minutes.
   - If an oral liquid or a powder is prescribed, add the dose to 4 to 8 oz of cold water or juice and sip slowly during a period of 5 to 10 minutes. Measure the dose accurately.

Activity D DOSAGE CALCULATIONS

1. 4 tablets in a day
2. 160 mL
3. 2 tablets
4. 4.8 mL

SECTION II: APPLYING YOUR KNOWLEDGE

Activity E CASE STUDY

1. The drip rate would be 42 drops/min.

   1000 mL/4hr = 250 mL/hr

   250 mL/hr × 1 hr/60 min = 4.2 mL/min

   4.2 mL/min × 10 drops/mL = 42 drops/min

2. Signs and symptoms a patient with fluid overload might exhibit include: headache, weakness, blurred vision, behavioral changes (confusion, disorientation, delirium, drowsiness), weight gain, isolated muscle twitching, hyponatremia, rapid breathing, wheezing, coughing, rise in blood pressure, distended neck veins, elevated central venous pressure, and convulsions.

SECTION III: PRACTICING FOR NCLEX

Activity F NCLEX-STYLE

1. **Answer: b**
   RATIONALE: When caring for a patient who needs to be administered magnesium, the nurse should confirm that the patient does not have a heart block or myocardial damage, because presence of these conditions contraindicates the use of magnesium. Potassium is contraindicated in patients who have untreated Addison disease. Sodium is contraindicated in patients who experience fluid retention. Calcium is contraindicated in patients taking digitalis, because there is an increased risk of digitalis toxicity when digitalis preparations are administered with calcium.

2. **Answer: a, b, d**
   RATIONALE: When caring for a patient who is being administered electrolytes and experiencing GI disturbances, the nurse should ensure that the patient takes the drugs with meals to reduce nausea. Meals should be served in

smaller quantities and more frequently. The nurse should also continue to monitor the patient for signs and symptoms of nausea. The nurse should not administer antacids to the patient. The nurse also need not encourage an increase in the patient's intake of fruit juices because these interventions will not help in reducing nausea, nor will they reduce the symptoms and other discomforts associated with GI disturbances.

3. **Answer: c**
RATIONALE: The nurse should know that if a patient's intake of protein nutrients is significantly less than is required by the body to meet energy expenditures, a state of negative nitrogen balance occurs. The body begins to convert protein from the muscle into carbohydrate for energy to be used by the body. This results in weight loss and muscle wasting. Metabolic acidosis is an adverse reaction to ammonium chloride and protein substrates. GI disturbances are likely to occur with the administration of electrolytes. Hypotensive episodes occur as adverse reactions to plasma protein fractions.

4. **Answer: c**
RATIONALE: When caring for a patient who is being administered fat emulsions, the nurse should monitor the patient's ability to eliminate the infused fat from the circulation because the lipidemia must clear between daily infusions. The nurse should not administer an IV solution, which is a little below room temperature. The IV solution should be administered at room temperature. Diarrhea is not known to occur with the use of fat emulsions, though the nurse must monitor the patient for difficulty in breathing, headache, flushing, nausea, vomiting, or signs of a hypersensitivity reaction. The nurse should monitor the patient for signs of hypernatremia if the patient is administered NaCl solution through the IV route. Hypernatremia is not known to occur with the administration of fat emulsions.

5. **Answer: a**
RATIONALE: When caring for a patient who is being administered plasma proteins, the nurse should monitor for adverse reactions such as urticaria, nausea, chills, fever, and hypotensive episodes. Flushing of skin is an adverse reaction to protein substrates and not plasma protein fractions. Dyspnea and wheezing are the adverse reactions to energy substrates.

6. **Answer: b, c, e**
RATIONALE: When caring for a patient on sodium electrolyte infusion therapy, the nurse should observe the rate of IV infusion as ordered by the PHCP every 15 to 30 minutes. The nurse should also observe the patient's condition for signs of pulmonary edema, especially if sodium is given via IV. Patients receiving NaCl by the IV route have their intake and output measured every 8 hours. When caring for a patient who is being administered magnesium, the nurse should inform the PHCP if the patient voids less than 100 mL of urine every 4 hours. Magnesium is eliminated by the kidneys, and so it is used with caution in patients with renal impairment. A microscopic filter is attached to the IV line when amino acid solutions are administered. The filter prevents microscopic aggregates from entering the bloodstream where they could cause massive emboli.

7. **Answer: b**
RATIONALE: The nurse should know if the patient has congestive heart failure before administering bicarbonate. Bicarbonate is used cautiously in patients with CHF or renal impairment and with glucocorticoid therapy. Bicarbonate is a pregnancy Category C drug and is used cautiously during pregnancy. Bicarbonate is contraindicated in patients with metabolic or respiratory alkalosis, hypocalcemia, renal failure, or severe abdominal pain of unknown cause, and in those on sodium-restricted diets.

8. **Answer: a**
RATIONALE: The nurse should check the patient's pulse rate at regular intervals, usually every 4 hours or more often if an irregularity in the heart rate is observed. Depending on the patient's condition, cardiac monitoring may be indicated so that it can continuously monitor the heart rate and rhythm during therapy. The nurse should discontinue the IV infusion immediately and contact the PHCP in case an extravasation occurs during administration. Potassium is irritating to the tissues and may also cause tissue necrosis. The nurse need not monitor the patient for nausea and vomiting, since they do not occur with a decreased or increased cardiac output. The nurse should not ensure a direct IV injection of potassium, as it can result in sudden death. Concentrated potassium solutions are for IV mixtures only, and should never be used undiluted.

9. **Answer: a**

   RATIONALE: When caring for an elderly patient who is being administered fluids, the nurse should carefully monitor the patient for signs and symptoms of fluid overload. The elderly are at an increased risk for fluid overload because of the incidence of cardiac disease and decreased renal function that may increase with age. The nurse observes the patient for difficulty in breathing, headache, flushing, nausea, vomiting, or signs of a hypersensitivity reaction when the patient is being administered lipid solutions. The nurse should monitor for signs of hypercalcemic syndrome and report the same to the PHCP when the patient is administered calcium. The nurse should test the patient's knee jerk reflex before each dose of magnesium.

10. **Answer: d**

    RATIONALE: The nurse should monitor the patient for systemic acidosis, which occurs due to the interaction of ammonium chloride and spironolactone. Respiratory depression, heart block, and systemic alkalosis are not known to occur due to the interaction of ammonium chloride and spironolactone. Prolonged respiratory depression and apnea occur when magnesium is administered with the neuromuscular blocking agents. When magnesium is used with digoxin, heart block may occur. Prolonged use of oral sodium bicarbonate or excessive doses of IV sodium bicarbonate may result in systemic alkalosis.

11. **Answer: b**

    RATIONALE: Depending on clinical judgment, 2 unsuccessful venipuncture attempts on the same patient warrants having a more skilled individual attempt the procedure.

12. **Answer: a**

    RATIONALE: Potassium and magnesium are the major intracellular fluid electrolytes.

13. **Answer: d**

    RATIONALE: Sodium and calcium are the major extracellular fluid electrolytes.

14. **Answer: b**

    RATIONALE: Potassium is the electrolyte necessary for the transmission of impulses and the contraction of smooth, cardiac, and skeletal muscles.

15. **Answer: a**

    RATIONALE: The use of furosemide (Lasix) can lead to hypokalemia.